TRANSGENDER
Mental Health

TRANSGENDER
Mental Health

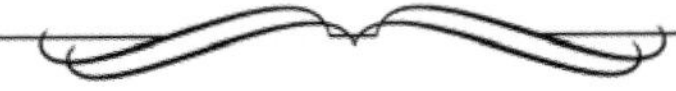

by

Eric Yarbrough, M.D.

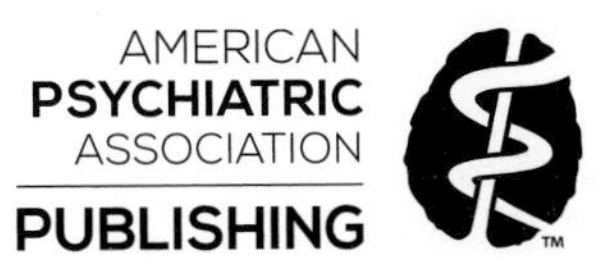

Note: The authors have worked to ensure that all information in this book is accurate at the time of publication and consistent with general psychiatric and medical standards, and that information concerning drug dosages, schedules, and routes of administration is accurate at the time of publication and consistent with standards set by the U.S. Food and Drug Administration and the general medical community. As medical research and practice continue to advance, however, therapeutic standards may change. Moreover, specific situations may require a specific therapeutic response not included in this book. For these reasons and because human and mechanical errors sometimes occur, we recommend that readers follow the advice of physicians directly involved in their care or the care of a member of their family.

Books published by American Psychiatric Association Publishing represent the findings, conclusions, and views of the individual authors and do not necessarily represent the policies and opinions of American Psychiatric Association Publishing or the American Psychiatric Association.

If you wish to buy 50 or more copies of the same title, please go to www.appi.org/special-discounts for more information.

First Edition

Manufactured in the United States of America on acid-free paper
22 21 20 19 18 5 4 3 2 1

American Psychiatric Association Publishing
800 Maine Ave. SW
Suite 900
Washington, DC 20024-2812
www.appi.org

Library of Congress Cataloging-in-Publication Data
Names: Yarbrough, Eric, 1979– author. | American Psychiatric Association Publishing, issuing body.

Title: Transgender mental health / by Eric Yarbrough.

Description: First edition. | Arlington, VA : American Psychiatric Association Publish ing, [2018] | Includes bibliographical references.

Identifiers: LCCN 2017055788 (print) | LCCN 2017056832 (ebook) | ISBN 9781615371891 (ebook) | ISBN 9781615371136 (pbk. : alk. paper)

Subjects: | MESH: Transgender Persons—psychology | Mental Health | Culturally Competent Care | Health Services Accessibility | Patient Advocacy | Case Reports

Classification: LCC RC451.4.G39 (ebook) | LCC RC451.4.G39 (print) | NLM WA 305.1 | DDC 616.890086/7—dc23

LC record available at https://lccn.loc.gov/2017055788

British Library Cataloguing in Publication Data
A CIP record is available from the British Library.

CONTENTS

ABOUT THE AUTHOR

Eric Yarbrough, M.D., is Director of Psychiatry, Callen-Lorde Community Health Center, New York, New York, and President of AGLP: The Association of LGBTQ Psychiatrists.

The author has indicated that he has no financial interests or other affiliations that represent or could appear to represent a competing interest with his authorship of this book.

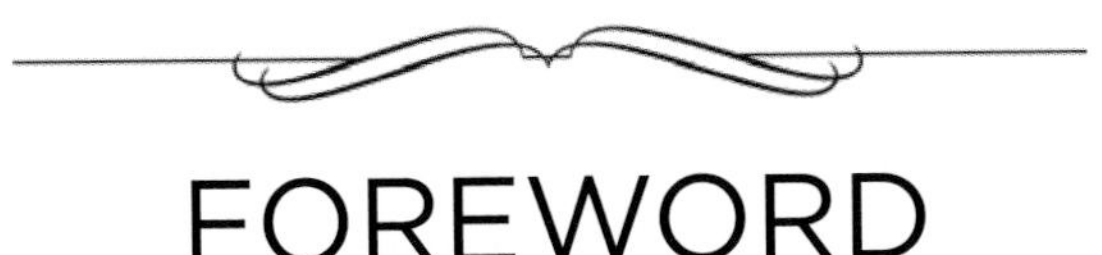

FOREWORD

ERIC YARBROUGH'S *Transgender Mental Health* feels like a watershed moment in the history of American psychiatry. It is being published at a time when transgender rights are a flashpoint in the so-called culture wars. State legislatures are passing and proposing "bathroom bills" to deny transgender people use of facilities matching their gender identity. There is uncertainty about the future ability of openly trans people to serve in the military. Many religious denominations are grappling with the question of how to integrate (or expel) transgender people of faith and their families. There are political (as opposed to medical) controversies about the age at which young people should have access to medical and surgical treatment.

This volume, published by American Psychiatric Association Publishing, moves away from psychiatry's historic pathologizing of trans individuals and instead seeks more accepting and respectful ways to improve their lives. It should be noted, however, that psychiatry's acceptance and respect were not always forthcoming.

In the nineteenth century, Krafft-Ebing's *Psychopathia Sexualis* labeled transgender presentations as forms of psychopathology (Krafft-Ebing 1886/1985). By the 1920s, however, European physicians began experimenting with gender reassignment surgery to change people's bodies rather than their minds. Yet this work became known to the general public only when international headlines trumpeted Christine Jorgensen's 1952 return from Denmark to the United States as a trans woman (Jorgensen 1967).

Although the account of Jorgensen's treatment was published a year later in the *Journal of the American Medical Association* (Hamburger et al. 1953), for almost three decades, most physicians and mental health practitioners were either oblivious about or critical of medical and surgical gender reassignment. In Green's (1969) survey, 400 physicians and psychiatrists criticized the use of surgery and hormones to irreversibly treat people suffering from what they perceived to be either a severe neurotic or psychotic, delusional condition in need of psychotherapy and "reality testing."

Professional perceptions would eventually change following the decision to include a diagnosis of *transsexualism* in the third edition of the American Psychiatric Association's (APA) *Diagnostic and Statistical Manual of Mental Disorders* (DSM-III; American Psychiatric Association 1980). The World Health Organization's (WHO) *International Classification of Diseases, Tenth Revision* (ICD-10; World Health Organization 1990) included diagnoses of *transsexualism* and *gender identity disorder of childhood* (Drescher 2010; Drescher et al. 2012). With diagnoses in both manuals, a growing international community of clinicians began offering medical and surgical treatment of gender dysphoric individuals (World Professional Association for Transgender Health 2011).

In 2007, APA announced the DSM-5 revision, the first to take place in the age of social media (Drescher 2010). Consequently, the process was highly scrutinized, with controversies emerging and reported on in the lesbian, gay, bisexual, transgender, and queer/questioning (LGBTQ) press (Chibbaro 2008; Osborne 2008) as well as in mainstream media outlets such as the *New York Times* (Carey 2008). LGBTQ activists called for the removal of gender diagnoses, just as homosexuality was deleted from DSM-II in 1973 (Bayer 1981, 1987; Drescher and Merlino 2007). Arguments for removal included societal intolerance of difference, the human cost of diagnostic stigmatization, using the language of psychopathology to describe what some people consider to be normal behaviors and feelings, and, finally, inappropriately focusing psychiatric attention on individual diversity rather than opposing the social forces that oppress sexual and gender nonconformity (Karasic and Drescher 2005).

On the other hand, there were also advocates for the transgender community who expressed competing concerns. For example, deleting the gender diagnoses from DSM-5 would lead third-party payers to deny access to medical and surgical care. In addition, transgender civil rights advocacy groups have used gender diagnoses successfully in court battles to improve access to care for incarcerated transgender prisoners in the United States, where denial of necessary medical care to incarcerated individuals is considered a "cruel and unusual punishment" in violation of the country's constitution (Alexander and Meshelemiah 2010). Thus, the challenge of the DSM-5 revision process was how to balance the conflicting issues of maintaining access to care, which required retaining a medical diagnosis, while reducing stigma associated with being labeled with a psychiatric diagnosis (Drescher 2010).

In 2013, the APA issued DSM-5 (American Psychiatric Association 2013), which revised the DSM-IV-TR diagnosis of *gender identity disorder* (American Psychiatric Association 2000) to a new diagnosis called *gender dysphoria*. In doing so, APA chose to preserve access to care but changed the name of the disorder and modified the criteria to reduce stigma. Among other things, this included separating the gender diagnoses from the sexual dysfunctions and paraphilias and narrowing the diagnostic criteria to reduce false positives (Zucker et al. 2013).

During the revision process, APA also issued two positions statements, one supporting access to care (American Psychiatric Association 2012a) and the other opposing discrimination against transgender individuals (American Psychiatric Association 2012b). APA also appointed a task force to review and recommend treatment guidelines for transgender individuals (Byne et al. 2012).

APA's decision had its intended effect of maintaining access to care. In May 2014, the U.S. Department of Health and Human Services reversed a longstanding 1981 ruling that classified gender reassignment as "experimental" treatment not reimbursable by Medicare (U.S. Department of Health and Human Services 2014). This reversal was based, in part, on the reasoning that DSM-IV-TR's gender identity disorder and DSM-5's gender dysphoria represented the view of American psychiatry that these disorders were medical conditions requiring treatment. Following that decision, many state Medicaid programs have begun to include some, if not all, transition services for eligible patients.

It should be further noted that at the time of this writing, WHO is revising ICD-11 for an anticipated publication date of 2018. WHO's Working Group on the Classification of Sexual Disorders and Sexual Health has recommended changing transsexualism to *gender incongruence* and moving the diagnosis out of ICD's mental disorders section into a new chapter called "Conditions Related to Sexual Health" (Drescher et al. 2012; Reed et al. 2016). At that juncture, retaining a mental disorder diagnosis in DSM-5 will no longer be necessary.

As medicine moves beyond a mental disorder model of gender variance, *Transgender Mental Health* is timely indeed. Dr. Yarbrough brings his experience and expertise from Callen-Lorde, one of the most gender-affirming treatment centers in the United States. He introduces mental health professionals to an "informed consent" model of care that includes respect for patient diversity, recognition of patients' felt identities, and abandonment of the historic gatekeeping role. Instead, clinicians are invited to empathize with the subjectivity of gender dysphoric or incongruent patients and to offer them treatments proven to reduce their suffering and despair. There is much to learn here, and it is hoped that this volume will fill a much-needed gap in the training of mental health professionals of all disciplines.

Jack Drescher, M.D.
New York, New York

REFERENCES

Alexander R, Meshelemiah JCA: Gender identity disorders in prisons: what are the legal implications for prison mental health professionals and administrators? Prison J 90(3):269–287, 2010

American Psychiatric Association: Diagnostic and Statistical Manual of Mental Disorders, 3rd Edition. Washington, DC, American Psychiatric Association, 1980

American Psychiatric Association: Diagnostic and Statistical Manual of Mental Disorders, 4th Edition, Text Revision. Washington, DC, American Psychiatric Association, 2000

American Psychiatric Association: Position Statement on Access to Care for Transgender and Gender Variant Individuals. Washington, DC, American Psychiatric Association, 2012a. Available at: www.psychiatry.org/File%20Library/Learn/Archives/Position-2012-Transgender-Gender-Variant-Access-Care.pdf. Accessed March 1, 2016.

American Psychiatric Association: Position Statement on Discrimination Against Transgender and Gender Variant Individuals. Washington, DC, American Psychiatric Association, 2012b. Available at: www.psychiatry.org/File%20Library/Learn/Archives/Position-2012-Transgender-Gender-Variant-Discrimination.pdf. Accessed March 1, 2016.

American Psychiatric Association: Diagnostic and Statistical Manual of Mental Disorders, 5th Edition. Arlington, VA, American Psychiatric Association, 2013

Bayer R: Homosexuality and American Psychiatry: The Politics of Diagnosis. New York, Basic Books, 1981

Bayer R: Politics, science, and the problem of psychiatric nomenclature: a case study of the American Psychiatric Association referendum on homosexuality, in Scientific Controversies: Case Studies in the Resolution and Closure of Disputes in Science and Technology. Edited by Engelhardt HT, Caplan AL. New York, Cambridge University Press, 1987, pp 381–400

Byne W, Bradley SJ, Coleman E, et al; American Psychiatric Association Task Force on Treatment of Gender Identity Disorder: report of the American Psychiatric Association Task Force on Treatment of Gender Identity Disorder. Arch Sex Behav 41(4):759–796, 2012 22736225

Carey B: Psychiatrists revising the book of human troubles. New York Times, December 18, 2008, pp A1, A20

Chibbaro L: Activists alarmed over APA: head of psychiatry panel favors "change" therapy for some trans teens. Washington Blade, May 30, 2008. Available at: www.thetaskforce.org/static_html/TF_in_news/08_0612/stories/28_activists_alarmed.pdf. Accessed December 7, 2017.

Drescher J: Queer diagnoses: parallels and contrasts in the history of homosexuality, gender variance, and the diagnostic and statistical manual. Arch Sex Behav 39(2):427–460, 2010 19838785

Drescher J, Merlino JP (eds): American Psychiatry and Homosexuality: An Oral History. New York, Harrington Park Press, 2007

Drescher J, Cohen-Kettenis P, Winter S: Minding the body: situating gender identity diagnoses in the ICD-11. Int Rev Psychiatry 24(6):568–577, 2012 23244612

Green R: Attitudes toward transsexualism and sex-reassignment procedures, in Transsexualism and Sex Reassignment. Edited by Green R, Money J. Baltimore, Johns Hopkins University Press, 1969, pp 235–251

Hamburger C, Stürup GK, Dahl-Iversen E: Transvestism; hormonal, psychiatric, and surgical treatment. J Am Med Assoc 152(5):391–396, 1953 13044539

Jorgensen C: Christine Jorgensen: A Personal Autobiography. New York, Paul S. Ericksson, 1967

Karasic D, Drescher J (eds): Sexual and Gender Diagnoses of the Diagnostic and Statistical Manual (DSM): A reevaluation. New York, Haworth, 2005

Krafft-Ebing R: Psychopathia Sexualis. Translated by Wedeck H. New York, Putnam, 1886/1985

Osborne D: Flap flares over gender diagnosis. Gay City News, May 15, 2008. Available at: http://archive.li/ppyBZ. Accessed December 7, 2017.

Reed GM, Drescher J, Krueger RB, et al: Disorders related to sexuality and gender identity in the ICD-11: revising the ICD-10 classification based on current scientific evidence, best clinical practices, and human rights considerations. World Psychiatry 15(3):205–221, 2016 27717275

U.S. Department of Health and Human Services: NCD 140.3, Transsexual Surgery, Docket No A-13-87, Decision No 2576. Washington, DC, Departmental Appeals Board, Appellate Division, May 30, 2014. Available at: www.hhs.gov/sites/default/files/static/dab/decisions/board-decisions/2014/dab2576.pdf. Accessed September 24, 2017.

World Health Organization: International Statistical Classification of Diseases and Related Health Problems, 10th Revision. Geneva, World Health Organization, 1990

World Professional Association for Transgender Health: Standards of Care for the Health of Transsexual, Transgender and Gender Non-Conforming People, 7th Version, 2011. Available at: www.wpath.org/site_page.cfm?pk_association_webpage_menu=1351&pk_association_webpage=3926. Accessed December 7, 2017.

Zucker KJ, Cohen-Kettenis PT, Drescher J, et al: Memo outlining evidence for change for gender identity disorder in the DSM-5. Arch Sex Behav 42(5):901–914, 2013 23868018

ACKNOWLEDGMENTS

I WOULD LIKE to acknowledge that this book would not have happened without the encouragement and forethought of Dr. Petros Levounis. It was he who saw the need for the American Psychiatric Association to have a book dedicated to the topic of transgender mental health.

Dr. Jack Drescher, who wrote the foreword for this book, has been a mentor, teacher, and supporter of my lesbian, gay, bisexual, transgender, and queer/questioning (LGBTQ) education since I was a medical student. I depended on him as an expert to fine-tune the details and provide a historical background to the topics included in this book.

My education regarding gender diversity started in college with my professor Dr. Katharine Stewart. Her courses were transformative, and she still is probably the best teacher I have known.

The members of AGLP: The Association of LGBTQ Psychiatrists provided me with the resources and supervision that have led me down my career path. It has been an organization near and dear to my heart for many years.

The following people provided me with emotional support and/or feedback regarding the contents of this book: Khaldun Ahmed, Erin Black, Kevin Donnelly-Boylen, Victoria Formosa, David Guggenheim, Bill Lubart, Fred Martin, Angeliki Pesiridou, Morris Roy, Abraham Scott, Asher Sullivan, and Kathleen Yount.

Last, I would like to thank the staff and patients at Callen-Lorde Community Health Center. My experience working with them has been invaluable, enlightening, and heartwarming. It is a unique place to work and serves as a reminder to me that there is reason for hope.

Part I

General Topics

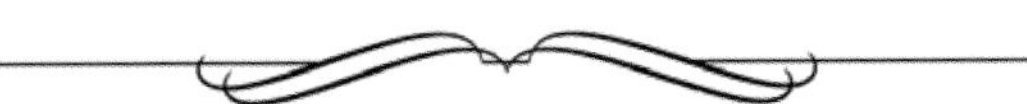

1

INTRODUCTION

> Gender is not something that one is, it is something one does, an act…a doing rather than a being.
>
> *Judith Butler*

PURPOSE

For better or worse, transgender and gender-nonconforming (TGNC) people are now in the midst of national political and social spotlights. For the first time in history, large portions of the world population are aware that gender diverse people exist. However, those who don't fit so neatly into the gender binary are marginalized and shunned from public society. Most cultures have little tolerance for individuals who don't follow general social gender norms.

The growing number of gender diverse people in the world is something of a misconception. Gender diverse people have existed as long as people have existed. The fact that greater society is now aware of them is mostly due to increasing safety and acceptance by communities. This was partly accomplished through advocacy organizations educating policy makers; research and scientific organizations educating clinicians; and, to a greater extent, the media of movies and television educating the general public. Regardless of the reason for this awareness, gender diverse people are now feeling more comfortable to come out and express their gender identity.

Now that so many people are aware of the TGNC population, there are more reactions to being around those who are gender diverse. Seeing people who are not like ourselves makes us question our own sense of self, and the presence of TGNC people has encouraged individuals to examine their own gender and the gender of others. Ideas about what is masculine and feminine are being called into question, and even people who do not necessarily identify as gender diverse are bending gender with the way they dress, how they talk, and the activities in which they participate. Society is being forced to look at the historical institution of gender now more than ever.

Despite the growing presence of gender diverse people in the media, the medical and mental health communities' responses have been lacking. Gender clinics sparsely populate large urban areas, and those clinics tend to be over capacity with referrals of gender diverse people seeking care. The great majority of patients needing treatment either get poor treatment from those who are not TGNC competent or simply don't seek services out of frustration and an inability to connect with clinicians who work with and understand gender diversity.

Given this information, the purpose of this book, above all else, is to increase access to care for TGNC people. The information in this book was selected in order to increase awareness and educate clinicians on how to address basic TGNC needs. My hope is that by reading this book, many mental health professionals, especially those who are timid about working with TGNC people, will feel more comfortable and confident in their ability to provide basic and safe care to those people who, at this time, don't have any good options.

This book is aimed at those mental health professionals who want to work with TGNC people but don't know how. Professional training programs provide little to no teaching regarding sexual orientation or gender diversity. By reading the chapters of this book, you will become familiar with the major topics, in both medical and mental health, that will start you on the path to creating a TGNC-competent practice.

The scope of this book is to target all mental health professionals, including psychiatrists, psychiatric nurse practitioners, psychologists, social workers, mental health counselors, art therapists, family therapists, pastoral counselors, and school counselors. The topics covered and the manner in which they are covered are meant to be both accessible and applicable to all of these professions. The amount of detail is intended to supplement the knowledge base and scope of practice of most mental health professionals. There are topics in this book that deserve more attention, and more details could have been put in each chapter to deepen the amount of information provided. However, this book is not meant to serve as a TGNC textbook. Many readers might wonder why I have glossed over certain subject matters and focused so much on others. My answer would be to redirect the reader back to my original goal: to increase access to care. The best way to increase access to care is to provide a simple yet thorough guide covering major topics that will apply to the everyday practice of most mental health professionals. This book functions as a highly accessible guidebook to help clinicians start their journey into the world of gender diversity. Hitting the largest audience possible is the best way to expand access to care.

The majority of mental health professionals are not trained to work with gender diverse people. This book is meant for them by increasing general awareness and providing a basic guidebook by which to start treatment with the TGNC community. In addition, there are many mental health clinicians who are already experts in TGNC care. Although they may find helpful information throughout the chapters, particularly those focused on medical and surgical options for care, for these clinicians, the book will likely serve as a general review and help them solidify their knowledge and basic understanding of TGNC-competent treatment. This book is written in a way as not to be too clinical. Individuals who are not mental health professionals and even those not in the medical community will be able to read and digest the information provided.

WHY NOW?

Although the medical practice of working with TGNC people has existed for the past 80 years, at this particular time in history two co-occurring gender-related events are taking place. The first event has to do with the individual TGNC patient. Practitioners in the medical and mental health fields are starting to recognize the needs of this group of patients, who have been neglected and marginalized in the past. The medical community prides itself in standard practices, and these need to be developed for gender diverse people in order to provide appropriate care. Clinics are starting to provide TGNC people with a wide range of medical and mental health services. Insurance companies, both private and public, are starting to pay for gender-affirming procedures, and TGNC patients now have access to possibilities that were not available to them before.

The second event involves culture. We are starting to see a more global shift regarding gender, gender roles, and gender diversity. The presence of gender diverse people in mainstream media has made the public aware of the variety of ways gender can present itself. People who identify as lesbian, gay, bisexual, transgender, or queer/questioning (LGBTQ) are making their presence known more in smaller communities, leading to an overall change in perception and getting those around them to think about gender and sexuality in a new way. Stereotypical roles of what it means to be a boy or girl, man or woman, are starting to be questioned. People have been departing from traditional gender norms in the way they dress, talk, act, work, and have sex. Stepping outside of the rules, or *gender bending*, is becoming more common. The long-held rules about what makes a person male or female are changing.

WHO AM I?

It might be difficult for a reader to trust the information in this book without a little background on me, the author. I am a cis white gay male (cis is explained in Chapter 2, "Understanding the Gender Spectrum") who grew up in rural Alabama. Because of where I grew up, the early parts of my life were largely devoid of diversity in many aspects, but I was lucky to have exposure to people in my life who had me questioning social norms from an early age. One elementary school teacher I distinctly remember identified as female but presented herself as traditionally male. She had a short haircut and wore button-up shirts with a tie and men's dress shoes. She was a woman of color in a mostly white part of the South. She was a wonderful teacher. Her presence in my life, along with that of many more of my early educators, created in me positive associations with those who didn't fit neatly into the boxes they were supposed to fit in.

While studying psychology in college, I was fortunate to have access to several classes on sex, sexuality, and gender. Deconstructing what constituted a man or a woman was a regular part of my homework, and my teacher, an out lesbian-identified cis woman, opened my mind to noticing the arbitrary rules that dictate so much of our lives and behavior. She challenged her students to look at gender diversity and primed me to be open to gender diverse patients. While in college, I worked on a suicide hotline, and there I was exposed to transgender-identified people (both staff and callers) as well as callers with chronic and persistent mental illness. Listening to their stories, I started to understand the positions they find themselves in, the ongoing struggle with the way society treats them, and their need for help coupled with their inability to locate services.

After medical school, I matched in my psychiatric residency in New York City. There, I started to come across more TGNC patients. Many of my fellow clinicians would shy away from taking these patients because they said they felt untrained and generally unprepared to treat them. Luckily again, as a medical student, I had joined the Association of LGBTQ Psychiatrists (AGLP), many of whom are TGNC experts. By attending their meetings and getting to know the organization's members, I was exposed to the basics of TGNC care and had mentors I could call for ongoing supervision. I fell in love with the organization so much that I joined the board and eventually came to serve as its president. Now I'm fortunate in that I can provide supervision and training regarding gender diversity to students, residents, and colleagues. If you are working in a clinic and say "yes" to one TGNC person, and that person has a good experience working with you, word of mouth quickly spreads, and both staff and other clinicians will refer TGNC people to you. With an open ear, an understanding mind, and a warm heart, you, too, can become the local expert.

My growing expertise with TGNC people got me connected to Callen-Lorde Community Health Center, where I now work as the Director of Psychiatry. Callen-Lorde is a Federally Qualified Health Center that focuses on the medical and mental health treatment of LGBTQ individuals. It is located in New York City and has more than 4,000 TGNC-identified patients.

This book is based largely on my life experiences working with TGNC people. Friends, colleagues, and patients have told me their stories, and I want them to know I have heard them. I have attempted to combine both the stories I have heard with the clinician's experiences I have had into a volume that can take other mental health professionals down a similar educational road. It is a road, if you keep your mind and heart open to learning, that will instill in you a sense of compassion, empathy, and duty to help TGNC people get the care and treatment they deserve.

INSTRUCTIONS

This book is meant to be read from cover to cover. It serves more as a guidebook rather than a reference or textbook. The topics covered in the earlier chapters will provide you with information that you will need in later chapters. The book is additive and works to build on each chapter. I would encourage you to start at the beginning and read through to the end. None of the chapters are too heavy in their treatment of the material, and this book should be an easy read for any mental health professional regardless of your specialty.

The questions at the end of each chapter are multilayered. Not only do they test your comprehension of the material you have read, but they will also provide further information and help you to see the complicated political, social, and cultural barriers most TGNC people experience when trying to get adequate care. Some of the multiple-choice answers may seem obvious, with even ridiculously wrong answers provided for distraction, but I assure you that most of the answers provided will describe experiences I have either witnessed myself or was told of by patients and colleagues. The wrong answers will teach you about what the medical and mental health community is doing wrong in much the same way the right answers will give you guidance.

REFERENCES

Each chapter includes only a select group of references. These references were picked not only to cite certain information provided in the book but also to serve as excellent resources for further learning in topics you will want to know more about. The references are largely new in that most of them were published post-2010. There are many excellent TGNC articles published prior to 2010, but I wanted to keep the research current. Keeping research current communicates to readers the contemporary nature of what they are reading and gives them more confidence, knowing they are being brought up to date on the most recent research and standards of care. The references are also multidisciplinary in that the authors are professionals from various mental health backgrounds, including psychiatrists, psychiatric nurse practitioners, psychologists, social workers, and counselors. The references will provide you with the voices of all types of mental health professionals contributing to TGNC knowledge.

CASES

The chapters include a collection of case presentations. These presentations are intended to solidify previous topics and help you apply what you have read to a clinical situation. The stories provided are real, although significantly disguised. Patient names, ages, gender identities, and locations have been shifted and merged with other cases to ensure confidentiality. The heart of each case, however, is a true story that has happened to a TGNC individual. Some of them are heartbreaking, and all of them will show you the definite need for TGNC-competent clinicians and access to care.

WORD CHOICES

This might be the most difficult and controversial topic to write about, but the word choices I made when writing this book were deliberate. The way people describe themselves, their identity, and their gender are very personal. Words that are appropriate in some groups may be not be appropriate in others. The word choices I have made serve as a representation of the majority of words both patients and staff have used in my work with them. This language will not be universal, and I dare say it may even be offensive to some. My intention with my wording is to convey the spirit of TGNC care I have both participated in and witnessed in my career.

The book is written through experiences that have taken place in the United States, although I have interacted with many colleagues and supervisors from other countries. That means the way I write about medicine and the way the cases are presented will be with a Western style and bias. TGNC care in other parts of the world might not describe gender diverse people the way I do or purpose treatment for them in the way this book is arranged. Practitioners should pay attention to cultural sensitivity, particularly when working with patients who grew up in other parts of the world.

Throughout the chapters, you will notice that sometimes I will say TGNC person/people and other times I will say TGNC patient. The world *patient* is used when the focus of the topic is on clinical interventions or clinical situations. People who are TGNC are not inherently ill, and they certainly do not automatically have a psychiatric disorder. TGNC people do, however, seek treatment, and my personal preference is to respect the clinician-patient relationship by using these word choices.

In the same vein, the DSM-5 (American Psychiatric Association 2013) diagnosis of gender dysphoria is used throughout the book as well. TGNC people are said to have "dysphoric" symptoms in relation to their body. This is not true for all TGNC people. Some TGNC people might have feelings about their gender and gender identity, but they are not dysphoric about their body, nor do they wish to seek treatment with gender-affirming procedures. There are many TGNC people who do have dysphoric symptoms and would very much like to make adjustments to their body through medicine or surgical means. The details of gender dysphoria will be explained more in Chapter 7, "The Gender Dysphoria Diagnosis," but it is essential to realize that the diagnosis of gender dysphoria was included in DSM-5 as a means to provide an avenue for care and treatment. Diagnosis is required by insurance companies for patients seeking to cover the cost of hormones and gender-affirming procedures. A growing number of mental health professionals do not believe that TGNC people have a mental illness, and the diagnosis of gender dysphoria remains a means to an end, with that end being access to care.

My use of the acronym TGNC throughout the book is on purpose as well. Transgender and gender nonconforming are two aspects of the gender spectrum. Persons who are gender nonconforming may not necessarily consider themselves transgender. Including the nonconforming part of TGNC is important so that you will remember that gender is on a spectrum and is not a binary concept. People don't just transition from male to female or from female to male. They may shift on the gender spectrum, but how and in which way is a personal decision.

LGBTQ stands for lesbian, gay, bisexual, transgender, and queer/questioning and will also make an appearance throughout the chapters. Individuals who are diverse on the spectrum of sexual orientation and gender frequently are grouped together historically, mostly in political ways. Gender and sexuality are two separate phenomena and should be treated as such; however, some things are unique and particular to both groups. These phenomena overlap and interact in complex ways. Internalized homophobia and internalized transphobia, which will be explained in Chapter 8, "Gender-Affirming Mental Health," are shared experiences among all LGBTQ people. LGBTQ is substituted for TGNC when a topic applies to the larger group.

The use of the word *therapist* as a substitute for *practitioner* will happen frequently. I am a psychiatrist, but this book is intended for all mental health professionals. Few areas in the book have information that will pertain only to psychiatrists. All psychiatrists are trained to be therapists, and many do only therapy in their full-time work. All psychiatrists, whether they are aware of it or not, are doing supportive therapy with all of their patients. When I use the term therapist, it pertains to all mental health professionals, whether a psychiatrist, psychologist, social worker, counselor, or case manager.

CAVEATS

Concept of Gender Binary

The later chapters in this book are heavily binary in that the material is organized on the basis of masculinizing and feminizing effects of treatment. It is important to note that when working with TGNC people, the focus of treatment should not be on the body. Gender is situated in the mind, and the body may be changed to reflect the mind on the basis of individual preference. The chapters that are structured in this binary way will help organize the reader's understanding of the material and make the information accessible. Information presented in either a masculinizing or feminizing section could apply to people at any point on the gender spectrum. Given that the hormones and surgeries have generally opposite effects, splitting the chapters was the best way to convey the material. Truly appreciating gender nonconformity means letting go of a gender binary and recognizing that we all fall on a spectrum.

Repetition

Some of the topics in this book will be repeated numerous times. As stated at the beginning of this introduction, TGNC people having access to care is the primary message that all chapters in this book will emphasize. Repeating topics is an effort to solidify this information in readers' awareness and help them to provide quality TGNC-competent care. Covering the same topics repeatedly is an effort to make sure the most crucial messages are the ones that readers remember the most.

Introductory Coverage

There are topics that will not be covered in this book in depth even though they are significant to the TGNC community. One such set of topics includes the knowledge that medical diagnoses such as sexually transmitted diseases and HIV affect the TGNC community disproportionately. Special topics of sex and sexuality have their own chapter (Chapter 12, "Sexuality"), which includes research devoted to studying sexually transmitted disease in the TGNC community. Medical and surgical topics are brought up throughout the chapters in this book, but some of the details about medicinal treatments were left out if they did not apply directly to mental health professionals. The material depth was selected because the book is intended to provide necessary information while not overwhelming the reader with details.

Exclusion of Children

This book is not meant for practitioners working with children and adolescents who are gender dysphoric. Although many of the topics can be used directly to treat both children and adolescents, the care of TGNC youth is its own unique field requiring special skill sets that are not covered in this book. Topics such as gender atypical children, puberty suppression blockers, and family interventions require their own chapters and case presentations. The subject matter in this book is for adults who have gender dysphoric symptoms, and the mental health professionals referred to in this book are those who work with adults. The diagnosis and treatment of TGNC children is in its infancy (no pun intended), and much research is needed to help understand at which point along the path of development interventions are needed. The vast majority of patients mental health professionals will see who identify as TGNC will be young adults or older adults who have known about their gender variance for many years.

CRISIS AND OPPORTUNITY

Mental illness is not the focus of this book, and it should not be the focus of treatment when working with someone who is TGNC. Treatment with TGNC people is about embracing the varied ways the world can express gender. Mental health professionals spend their careers diagnosing people and assigning them treatments depending on the symptoms they are presenting with. It is a fortunate position to be in when working with TGNC people because the focus of treatment is not about treating gender diversity. It is about accepting gender diversity.

The TGNC population does have disproportionate amounts of depression, anxiety, trauma, substance abuse, and suicide attempts. Much of the discrepancy when compared with the general population can be explained by transphobia and stigma. Gender diverse people are ingrained with negative images and ideas about themselves from an early age. Over time, this negativity turns into internalized transphobia. Internalized transphobia can lead to a myriad of symptoms.

All mental health diagnoses aside, working with TGNC people is an opportunity to focus on positive treatment options for people to better express themselves externally on the basis of their internal gender identity. Providing space for gender diverse persons to express themselves and, over time, discover who they are is an extremely rewarding opportunity.

CONTENTS OF THIS BOOK

The contents of this book are broken down into four major parts. The first part focuses on general topics with TGNC people such as understanding gender diversity. The second covers mental health–related topics, including diagnosis and mental health particulars related to gender diverse people. The third part focuses on medicinal or hormone treatment options as well as general primary care topics. The last part discusses surgical gender-affirming procedures as well as nonsurgical interventions.

Part I: General Topics

The main focus of this part is general TGNC topics. Chapter 2, which is probably the most important chapter, covers the gender spectrum. If a clinician is unable to grasp the idea of the gender spectrum and the range of gender variance present in patient populations, then I would hazard to say that person is not cut out for working with TGNC people.

After this discussion of the gender spectrum, a brief history of TGNC people throughout time will be covered. Chapter 3, "Historical Background," initially focuses on historical figures and then shifts to the history of TGNC care and gender-affirming procedures. It is a brief overview and will cover only the highlights of TGNC culture and medicine throughout the years.

Following TGNC history, a guidebook of sorts introduces practitioners to ways to create a TGNC-friendly clinic. It isn't enough to say one is TGNC competent; clinicians must show competence through the way they set up their office, organize their medical records, and train their staff. Chapter 4, "Establishing a TGNC-Friendly Clinic," is a step-by-step guide to help all clinics adjust in order to make room for gender diverse people.

With Chapter 5, the focus shifts to advocacy. Frequently more important than providing mental health specific treatment, advocacy is a way that mental health professionals can assist their TGNC patients the most. It is fortunate that mental health professionals have taken on the role of advocate within the realm of TGNC medicine. Although not all TGNC people will require mental health treatment for mental illness, most will require advocacy from their mental health team. Mental health professionals are, above other medical professionals, able to understand the social and cultural implications of being gender diverse. It is through this understanding that they can identify when social injustices have occurred and advocate for change to better support their TGNC patients' lives.

Specific to advocacy, letter writing for gender marker changes and gender-affirming surgeries (Chapter 6, "Letter Writing") will most certainly be part of the treatment all mental health professionals will provide to their TGNC patients. Knowing the specifics of what is needed in these letters can be confusing, but it becomes easy once the necessary formula and background of these letters are understood. By making more clinicians available to write letters of support for gender-affirming procedures, we are increasing access to care in places where it is needed most.

Part II: Mental Health–Related Topics

This part is dedicated to mental health factors in TGNC care. The first chapter in this part, Chapter 7, "The Gender Dysphoria Diagnosis," focuses on understanding the diagnosis and history of gender dysphoria. Because this is a relatively new diagnosis to DSM, knowing the criteria and history behind the diagnosis is needed in order to provide TGNC-competent care.

Chapter 8, "Gender-Affirming Mental Health," gives an overview of mental health treatment specific to TGNC care. Most mental health professionals will be familiar with the material in this chapter but may not understand how it applies to gender diverse people. Although volumes could be written about this topic in particular, I've attempted to condense the information to make it accessible and to provide a general overview for clinicians who are starting work in TGNC mental health. Although this is the only topic labeled specifically as mental health treatment, every chapter in the book pertains to the biological, psychological, and social aspects of TGNC care.

Next is Chapter 9, "Transitions and Detransitions." Neither of these transitions has a direction, nor do they have a direct finish line. The goal is self-expression and alignment of the body and mind if preferred. Looking at experiences people have when transitioning will help clinicians prepare future patients for what to expect when navigating gender diversity and change. The vast majority of people who transition in some way are very satisfied with their results; however, it would be an oversight not to mention that some people may want to detransition. Detransitioning doesn't necessarily mean that someone stops identifying as transgender. It is a bit more complicated than that. The chapter provides general guidelines clinicians can use when encountering individuals who report that they want to detransition.

Chapter 10, "Families," provides guidance in understanding ways in which families and families of support are necessary. Some TGNC people are estranged from their biological family and depend on close friends or a "family of choice" for support. For those TGNC people who are still connected with their biological family, having family meetings and providing information sessions to family members can be complicated. Trying to get families to accept and support their loved ones for who they are while navigating their own personal feelings is a common task for most LGBTQ mental health professionals.

Gender diversity can manifest in a variety of ways, and many TGNC people have histories of trauma. These trauma histories, specifically repeated traumas, can create symptoms of dissociation. Some patients may have dissociative identities with varying gender presentations. Chapter 11, "Plurality," will help clinicians navigate multiple identities or alters and provide safe and affirming care.

The last chapter in Part II is Chapter 12, "Sexuality." Sex and sexuality are topics that mental health professionals are generally comfortable talking about. Understanding the diverse ways in which sexuality and gender diversity exist and looking at each person individually are critical elements in providing TGNC-competent care. Sexuality is a topic that can be sensitive for TGNC people given the dysphoria they may have with their bodies.

Part III: Primary Care and Hormone Treatment

In Part III, the focus switches from mental health to physical health. Three chapters provide an overview of general physical health with people who are TGNC (Chapter 13, "Primary Care") as well as masculinizing and feminizing hormones (Chapter 14, "Transmasculine Hormones," and Chapter 15, "Transfeminine Hormones"). You may ask why mental health professionals need to know some of the specifics of medicinal treatments available to TGNC people. The main reason is that so many other medical professionals do not. We can best provide safe and effective care if we address all aspects of our patient's needs—social, psychological, and physical. Even if you are working alongside open-minded and well-meaning primary care clinicians, they may not be aware of the nuances involved in TGNC care. Many are willing to alter their practice and meet patient needs with a little advocacy on the part of the mental health clinician.

By the end of Part III you will understand what basic physical problems TGNC people face. In addition, you will be able to provide information to future patients about what to expect from hormone or medicinal treatments. The process of change when someone is taking hormones can be long and also dramatic. Clinicians need to be prepared to have discussions about their patients' bodies and minds following the initiation of hormone treatment.

Part IV: Surgical and Nonsurgical Gender-Affirming Procedures

In this last part, all major gender-affirming procedures will be discussed. Top and bottom surgery (Chapters 16–19) will be looked at through masculinizing and feminizing lenses. It is necessary for all mental health professionals who plan to work with TGNC people to know the information in these chapters. If clinicians do not understand the general details of gender-affirming procedures (including nonsurgical options covered in Chapter 20, "Other Gender-Affirming Procedures"), they will not be able to write letters of support or assess their patients for capacity. Many TGNC people will know more details about the surgical procedures than their mental health providers do, but it is good clinical practice to provide our patients with psychoeducation and understanding of what procedure they have selected and the potential physical and mental implications both presurgery and postsurgery.

FINAL REMARKS

You are about to start on a journey to become a TGNC-competent clinician. Provided for you in these chapters are my best organization and presentation of the material that is absolutely necessary to know when working with someone who is TGNC. Each chapter will provide you with references for further reading. How deep you delve into the world of gender diversity will depend on your interest in and desire to provide care for gender diverse people.

The study of TGNC people remains in its infancy. The recommendations and suggestions in this volume will change over time as more knowledge and understanding are acquired. There may be many who don't agree with the recommendations I have to offer, and I would encourage you to get as much information as you can from as many sources as possible. Others will have insight into topics and experiences that I might be blind to. Other references have already been written from medical and social perspectives, and they deserve your attention should you wish to get more details. The focus of this volume will be ultimately on the mental health of TGNC people.

As you gather information from this and other volumes, your understanding of and ability to work with gender diversity will increase. You will probably interact with other clinicians who have no knowledge or understanding of TGNC care. Some may even be hostile or discriminatory toward TGNC individuals. I would encourage you to approach the lack of education in others just as you will with yourself as you read this book. You will be new to this material just as others will be new to it. By learning ourselves, we can teach others. If you are to have any hope of getting other clinicians on board with TGNC care, you will need to approach them in a nondefensive and noncritical way. Clinicians should be encouraged to learn, not be critiqued for their lack of knowledge, especially when they are seeking out that knowledge.

All of us, no matter where we fall on the gender spectrum, should approach each other with new eyes, appreciating the individual nature and expression each of us possesses. Only by truly seeing each other and supporting each other can we start to provide a fertile ground for learning and nurture a larger and more general understanding of gender diversity. By approaching individuals this way, we can engender and foster mental health care that will embrace gender diversity and help us to provide the most compassionate care possible.

REFERENCE

American Psychiatric Association: Diagnostic and Statistical Manual of Mental Disorders, 5th Edition. Arlington, VA, American Psychiatric Association, 2013

2

UNDERSTANDING THE GENDER SPECTRUM

I believe gender is a spectrum, and I fall somewhere between Channing Tatum and Winnie the Pooh.

Stephen Colbert

WORKING WITH TRANSGENDER and gender-nonconforming (TGNC) patients starts with an exploration of the self. Not all mental health professionals have personally dealt with mental illnesses of their own, such as major depression, generalized anxiety, bipolar disorder, and even schizophrenia, but it is certain that all mental health professionals have a gender by which they identify. At birth, we are assigned a sex. Having a penis puts you in the male category, and having a vagina puts you in the female category, with a blue or pink blanket swaddled around you not long after you are born. From birth until age 3, when we begin to develop our own ideas about gender, we are bombarded with gender stereotypes that conform us to culturally expected norms.

Consider what makes a baby look more stereotypically like a boy or a girl. It is usually the clothing the parent puts on the child or the toys the baby is given to play with. Babies are generally gender neutral, and our perception of their gender is shaped by cultural norms (see the section "Gender" below). Many of us have access to our baby pictures, and we can deduce that the concepts of *boy* and *girl* were placed on us well before we knew our own gender or sex. Mental health professionals who want to work with gender diverse people must first explore what gender means to themselves and understand where they fall on the gender spectrum. Only by doing so can we be open to the experiences and expressions of our gender diverse patients.

GENDER

Gender is different from sex (Figure 2–1). Gender refers to our internal thoughts about who we are, and it starts to develop between the ages of 3 and 5. It is the way we see ourselves as male, female, or anywhere in between. It affects how we walk, talk, and carry ourselves. It affects how we dress, what jobs we aim for, and how we plan for the future. It affects our sexual orientation and sexual behavior. Gender is the first major factor other than the color of our skin that will touch and shape our entire lives.

Generally, the sex we are assigned at birth and the gender we come to identify as are congruent. Although this is usually true, the majority of us don't fall into all the stereotypes assigned to male and female by society. According to these stereotypes (Figure 2–2), men are supposed to be strong, unemotional, aggressive, and powerful. Men like sports and are good at math. Women are soft, emotional, and passive. They like to cook, wear makeup, and raise children. These are examples of primitive views of gender and sexuality that society continues to slowly move away from. Do all men hunt and all women gather? What constitutes masculinity? Although many people might be quick to dismiss overarching and inflammatory concepts of gender, many people still hold fast to these concepts and pass them along to their children.

As previously stated, the understanding of gender begins with the treating clinician. The world is dichotomized into male and female, boy and girl. Working with TGNC patients requires clinicians to break down the rigid views of gender they have carried since childhood. We have to start viewing gender as a spectrum by seeing maleness in the feminine and femaleness in the masculine.

GENDER STEREOTYPES

Start by looking at your own beliefs. Imagine in your mind a typical man. What makes someone masculine? What makes someone male? There might be many overlapping traits, but are all the identifiers the same? A good concept to examine is what physical qualities make someone male. What general shape do you place on a male or masculine figure? Most would agree it is in the form of an upside-down triangle (Figure 2–3). The shoulders are broad and the waist is small. Men are seen as top heavy and moving in a more lumbering way. Not all men have this basic shape, but you still might refer to them as masculine or male.

What other cues do you look for when deciding if someone is male? Maybe you'll look at the face (Figure 2–4). The spread of the brow, the thickness of the nose, and the prominence of the jaw might give you signals. Your

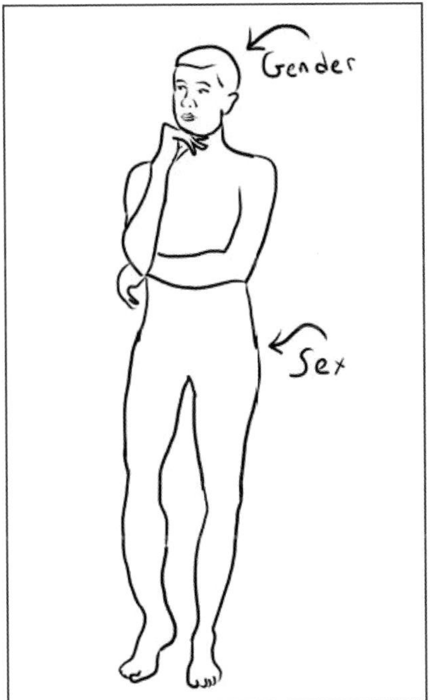

FIGURE 2–1. Sex is associated with the body, and gender is associated with the mind.

version of a male might even include a beard. Is a beard required to make a male masculine?

Not all men are the shape of an upside-down triangle. Some men might have facial hair, but many do not. The shape of a man's face can be as diverse as fingerprints. Yet despite the spectrum of male presentation, you still would refer to these characteristics as belonging to men, as being male or even masculine.

What about behavior? Is someone the take charge type? Do they tend to lead? Are they bad at asking for directions? Are these aspects male, masculine, or both? What aspects of ourselves do we identify as masculine or feminine? Do these characteristics make us any more male or female? The world is made up primarily of two sexes but a whole spectrum of genders. It will be freeing for us not only to think of TGNC patients having a divergence of gender but also to appreciate that everyone falls on a spectrum of gender identity from the masculine to the feminine. Gender is a spectrum much in the same way that Alfred Kinsey pointed out the spectrum for sexual orientation, sexual fantasy, and sexual behavior (Kinsey et al. 2010). *Letting go of the*

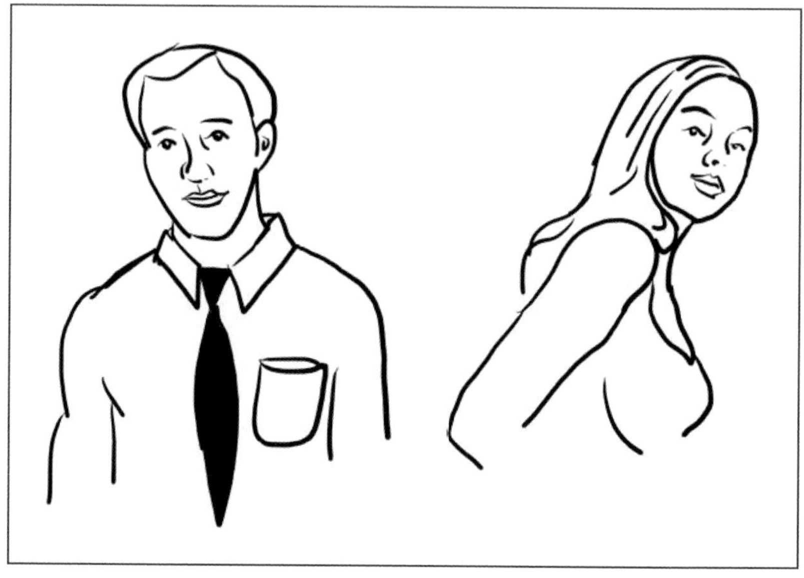

FIGURE 2–2. Many cues lead us to decide if someone is male or female.

gender dichotomy is an essential first step for clinicians when working with TGNC patients. It is the most important concept in this book.

GENDER AND OUR PATIENTS

What gender cues do we look for when we meet a patient for the first time? And how much of what we pick up on is conscious or unconscious? Although many people continue to hold on to the primitive views of gender identity and expression listed in the previous section, the mental health clinician needs to start understanding the more subtle stereotypes etched in his or her own mind. Take, for example, fingernail polish. Painting one's fingernails has been thought of as traditionally feminine in modern Western culture. However, in many subcultures throughout time such as ancient Babylonia, men would wear fingernail polish. Some men in entertainment do today. These same males and others might pierce their ears or wear makeup. When we see a patient with fingernail polish, earrings, and makeup, do we automatically assume that person is female? It might depend. There are other cues we look for even in the instant when we assign male or female to an individual: hair length, height, muscle mass, and body shape all contribute to our automatic assessment of boy or girl.

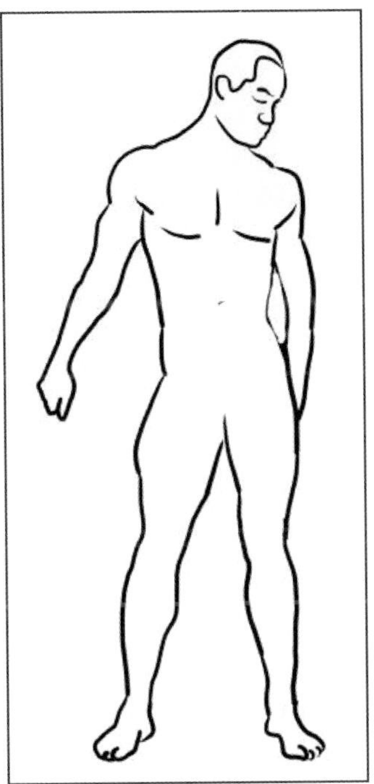

FIGURE 2–3. Being male is generally associated with a stereotypical shape.

As mental health professionals, it is important for us to be aware of our own automatic thinking when working with TGNC patients. Being aware of our own automatic thoughts is the best way to move beyond them. When addressing a patient by a pronoun, the only cue you should be certain of is that person's verbally expressed desire to be called by that pronoun. There are patients who look male, dress masculine, and act in a manly way but still might identify as a female on the inside and want to be called *she* and *her*. In working with TGNC patients, the mental health professional needs to be ready to work with the whole spectrum of gender identity and be prepared to encounter TGNC patients in various stages of transition and development. The quicker we can let go of our own rigid views of gender, the better equipped we will be to serve our TGNC patients in the most supportive way.

BINARY AND NONBINARY GENDER

Accepting that gender doesn't exist as a dichotomy, we can start to see the varied ways patients can present in a collage of gender presentations. Some

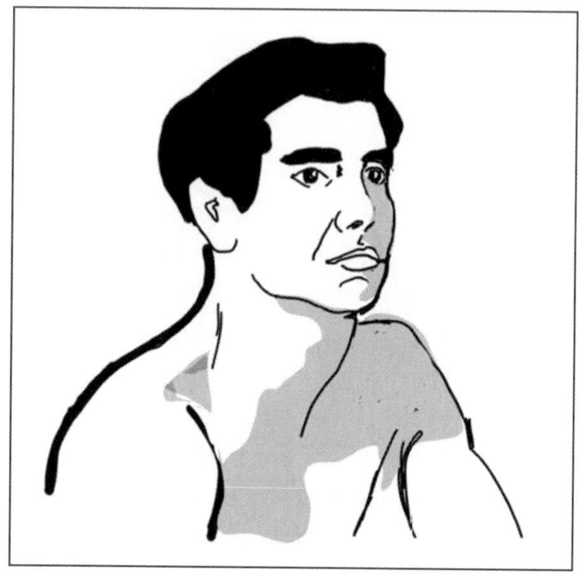

FIGURE 2–4. Facial cues further direct us in assigning gender.

patients might see themselves as existing both as male and female at the same time. They might go by the pronouns *he* and *him* as well as *she* and *her*. There are other patients who are nonbinary and say they belong to neither male nor female genders and prefer pronouns such as *they* and *them*. These patients might label themselves as gender nonconforming. Being TGNC doesn't mean that people are still required to be either male or female. Their gender can be male, female, both, or neither. Most people have aspects of themselves that are gender nonconforming in some way.

Many mental health professionals might find this concept difficult to understand or accept. In working with the TGNC population, it is necessary to continually question our assumptions about gender and sexuality so that we don't place our patients into gender boxes they don't belong in. Being nonbinary is just another way of expressing gender without conforming to traditional gender views.

PRONOUNS

Just as there are countless gender identities, there are countless gender pronouns (Figure 2–5). Throughout modern history, gender pronouns have been examined, and many people wish to change or do away with them. Some people, in the past, have tried to combine *him* and *her* into *hir* or *he*

Subject	Object	Pronoun	Pronunciation
She	Her	Hers	As it looks
He	Him	His	As it looks
They	Them	Theirs	As it looks
Ze	Hir	Hirs	zhee, here, heres
Ze	Zir	Zirs	zhee, zhere, zheres
Xe	Xem	Xyrs	zhee, zhem, zheres

Example Sentences by Pronoun

- They – "They came into the clinic reporting that their depression had worsened."
- Ze – "Could you please tell zir when zirs appointment is?"

FIGURE 2–5. Example of pronouns and how they are used in speech.
Source. American Psychiatric Association 2017.

and *she* into *s/he*. Some pronouns have also been created that are new altogether, such as *ze* and *zir*. These pronouns are free of gender stereotypes and may be used by some patients. Making space for patients to express themselves in this way may be one of the most healing interventions you provide as a mental health professional. Using appropriate pronouns conveys to patients, at the very minimum, that you have heard them and recognize them for who they are.

The subject of pronouns is extremely important when addressing TGNC patients, and using the correct pronoun is the most basic level of respect we can provide to our patients. As easy as this might seem, it continues to be the hardest lesson to teach many practitioners in the medical and mental health community. Doctors, nurses, social workers, case managers, and hospital staff frequently misgender patients and refuse to respect TGNC patients' pronouns. Imagine you are a patient dealing with an acute psychiatric illness, such as a psychotic break, with all the stress of being admitted to the hospital. While you are suffering from symptoms, the hospital staff who are there to help you refer to you by the wrong name and gender, further triggering your stress levels. It's not a mystery why so many TGNC patients are skeptical and afraid of the medical and mental health care systems.

MISGENDERING

Misgendering patients is referring to them by a pronoun they do not use. This experience for a TGNC patient can range from anxiety provoking and uncomfortable at best to traumatizing and triggering at worst. Given how ingrained gender is in our everyday speech and automatic assumptions, it's understandable that individuals who don't fall into stereotypical gender norms might make clinicians uncomfortable that they will make a mistake by calling someone by the wrong pronoun. This will definitely happen at some point when working with the TGNC population. When you do misgender a patient, the appropriate way to handle it is to apologize and thank the patient for correcting you. If you go further than that and make a big deal of the situation, it will only lead to the patient feeling more uncomfortable and keeps the spotlight on their gender identity.

CISNORMALITY

The word *transgender* is considered by many to be a misnomer because it implies that the person transitions from one gender to the other. Many who are TGNC would say they are simply expressing the gender they have always known themselves to be. Others might embrace the term transgender because it might imply transitioning physically from one gender to the other both medically and surgically. There are as many views of the terminology of TGNC as there are people on the spectrum, which includes everyone.

One term that is generally accepted is the idea of cisgender. In chemistry, the prefix *cis* is used to designate chemical bonds that are located on the same side of a chemical structure, whereas the prefix *trans* designates opposite sides (Figure 2–6). As an adjective, the term cis can be used to describe gender identity. Almost all babies are assigned a sex—male or female—at birth. When this assigned sex at birth aligns with the gender by which an individual identifies, we refer to that person as *cisgender*. A person assigned male at birth who identifies as male would be referred to as a *cis male*, and a person assigned female at birth who identifies as female would be referred to as a *cis female*.

Some babies may not necessarily be assigned a sex at birth because they have ambiguous genitalia. This might be due to a number of genetic phenomena. The old term for this type of individual would have been *hermaphrodite*, but the current term is *intersex*, also known in DSM-5 as the gender dysphoria specifier *with a disorder of sex development* (American Psychiatric Association 2013, p. 453). Intersex is not the same as transgender or gender nonconforming. Typically, intersex persons identify their gender as they age, and they are assigned a sex on the basis of their gender identity. In the past, they were sometimes assigned a presumptive sex and were given sur-

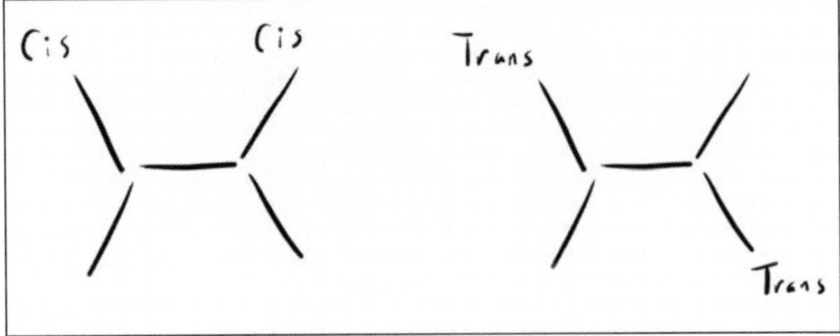

FIGURE 2–6. **In chemistry, cis bonds are on the same side, and trans bonds are on the opposite side.**

gical procedures as an infant to align their genitalia with the assigned sex. History has taught us that an assigned sex and gender identity do not always match up (Colapinto 2001). This created problems later on because the assigned sex and gender didn't always match up (Colapinto 2001).

People who are cisgender naturally see the world through a cisgender lens. Being *cisnormative* is having automatic expectations about the gender identity of people based on their sex assigned at birth. Expecting everyone to follow classic gender stereotypes is an example of cisnormativity. Assuming that all people are cisgender is another example. In order to be empathic with TGNC patients, it is necessary to view the world through the lens of gender diversity.

SEXUAL ORIENTATION

Many people confuse sexual orientation and gender identity (Figure 2–7). They believe that if a man is attracted to another man, then that means he really wants to be a woman. They also might say that women who identify as lesbian really want to be men. Gender identity is the way one views oneself as male, female, or in between. *Sexual orientation* is the sexual attraction someone has toward a gender and/or sex. Just as gender identity is on a spectrum, so is sexual orientation. Many people understand the spectrum of heterosexual, bisexual, and homosexual, but it is possible that people can also be attracted to both genders within the same person or the lack of gender within a person. Just as gender can be binary or nonbinary, attraction can be directed toward a gender binary or nonbinary. There are people who label themselves as pansexual who might be attracted to persons who are cis male, cis female, trans male, trans female, gender neutral, gender nonconforming, and any other of a host of gender identities.

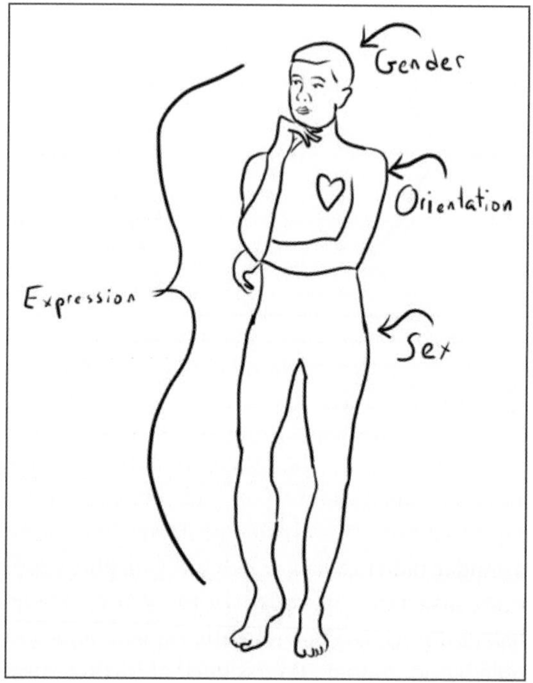

FIGURE 2–7. Sex, sexual orientation, gender, and gender expression should be thought of as separate characteristics.

The thing to remember when it comes to both gender identity and sexual orientation is that how patients define themselves is much more important than being able to place them in a box or category. Identifying someone's gender identity or sexual orientation for them is generally not helpful. It is a personal understanding that can be identified only by the patient.

HOW COMMON IS GENDER DIVERSITY?

There might be a perception that the presence of TGNC people is new and that gender diversity is a fad. In Chapter 3, "Historical Background," I will delve into evidence of how gender diverse people have existed throughout recorded history. The likely reason that TGNC people are coming into the public awareness more often lately is that it is now safer for people to identify as TGNC. Although it is by no means a safe world for those who are gender diverse, there is a growing number of people who are supportive of gender diversity, allowing individuals who previously had to hide their gender identity to now tell others.

The Williams Institute published a report in 2016 that identified the TGNC population in the United States to be about 1.4 million people (Flores et al. 2016). That is roughly 1 out of every 200 adults. Clinicians may say that they have never worked with a TGNC patient, but there is a great likelihood that they have. TGNC persons may not identify themselves as transgender to a clinician unless they know they are in a safe place to do so. To put this in perspective, about 2%–5% of the United States population has red hair. For every four to eight redheads you've seen, you have probably also come across someone who is TGNC.

SUMMARY

Understanding gender diversity as a spectrum is one of the first and most important steps a clinician needs to take when working with TGNC patients. Our concepts of what is masculine and feminine are largely culturally ingrained, and people are forced, sometimes uncomfortably so, into gender boxes from birth. Every human has gender diverse behaviors and uniqueness that do not make them solely male or female. All people fall somewhere on the gender spectrum. Knowing that gender is not a dichotomy will help clinicians appreciate those patients who are more gender diverse. Being aware of our own gender stereotypes will help prevent subjecting our patients to those same stereotypes. Respecting our patients' pronouns and where patients fall on the gender spectrum will help us to provide a basic safe space for care so that treatment and healing can begin.

Key Points

- Sex refers to anatomy. Gender is in the mind.
- Gender is not a dichotomy but exists as a spectrum.
- People can identify as male, female, both, neither, or anywhere on the spectrum.
- Clinicians must be aware of their own gender stereotypes when working with TGNC patients.
- Clinicians should respect patient pronouns.
- *Misgendering* is calling a person by the wrong pronouns.
- *Cisgender* refers to persons whose sex assigned at birth and gender identity are congruent.

- *Intersex* refers to people born with ambiguous genitalia and is not the same as TGNC.
- There are approximately 1.4 million TGNC people living in the United States.

QUESTIONS

1. You are scheduled to see a patient for the first time. The front desk staff calls you and says Mr. Smith is waiting for his first appointment. When you go out to the waiting room, the only person you see is a woman with long hair, wearing an ankle-length dress and makeup and carrying a handbag. You say, "Mr. Smith?" The patient replies, "I go by Ms. Smith, actually." What is the most appropriate response?

   A. "Oh, I'm so sorry! You're the first transgender patient I've worked with. The front desk staff said your name is Mr. Smith. I've made a horrible mistake."
   B. Ignore her remark and direct her to your office.
   C. Say, "I'm sorry about that; thank you for correcting me."
   D. Take her to the front desk staff and tell them the mistake they made. Explain to Ms. Smith in front of the office staff that it is their fault.

2. What should you call a person who is assigned female at birth and identifies as female?

   A. Trans woman.
   B. A cis female.
   C. Gender binary.
   D. Cogender.

3. Timothy is a 24-year-old man of trans experience who has been seeing you in an outpatient clinic for treatment of panic disorder. He sees you weekly for psychotherapy and has recently started to talk about his sexual orientation. He asks you if it is normal for a trans man to be attracted to gay men and wants to know how he should identify regarding his sexual orientation. What is your response?

   A. If he identifies as male and is attracted to men, he must be a gay man.

B. If he was assigned female at birth and is attracted to men, he is straight.
C. You don't know at this point, and you'd have to ask more questions about his behavior to give an appropriate response.
D. Sexual orientation and gender identity are separate. What is important is how he identifies himself, and you can help him explore this topic in your sessions.

4. The estimated population of TGNC people in the United States is approximately 0.6%. Why does it seem that there more TGNC people today than ever before?

   A. Research is better able to identify people who are TGNC because researchers have a better understanding of what questions to ask.
   B. Gender diverse people feel safer identifying as TGNC because society has become more aware of the gender spectrum.
   C. Growing awareness of gender diversity may help isolated people better explain their gender diverse feelings, whereas before, these feelings were suppressed.
   D. All of the above.

5. People who feel they don't really fit into traditional gender stereotypes and exist outside the realm of what most people would say is male and female may identify as

   A. Gender nonconforming.
   B. Pansexual.
   C. Cisgender.
   D. LGBT.

ANSWERS

1. **The correct response is option C.**

   When you misgender a patient, and it will happen at some point, it's best to apologize and thank them for correcting you. Addressing the issue further will only make the patient feel uncomfortable and put too much emphasis on their gender identity when they are probably coming to see you for some other concern. It's appropriate to correct the front desk staff but in a private place away from the waiting room and preferably not in front of the patient.

2. **The correct response is option B.**

   Someone who is assigned female at birth on the basis of primary sex characteristics and identifies as female is called a cis female. Someone who is assigned male at birth on the basis of primary sex characteristics and identifies as female is a trans female.

3. **The correct response is option D.**

   Sexual orientation and gender identity are separate. How people identify their gender or sexuality is personal and can be done only by the individual. Clinicians giving their opinion on how someone should identify is not typically helpful. Timothy should be encouraged to explore and identify himself on his own terms.

4. **The correct response is option D.**

   Gender diverse people have always been around in some form. Although there are technically more people now identified as being TGNC, this is likely due to improvements in research, safety, and awareness.

5. **The correct response is option A.**

   People will ultimately identify their own gender, and those who fall outside of the gender spectrum and don't conform to gender stereotypes may identify as gender nonconforming.

REFERENCES

American Psychiatric Association: Diagnostic and Statistical Manual of Mental Disorders, 5th Edition. Arlington, VA, American Psychiatric Association, 2013

American Psychiatric Association: A Guide for Working With Transgender and Gender Nonconforming Patients. Arlington, VA, American Psychiatric Association, 2017. Available at: www.psychiatry.org/psychiatrists/cultural-competency/transgender-and-gender-nonconforming-patients/definitions-and-pronoun-usage. Accessed December 12, 2017.

Colapinto J: As Nature Made Him: The Boy Who Was Raised as a Girl. New York, Harper Perennial, 2001

Flores AR, Herman JL, Gates GJ, Brown TNT: How Many Adults Identify as Transgender in the United States? Los Angeles, CA, The Williams Institute, 2016

Kinsey A, Pomeroy W, Martin C: Sexual Behavior in the Human Male. Bronx, NY, Ishi Press International, 2010

3

HISTORICAL BACKGROUND

> I defy any doctor in the world to prove that I am not a woman. I have lived, dressed, acted just what I am, a woman.
>
> *Lucky Hicks Anderson*

THE HISTORY OF transgender and gender-nonconforming (TGNC) individuals in the world is exceptionally vast. The term *transgender* was first used by Virginia Prince in the 1970s (Drescher 2010), but many people are not aware that gender diverse people have been present for centuries. In this chapter, I will cover the basic highlights of TGNC culture and medical treatment, but this will not do justice to the rich history covered by other authors in books dedicated to this subject (Meyerowitz 2009). The people and topics in this chapter are an attempt to provide a more diverse and accurate view of the TGNC world. So much of lesbian, gay, transgender, and queer/questioning (LGBTQ) history has been told through the stories of cis white people. People of color have been typically overlooked despite their major contributions to the development of what we now know as TGNC medicine.

The historical figures in this chapter will provide an introductory understanding necessary to appreciate the struggles faced by the TGNC population and hopefully will provide the reader with a level of empathy when working with TGNC patients. After exploring how long TGNC medicine and surgery have been around, you'll likely become more comfortable, trusting in the knowledge that has been gained through the evolution of TGNC care and using this information to provide better care to gender diverse people.

It is our responsibility not only to know TGNC history when working with gender diverse patients but to provide this historical perspective to our patients and their families, students, and colleagues who may not be aware.

Knowing the history of what our predecessors did will help us provide better consultation and options to our TGNC patients in the future.

HISTORICAL FIGURES

People have been bending gender, or stepping outside of the traditional gender dichotomy, as long as there has been a sense of man and woman. Gender diverse people are not a new phenomenon but have been around for much of recorded history. It may not be that all the individuals mentioned in this chapter would have identified as TGNC, but they represent a collection of nonbinary people who have broken the mold of what society has traditionally viewed as male and female. It is unclear how these people would have identified regarding their pronouns, so I have deferred to pronouns used in other historical texts. The nonbinary people throughout history are too numerous to name here, but the following are some of the more well-known examples.

As early as 218 A.D., the Roman Emperor Elagabalus was already bending gender rules. Although history is not clear, Elagabalus was said to have had relationships with both men and women, and he frequently wore his makeup, hair, and clothing in a feminine way. Some have even said that he attempted to find someone to perform gender reassignment surgery in order to make his body more female in appearance. Ultimately, at the young age of 18, he was assassinated.

Joan of Arc is a widely known fifteenth-century French historical figure who was known to have a proclivity for masculine clothing, particularly military clothing. Although the reasons for her preference for male attire are not entirely known, she is one of the most well-known early figures to have dressed outside of the cultural norm.

A lesser-known French citizen of the nineteenth century, Le Chevalier D'Eon de Beaumont, was a diplomat, soldier, and spy under King Louis XV. She spent the majority of her life and work living as a woman and asked to be officially recognized by the royal court as female, which was granted. Stories suggest that she may have been intersex and even claimed herself that she had been raised as a female. After her death, doctors found her to have male genitalia.

There are documented accounts of TGNC people in early American history. Albert Cashier was one of the first historically documented trans men. He was born Joanne Hodgers in 1843 but quickly started to identify as male and was already known as Albert when he enlisted in the Union Army and fought in the Civil War. He lived to the age of 71 and continued to wear male clothing up until he was admitted to a hospital in late life because of failing health. Once his caretakers discovered him to be female-bodied, they forced him to wear women's clothing until he died.

Lucy Hicks Anderson was an African American woman of trans experience. The concept of being a transgender woman was not common knowledge until recently, and she may have identified as transgender if she were alive today. Lucy lived in the early twentieth century in the United States and was married twice. She was convicted of perjury after it was found that she was born male. The charge of perjury was based on the facts that she had married a man and was assigned male at birth. She was best known for her statement regarding her gender identity, "I defy any doctor in the world to prove that I am not a woman. I have lived, dressed, acted just what I am, a woman" (Leonard 2017).

There were two men of trans experience who were musicians during the twentieth century. One was an African American gospel singer named Willmer "Little Ax" Broadnax, and the other was a jazz musician named Billy Tipton. Both had successful music careers, and the majority of people who knew them were unaware of their gender identity.

There are other examples of TGNC individuals within mainstream American culture. Another musically inclined person of trans experience was Angela Morley, an Emmy-winning and Oscar-nominated composer who transitioned in the later part of her life to female. Renée Richards was a tennis player in the 1970s who transitioned to female during the middle of her career. It took a Supreme Court ruling before she was allowed to play as female because of the genetic testing that was involved. From 1960 to 1980, Virginia Prince published 100 editions of a magazine called *Transvestia* and lived her life as a female. Although she started a society for cross-dressers, she identified as female, went by feminine pronouns, and helped popularize the word *transgenderism* (Drescher 2010).

GENDER SPECTRUM

While gender diverse people were slowly being incorporated into mainstream culture, the beginnings of TGNC medicine started with people who conceptualized gender as being more than a physical characteristic. Many German thinkers prior to World War II were writing about and studying the gender of the mind and its relation to the body. Early writers began to understand that the two were somehow intertwined but also existed separately.

Karl Heinrich Ulrichs is thought by some people to have likely started what is now known as the gay rights movement in the latter part of the nineteenth century. As a cis gay male, he was a writer who contributed a great deal to the study of sexuality. He was most noted for his view that homosexuals were potentially a "female psyche caught in a male body" (Group for the Advancement of Psychiatry, LGBT Issues Committee 2015). A precedent was written establishing that the gender of the mind can exist separate from the sex of the body. For better or worse, Ulrichs's theories also created an overlap between sexual orientation and gender identity. Although separate from each other, gender and sexuality are connected in a multidimensional and individualistic way. The two are frequently confused by mainstream culture and remain tied together politically in the acronym LGBTQ.

In 1919, Magnus Hirschfeld opened the Institute of Sexology in Germany. This center of research was dedicated to studying both sexuality and gender. Hirschfeld was a physician who advocated for the rights of LGBTQ people, and his research gave birth to the study of gender. The Institute of Sexology both employed and studied those with diverse sexual orientations and gender identities, and Hirschfeld himself was the first person to distinguish the differences between homosexuality and transgenderism (Drescher 2010). Hirschfeld also used the term *transvestite,* and his work inspired many other pioneers in the field of TGNC medicine. Unfortunately, he was living in Germany during the rise to power of the Nazi party. Being Jewish, he had to flee the country, and much of his research was destroyed by Nazi book burnings. It's unclear if his research was destroyed primarily because he was Jewish or if many individuals in the new regime had visited the Institute of Sexology and wanted to destroy notes that had been taken about them.

Havelock Ellis was a colleague of Hirschfeld's who helped him develop the separation of gender from diverse sexual orientations. He used the term *eonism* to describe people who are today known as TGNC. The word was named after the Chevalier d'Eon mentioned in the previous section. Although Ellis and Hirschfeld's research in gender studies helped expand the knowledge of TGNC people, clients of the Institute were still referred to as "deviant," and the focus was generally on understanding gender diversity from the viewpoint that it was ultimately a pathology.

Eugen Steinach was an endocrinologist whose work focusing on sexual behavior was more on the biological side of research during the early twentieth century. Steinach transplanted testes from male guinea pigs into female guinea pigs and found that the female guinea pigs with the implanted testes developed typical male behavior. In particular, they attempted to mount other females. As a result of this research, Steinach linked the sexual hormones, primarily testosterone and estrogen, to sexual behavior. His work led to our modern understanding of hormones and how they affect our body and behavior.

PSYCHOANALYSIS

Psychoanalysis has provided help and treatment for many patients for the past 100 years. Its relation to gender and sexuality, however, has been complicated. Although many people would say the goal of psychoanalysis is understanding and exploration, patients who had a diverse sexual orientation or gender identity were frequently pathologized, and attempts were made to correct their "perversion." In general, some psychoanalysts have attempted to be compassionate in their interpretations and treatments, but psychoanalysis may have further propagated the idea that gender diverse people were suffering and that something had gone wrong in their development. It was a psychoanalyst, Robert Stoller, who coined the term *gender identity* (Stoller 1964). Although there have been many sympathetic psychoanalysts who have worked with TGNC people, the focus of treatment was, and sometimes still is, to "cure" the TGNC person. Attempting to "cure" people of their diverse gender identity is called *conversion therapy* and is now widely seen as unlikely to succeed and even unethical by some clinicians and state laws. The damage of the relationship between those persons who are TGNC and psychoanalytic thought is still being repaired, and the focus of psychoanalysis and psychotherapy has turned to accepting those who fall across the gender spectrum by providing gender-affirming treatments (Drescher and Haller 2012).

TGNC MEDICINE AND SURGERY

After all the groundwork was set regarding the separation of the gender of the mind and the sex of the body, individuals who were TGNC started to have access to medical and surgical treatments that would align their gender identity and physical self. There were pioneers who created gender-affirming techniques and brave individuals who took the first steps in transition, helping pave the way for many of the services available to TGNC people today.

Gender-affirming surgical techniques were developed during the first half of the twentieth century, and there are debates over who was the first person to receive gender-affirming surgery. Magnus Hirschfeld advocated for surgery with two of his clients. The first was Dörchen Richter, who received gender-affirming treatments, including orchiectomy (removal of the testes), penectomy (removal of the penis), and vaginoplasty (construction of a vagina). Lili Elbe, whose story was made famous in the novel and film *The Danish Girl,* also received surgical intervention around this time (Goddard et al. 2007).

Michael Dillon was a physician and a man of trans experience. In the 1930s, he started to take testosterone, and after being admitted to a hospital secondary to falling and hitting his head, he was able to talk a plastic surgeon colleague into performing a double mastectomy. The surgeon also helped him change his gender on his birth certificate. At this point, Dillon was placed in touch with Dr. Harold Gillies, who performed the first phalloplasty, which consisted of several operations (for details of the procedure, see Chapter 18, "Transmasculine Bottom Surgery"). Eventually, Dillon had to leave England because of the rumors that started to circulate about him and his gender identity. Not only did Dillon make history by receiving the first phalloplasty, he also befriended a racer and pilot named Roberta Cowell and performed an orchiectomy on her in 1948 before even graduating from medical school. Roberta Cowell was known to be the first British woman of trans experience to receive gender-affirming surgery. Also of note was Alan Hart, a physician who specialized in radiology and helped modernize the detection of tuberculosis. In 1917, he became the first trans man to receive a hysterectomy (Riverdale 2012).

By the 1950s, several people had already undergone gender-affirming surgeries, although the process was largely underground and out of the public eye. Christine Jorgensen, a veteran from New York City, had already started estrogen and sought gender-affirming vaginoplasty outside of the United States. When she returned to the United States, she received unprecedented publicity about her gender-affirming procedure on the front page of the *New York Daily News*. The headline read, "Ex-GI Becomes Blond Bombshell." This brought the idea of gender-affirming surgery into the mainstream, and awareness about TGNC people started to rise.

THE GENDER REVOLUTION

By the middle of the twentieth century, TGNC people started to obtain access to hormones and surgical procedures. Clinics started to open, and a specialty dedicated to TGNC people was born. It was during this time that the dichotomy of gender being only male or female was brought to question. The scientific understanding of how to prescribe hormones and accomplish gender reassignment was rudimentary at best; however, some of the techniques that were developed early on still exist and are widely used today.

Harry Benjamin is probably the most widely known pioneer in the use of hormones with the TGNC community. A younger colleague of Magnus Hirschfeld, Benjamin dedicated much of his life to working with TGNC people, and the Harry Benjamin International Gender Dysphoria Association was founded and named after him in 1979. This organization later became what we know today as the World Professional Association for Transgender Health (WPATH). Reed Erickson, a patient of Harry Benjamin's, was a philanthropist and a man of trans experience. He founded the Erikson Education Foundation, which funded research to study TGNC people and sponsored symposia. Erickson's generosity helped lay the foundation for WPATH.

Although many researchers had good intentions, some of the research and treatments led to controversy. John Money was a psychologist and sex researcher who helped start the Johns Hopkins Gender Identity clinic in 1965. The majority of his career was dedicated to the study of gender and sexuality, and he was the first person to describe the term *gender role* (Drescher 2010). One consulting case he was particular known for was that of David Reimer. Reimer, at the suggestion of Money, was raised as a girl following a botched circumcision that destroyed his penis. Reimer's transition to female was initially called a success, and common practices around assigning gender at birth, especially with intersex people, were based on this case. This led to unnecessary surgeries on intersex infants for decades. By his teenage years, Reimer started to identify as a male and suffered from depression for years after learning about his history. He ultimately committed suicide at the age of 38 (Colapinto 2001).

STONEWALL RIOTS

Although research and medicine were partially open to understanding and accepting TGNC people, society continued to discriminate against those who were gender diverse. During the 1960s, police raided places where LGBTQ people were known to socialize and harassed and arrested them. The Stonewall Inn was a known LGBTQ social hangout and bar in Greenwich Village, New York City. One night in 1969, the patrons of the bar reached their frustration limit with the police raids and fought back, leading to riots. Two notable people present at the riots were Sylvia Rivera, a transgender woman of color, and Marsha P. Johnson, her friend who was gender nonconforming. The riots that resulted from Stonewall helped propagate a social revolution around LGBTQ rights, and pride events around the United States are typically held at the end of June to mark the anniversary of the riots. Sylvia Rivera was a lifelong supporter of LGBTQ rights and helped found the organization Street Transvestite Action Revolutionaries (STAR). The focus of this organization was to help homeless TGNC women of color.

BACKLASH AND MAINSTREAM ACCEPTANCE

Between the 1970s and 2000, a political and social backlash halted much of the progress that had been made. The gender-affirming clinics that had opened in many parts of the country were closed down. Research and treatment regarding gender dysphoria went on hiatus. HIV and AIDS started to make a devastating presence in the community, and the tension between the LGBTQ community and the larger cis straight world started to grow. For many TGNC people, this was a time when finding gender-affirming treatments was nearly impossible. In this time of quiet, however, there were shifts in perspective taking place. Slowly, the idea of gender diversity as a pathology was changing. The groundwork for future TGNC-affirming care was being laid (Denny 2004). The situation began to improve in the 2000s, when the acceptance of LGBTQ people into mainstream media helped familiarize the general population with gender diverse people. Although not explicitly transgender, performers such as Grace Jones and David Bowie were two examples of mainstream individuals who presented in nontraditional ways. This acceptance of gender diverse people over time has led to clinics opening their doors once again to offer gender-affirming treatments.

RECENT HISTORY

In the past two decades, there has been an increase in services available to LGBTQ people. Clinics that identify as trans affirming are opening in larger cities around the United States and in many parts of Europe. Places such as Fenway Health in Boston, the Mazzoni Center in Philadelphia, Lyon-Martin Health Services in San Francisco, and Callen-Lorde Community Health Center in New York City all offer services specific to the LGBTQ community. These are multidisciplinary facilities offering medical and mental health treatments. They create a safe environment with affirming clinicians who provide high-quality care to those individuals most in need.

The specialty of gender-affirming surgery is also starting to blossom. Pioneers such as Marci Bowers and Christine McGinn not only specialize in gender-affirming procedures but identify as transgender themselves. Marci Bowers, in particular, is widely known to be the first out transgender-identified surgeon. For many gender diverse people, having a surgeon who identifies as TGNC can be very powerful and comforting.

Decades-old techniques are starting to be perfected as more procedures are done. Public insurance, such as state Medicaid programs, is now paying for gender-affirming procedures—giving access to many individuals for whom surgical options were previously unavailable because of the high cost—largely because the Department of Health and Human Services stopped labeling these procedures as "experimental" (U.S. Department of Health and Human Services 2014). Research has continued to expand, and journals such as *LGBT Health* and *Transgender Health* publish scholarly articles dedicated to the understanding of TGNC people.

Organizations such as the Gay and Lesbian Medical Association (GLMA), the Association of LGBTQ Psychiatrists (AGLP), and the United States Association for Transgender Health (USPATH) bring together clinicians who advocate for universal standards of care and civil rights concerns regarding the LGBTQ population. The Human Rights Campaign (HRC) is a nonprofit organization dedicated to advocacy for persons who are LGBTQ, and Peggy Cohen-Kettenis and Norman Spack have opened clinics devoted to the study and care of children who are gender diverse.

SUMMARY

Gender diverse people have been present as long as the concept of gender has existed. Although the names mentioned in this chapter are some of the most notable, there are many other gender diverse people who have lived throughout history. Concepts of what is male and female have slowly developed throughout time, but only in the past century have the ideas of gender and sex started to separate. As the concept of gender of the mind developed, so did the concept of the gender spectrum. Understanding of the gender spectrum helped pave the way for treatment for persons experiencing symptoms deriving from a disconnect between the gender of the mind and the sex of the body. Even though a great deal of progress has been made, we are still at the start of understanding the gender spectrum, and the gender revolution will continue to challenge gender stereotypes that have for so long been in place.

Key Points

- The presence of transgender and gender nonconforming people has been documented throughout history.
- The idea that a gender of the mind exists separately from a sex of the body started with Karl Heinrich Ulrichs in the late 1800s.
- Prior to World War II, many European clinicians had already started to study and treat patients with gender dysphoria.
- Historical stigmatization and pathologizing of gender diversity have made it difficult for the TGNC community to trust the larger medical field.
- Gender-affirming surgical procedures started in the early twentieth century.
- Gender-affirming clinics and organizations are just now starting to become more common.

QUESTIONS

1. What is the historical significance of Dr. Michael Dillon?

   A. He performed the first phalloplasty procedure.
   B. He defined the gender spectrum.
   C. He opened the first sexology clinic.
   D. He received the first phalloplasty procedure.

2. Who was responsible for bringing gender-affirming surgery into conscious awareness in the United States?

   A. Magnus Hirschfeld.
   B. Harry Benjamin.
   C. Christine Jorgensen.
   D. Roberta Cowell.

3. You have been working with a cis woman named Janet for the past 2 years. She has a cis male child who recently had a botched circumcision in which the baby's penis was completely destroyed. A pediatrician involved in the case suggested raising the child as a girl. From what we know of the Reimer case, what would you suggest to Janet?

   A. Raising the child as a girl will probably lead to no major difficulties.
   B. Raising the child as a boy will probably lead to no major difficulties.
   C. The child's long-term gender identification is unclear.
   D. Tell Janet you don't wish to offer any sort of opinion on the case.

4. Ali is an adolescent boy of trans experience you've been working with in psychotherapy, providing gender-affirming treatment. He tells you that he was reading an article about transgender rights and saw mention of the Stonewall Riots. What do you tell him when he asks what made the Stonewall Riots significant?

   A. They helped propagate the LGBTQ civil rights movement.
   B. They made same sex marriage legal.
   C. They occurred in New York City.
   D. They argued for insurance to pay for gender-affirming procedures.

5. Who is the first openly TGNC-identified surgeon in the United States?

    A. John Money.
    B. Marci Bowers.
    C. Sylvia Rivera.
    D. Reed Erickson.

ANSWERS

1. **The correct response is option D.**

2. **The correct response is option C.**

3. **The correct response is option C.**

    This is a complicated case, and raising the child as a boy or as a girl would probably lead to some difficulties. You are aware of what happened with the Reimer case, in which a boy with a botched circumcision was raised as a girl and transitioned back to being a boy. It's probably unclear how the child with identify at this point.

4. **The correct response is option A.**

5. **The correct response is option B.**

REFERENCES

American Psychiatric Association: Position Statement on Access to Care for Transgender and Gender Variant Individuals. Washington, DC, American Psychiatric Association, 2012. Available at: www.psychiatry.org/File%20Library/Learn/Archives/Position-2012-Transgender-Gender-Variant-Access-Care.pdf. Accessed March 1, 2016.

Colapinto J: As Nature Made Him: The Boy Who Was Raised as a Girl. New York, Harper Perennial, 2001

Denny D: Changing models of transsexualism. J Gay Lesbian Psychother 8(1/2):25–40, 2004

Drescher J: Transsexualism, gender identity disorder and the DSM. J Gay Lesbian Ment Health 14(2):109–122, 2010

Drescher J, Haller E: Position Statement on Access to Care for Transgender and Gender Variant Individuals. Arlington, VA, American Psychiatric Association, 2012

Goddard JC, Vickery RM, Terry TR: Development of feminizing genitoplasty for gender dysphoria. J Sex Med 4(4 Pt 1):981–989, 2007 17451484

Group for the Advancement of Psychiatry, LGBT Issues Committee: LGBT Mental Health Syllabus, 2015. Available at: http://www.aglp.org/gap/6_transgender. Accessed April 29, 2017.

Kinsey AC, Pomeroy WB, Martin CE: Sexual Behavior in the Human Male. Philadelphia, PA, WB Saunders, 1948

Leonard K: Anderson, Lucy Hicks [Tobias Lawson] (1886–1954). African American History in the American West: Online Encyclopedia of Significant People and Places. Blackpast.org. Remembered and Reclaimed, 2017. Available at: www.blackpast.org/aaw/anderson-lucy-hicks-1886-1954. Accessed April 29, 2017.

Meyerowitz J: How Sex Changed: A History of Transsexuality in the United States. Cambridge, MA, Harvard University Press, 2009

Riverdale J: A brief history of FTM trans civilization. TransGuys.com. October 29, 2012. Available at: http://transguys.com/features/ftm-trans-history. Accessed April 29, 2017.

Stoller RJ: A contribution to the study of gender identity. Int J Psychoanal 45(2–3): 220–226, 1964 14167035

U.S. Department of Health and Human Services: NCD 140.3, Transsexual Surgery, Docket No A-13-87, Decision No 2576. Washington, DC, Departmental Appeals Board, Appellate Division, May 30, 2014. Available at: www.hhs.gov/sites/default/files/static/dab/decisions/board-decisions/2014/dab2576.pdf. Accessed March 22, 2015.

4

ESTABLISHING A TGNC-FRIENDLY CLINIC

...Queer spaces facilitate a queer sexuality that is flexible and fluid. And, with this sexual landscape of flexibility is spaciousness for the inclusion of transgender bodies and sexualities.

Amy Stone

A RECURRING THEME in the chapters of this book is the continued lack of access to trans-competent care in the medical and mental health community. Transgender and gender-nonconforming (TGNC) people have few places to seek treatment that provide knowledgeable professionals, respectful staff, and a safe environment. Finding a gender-affirming clinician can be difficult, let alone finding a clinic that specializes in TGNC care. There are only a handful of TGNC specialized clinics around the world. Now, more than ever, there is a need for more clinicians who are TGNC competent working in gender-affirming settings.

Learning all the medical, surgical, and mental health treatment options available to TGNC people is pointless if the space in which treatment is provided is not welcoming to a gender diverse population. Space is not limited just to physical structure. The staff, clinicians, and security personnel all participate in making an environment safe and friendly to TGNC people. The main two reasons why some TGNC people choose not to seek medical care are a lack of trans-competent providers and a fear that once they do seek treatment, they will be discriminated against by staff and clinicians.

Every clinic needs to make some changes in order to be more inclusive of TGNC patients. How many changes are made is correlated with how trans-friendly a treatment facility wants or needs to be. If the goal is to be more open

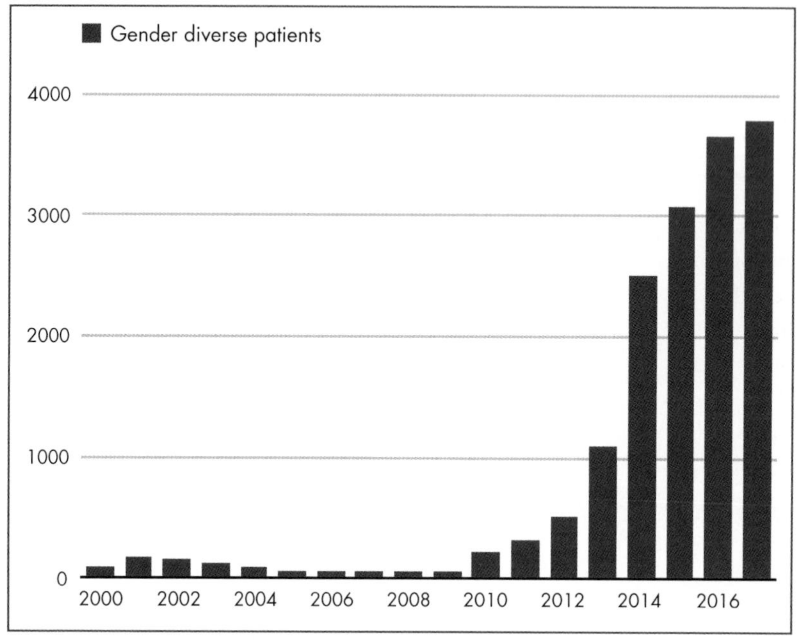

FIGURE 4–1. Increase in number of transgender patients at Callen-Lorde Community Health Center from 2000 to 2017.
Source. P. Carneiro, personal communication, January 9, 2018.

to taking TGNC patients, then a thought experiment will help identify areas where alterations are needed. This chapter will function as that thought experiment. Imagine the core aspects of finding a TGNC-competent mental health professional: the experience of making an appointment, walking into the clinic, meeting your clinician, reading your patient chart, and getting connected with other services. Doing this will provide a guide to changes that need to be made to a clinic in order to make it a safe place for TGNC people to visit.

HOW DO PATIENTS FIND YOU?

The number of identified TGNC patients has increased dramatically over the last decade (Figure 4–1). However, just because the number of transgender patients has increased doesn't mean that the transgender population has increased. These concepts are separate.

TGNC patients now have treatment options that weren't available to them before. Their options range from having a competent mental health provider to medicinal and surgical treatments. Until recently, professional treatment was not considered safe for TGNC patients. Up to 33% of TGNC people have identified having at least one negative experience with a health care professional regarding their gender diverse status (James et al. 2016). TGNC individuals have even avoided HIV testing because clinics are seen as not trans-friendly (Sevelius et al. 2014).

How TGNC patients find you will depend on where you practice. In many urban settings, particularly if you are part of a large clinic, there are lesbian, gay, bissexual, transgender, and queer/questioning (LGBTQ) centers that identify safe spaces and providers. Groups may meet in these centers, and through word of mouth, members of the TGNC population will spread information regarding which local clinicians are most knowledgeable and friendly in providing competent care. However, just because providers are listed as "LGBTQ" doesn't mean they are knowledgeable in providing services the TGNC community needs. There are also underground Internet networks unavailable to clinicians where patients may post information about their experiences with providers.

If you are located in a more rural setting, you might also get patients by word of mouth, but advertising may be essential. Some clinicians now post online through organizations, labeling themselves as LGBTQ competent. This label is the first step in making it easier for patients to schedule an appointment, and the more information you provide, the easier it will be for potential patients to know you understand their needs. TGNC patients want mental health care that is of high quality just as any other patient would, and they will want to know their clinician can help provide additional services they may require. For example, TGNC patients may need a clinician who is knowledgeable about how to help them legally change their name or gender markers. They may want a clinician who understands the ins and outs of hormone treatment. They may also want a clinician who knows how to write mental health letters required for surgical procedures. Listing these items and having that knowledge base will elevate a clinician from being LGBTQ competent to being more of an expert.

IS IT SAFE?

Most clinicians have blind spots when empathizing with TGNC patients and how they access care. In what part of town is the private office or clinic located? There are pockets of LGBTQ-friendly places in the world, and the TGNC community is generally aware of these locations. These pockets are usually full of a population in which diverse gender identity and sexual orientations are commonplace. Walking in and out of an LGBTQ-identified office in these areas would likely not be cause for alarm. However, imagine being located in an unsafe neighborhood where TGNC people are frequently attacked and even killed simply for walking down the street. It is important to remember that safety is a major factor for TGNC patients seeking care.

Clinicians who are known to be LGBTQ competent will quickly make a name for themselves in the TGNC community, especially in a rural area. Although this might increase business in some ways, a rural location might start to have a negative impact on both the clinician and the patients who seek treatment. Once your practice has a reputation of being LGBTQ friendly, patients may be outing themselves by parking in front of your office and walking in the door. Although having the reputation of being the local LGBTQ shrink or the "queer doc" might be a badge of pride for some, it's worth considering the negative implications of this reputation for your patient population.

Security guards or officers are located in hospitals and also frequently in large clinics. Having security also has its pros and cons. TGNC people can have a wide range of mental illness just like the larger population. Some TGNC people have serious mental illness. When working with serious mental illness, the presence of a security guard can provide a sense of comfort to the staff, clinicians, and patients in the waiting room. The potential trouble with having a uniformed security guard is the interaction the guard might have with a TGNC patient, especially one who is very symptomatic. The guard might approach a patient who is getting loud in the waiting room, arguing with a staff member, or showing signs of escalation. When patients are at their most vulnerable, the authoritative presence of a security guard could make things worse, and the patient may be misgendered (referred to as the incorrect gender) or even reminded of a previous trauma from interactions with security. Patients need to become familiar with your security staff and learn to trust them over time. Security should be trained on the correct use of pronouns, the basics of TGNC care, and the potential triggers that could take place in security-patient interaction.

The local police can also be a blessing or a curse. Mental health clinicians frequently work closely with law enforcement services when hospitalizing a patient. Having compassionate police officers present when patients are very ill can make a difficult situation safer. However, many officers are not familiar with TGNC individuals, and, even worse, some are outwardly prejudiced and hostile.

When working with police on a patient hospitalization, don't hesitate to take charge of the situation. Encourage the police to stay outside the office where the patient is located. If they must enter the room with emergency medical services (EMS), try to limit how many officers are in the room at once. TGNC patients, for many reasons, often have had traumatic interactions with law enforcement. The police can offer valuable help and provide safety, but only when they are understanding of the patient's psychiatric needs. If possible, have another staff member or colleague inform both the police and EMS of the patient's name, pronouns, and psychiatric need. This can happen before they enter the room to interact with the patient. In addition, having a list of medications, the patient's address and insurance information, and a letter providing all this information to the emergency department staff will help those staff provide the best possible care when hospitalization is required.

FRONT DESK STAFF

The front desk staff could end up being the first aspect of your practice or clinic that needs to be worked on. The first interaction a patient may have with you is through your front desk (Figure 4–2). These staff members will ask for the patient's name and may potentially use incorrect pronouns. If the front desk isn't prepared to interact with TGNC patients in a respectful way, the hopes of having a positive interaction with patients once they are in your office diminishes, and patients may leave without receiving care (Callahan 2015). Something as simple as using an incorrect name in a large office waiting room may out your patient as TGNC (Pandya 2014). Staff should be advised about how to identify the patient's name, potentially different billing name, and pronouns. They should also be advised about potential services that patients might be asking about, such as letters of documentation around name changes, gender marker changes, hormones, and surgery. When a TGNC person approaches the front desk about these services, staff should be ready to respond without needing an explanation from the patient.

In a warm and empathic environment, the front desk staff can create a safe environment and help TGNC patients feel at ease. The patients will likely get to know the staff over time, and it's not uncommon for them to feel more comfortable sitting in the clinic waiting room than anywhere else they go during the week. Where else can a TGNC person find a room full of respectful staff members and other patients who share many of their experiences? Given all these scenarios, some practitioners and advocates would say that cultural competency around TGNC topics should be mandated (Robinson 2010).

SIGNAGE

Working with the continued thought experiment of identifying ways to make your clinic TGNC friendly, ask yourself, "What cues could be added to an office or clinic that would signal to TGNC patients that they are in a friendly environment?" Treatment of TGNC patients doesn't happen only in

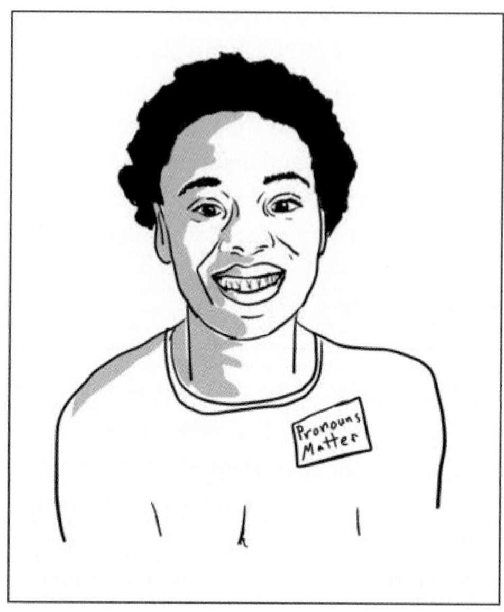

FIGURE 4–2. Front desk staff can communicate acceptance before treatment even begins.

the office; culturally sensitive treatment starts when patients walk into the lobby. Most lobbies have brochures set out, and these brochures can be about a range of topics helpful for any patient, including mental illness, work programs, and local social services. TGNC patients may need additional services. Having flyers or handouts specific to their needs will further communicate that they are welcome in a clinic that is TGNC competent. Although this might seem like a small gesture, TGNC people have been marginalized and ignored for years, and small efforts can go a long way toward building an inclusive and welcoming environment.

TGNC patients will need a variety of social supports. They may need access to a lawyer for name or gender marker change applications. Outside support groups, LGBTQ centers, and social clubs may all be represented in flyers. For clinics with a large number of TGNC patients, video recordings or handouts explaining clinic policies about TGNC-specific evaluations can both help clinic flow and provide visibility to TGNC people in the clinic waiting room.

The LGBTQ community has been identifying "safe" clinicians for years by word of mouth, and a pride flag sticker placed on the door or in the waiting room is a subtle symbol to patients that they are in the right place. The TGNC community has its own pride flag as well, consisting of five horizontal lines with light blue on the outside, white in the middle, and pink in be-

ALL GENDERS WELCOME
Trans Day of Remembrance
TGNC Pride
Pronouns Matter

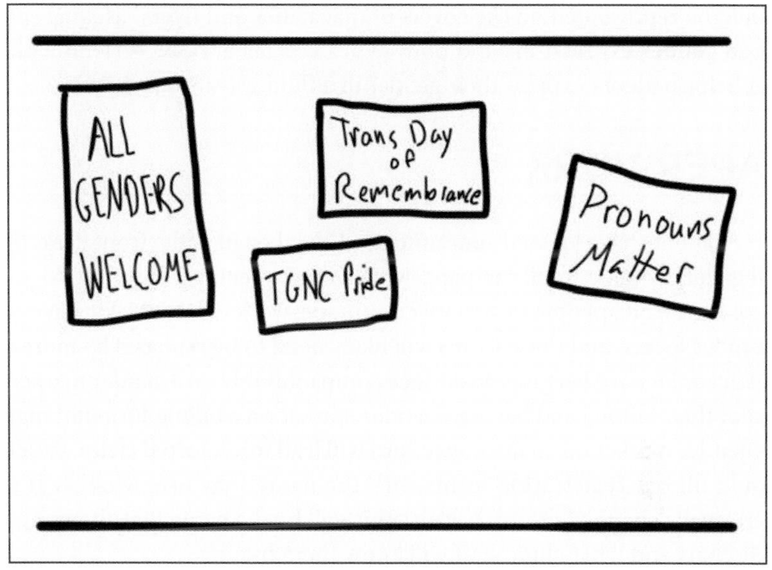

FIGURE 4–3. Gender-affirming signs around a clinic will help make gender diverse people feel welcome.

tween. The colors are blue for boys, pink for girls, and white for intersex. Also of note, the flag is the same pattern going up and down, so whichever way it is held, it will be held the right way. This is a powerful statement considering how TGNC individuals have been told most of their lives that they are not talking, walking, dressing, acting, or living like they should.

Signs about the importance of pronouns should be used when possible (Figure 4–3). Some clinics have stickers available at the front desk for patients to write the pronouns they use so they aren't misgendered when interacting with staff. Stickers with pronouns are generally worn around the lapel area. Staff are also encouraged to wear stickers and buttons identifying their pronouns to further normalize pronoun use within the clinic culture. Signage about pronouns communicates to both staff and patients that pronouns are important. Any clinic that focuses on the treatment of the LGBTQ population should have affirming signage up throughout the clinic.

Think about the clinic layout and bathrooms as well. Individual bathrooms are ideal, with signs that communicate that they are gender neutral. Avoid having male and female restrooms if possible. Finally, don't forget about the magazines lying around. There are a number of publications that focus on the queer community, such as *Out* and *The Advocate,* and having a subscription or two in the waiting room will only further communicate that you are creating a safe space for patients. People of all gender identities should be represented on the covers of magazines and flyers. Making space for all gender expressions and body types creates a TGNC-friendly place that helps patients express their gender in a fluid way (Stone 2013).

PAPERWORK

After patients have located your office and checked in at the front desk, they will generally need to fill out paperwork prior to seeing a clinician. Making space for TGNC people in general clinic paperwork can be tricky when you use older forms, and these forms will likely need to be replaced by more sophisticated record keeping. Insurance companies rely on a gender marker as part of their billing, and having a gender marker on a billing form not match the gender marker on an insurance card will lead to a rejected claim. Patients should fill out registration forms with the name they use, whether it has been legally changed or not, because this will be the name that shows up on their chart and what clinic staff will know them by.

Forms will also ask about the sex of a patient. The concept of sex is being supplemented with gender or gender identity, and at the very least, forms should provide options of male, female, or other. Although these options just start to capture the gender spectrum as opposed to a gender binary, they can create some confusion for clinical staff. Would a man of trans experience mark down *male* or *other* on his intake form? If he marks down male, will the clinician know to ask about female body parts during an examination? There will come a point in the registration and visit when patients will be required to "out" themselves as TGNC. Although the complexities of a person's gender identity need not be known by administrative staff, clinical staff must be alerted so they can take an appropriate history and provide safe treatment.

Forms may have options besides *other*, including *transgender* and *gender nonconforming* (Figure 4–4). Some forms might use *MtF* or *FtM* to signify male to female or female to male. Certain social media sites now offer more than 50 gender options, which might be a bit complex for a clinic registration sheet. Having a blank line to let patients write in their identity makes the form easier to read and provides no restrictions.

For billing purposes, a separate form is needed at registration to include the name and gender marker that will be provided to insurance companies (Figure 4–5). The patient doesn't want to see a rejected insurance claim any more than the clinic does, so be transparent about what the billing name and gender marker will be used for. Both will need to be updated if they are legally changed, and patients should be made aware of the importance of keeping this information up to date. Avoid using terms such as *birth name*. Using the term

☐ Male

☐ Female

☐ Transgender

☐ Nonbinary

☐ Intersex

☐ Other: ______________
(specify gender)

FIGURE 4–4. Registration forms should contain more options for gender than just male or female. A blank space for people to identify their gender is more inclusive.

birth name can bring up a host of feelings, including those of being invalidated. Some TGNC people might be so traumatized by early experiences that recalling their name assigned at birth induces a physiological stress response.

The last item on a registration form that may need to be altered is family contacts. Keep in mind that many in the TGNC population might be estranged from their family because of a number of possible circumstances. A list of social supports and their relation to the patient is necessary, but it need not involve the patient's biological family and may instead include a family of choice (see Chapter 10, "Families").

ELECTRONIC HEALTH RECORD

Unless they are in private practice, most clinicians don't have the ability to alter their electronic health record. Not being able to alter fields is a major disadvantage of an electronic record compared with a paper charting system. Whatever system you use, you'll have to work within the parameters

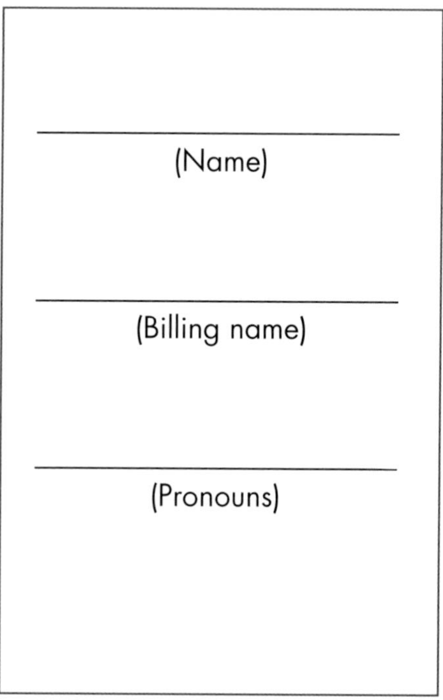

FIGURE 4–5. It is important for a patient record to have name options for individuals who are gender diverse.

available to note three specific gender fields: gender pronouns, sex assigned at birth, and legal sex (Deutsch and Buchholz 2015).

Discussing gender identity should be part of any initial general medical exam. If possible, have a field easily accessible for identifying the pronouns a patient uses. To decrease the possibility of a patient being misgendered, the chart should identify the patient's chosen name and should also include gender identity. The patient's legal name is important for billing. Birth sex is important for medical matters. In order to guide the medical history and physical exam, the clinician should be aware if the patient was identified as male or female at birth. Government identifications require a person to choose between M or F.

Every clinic will handle patient identification concerns in their own way depending on the system they use. If additional fields are not available to you, consider an asterisk (*) after the name to signify that more detailed information is located elsewhere in the chart. Having information appear if you hover a cursor over a patient's name or gender identity is another option (Deutsch and Buchholz 2015).

Electronic prescriptions create their own scenarios because generating or faxing a document will require your electronic record to pull information from the patient's legal name, not the chosen name. Few medical records are sophisticated enough to do this, and programmers should consider expanding these possibilities as new systems are created.

DOCUMENTATION

After the first visit from a patient, the first note you should write is generally an evaluation. Whether this evaluation is a psychosocial assessment, psychiatric evaluation, or general session note, a gender identifier typically appears in the first sentence. There are ways to communicate in your charting the gender identity of a patient. Different terminology can be used depending on the gender identity, birth sex, and surgical status of the patient. From a psychological perspective, it is important to identify in the opening line if the person is cis or trans. A person who was born male at birth but whose gender identity is female may be identified in charting in various ways:

- Woman of trans experience
- Affirmed female
- MtF transgender

Clinicians and patients may have their own preferences for identification. The second and third examples mentioned above use the term "female." *Woman of trans experience* is a more affirming label. *Affirmed female* has been suggested; this description comments on the medical and surgical status of the patient (Spack 2009). Identifying the patient as being *of trans experience* doesn't communicate a history of any hormonal or surgical treatments. When writing about your patients, naming their gender identity is more important that labeling patients as transgender. For your own clinical understanding of the patient and to provide better treatment, naming the patient's gender in the opening line will help provide more affirming treatment. All that being said, you may encounter patients who are at different stages and may be ambivalent about their identities. Be respectful and use terms such as *gender diverse* if there is uncertainty on the part of the patient as to their gender identity.

SOCIAL SERVICES

Depending on the size of your clinic, the need for social services can vary. A clinician who can spend an hour weekly with each patient will likely have the time to discuss the various social aspects of the patient's treatment plan. However, acquiring the necessary expertise in TGNC social services and having the time to help with TGNC-specific paperwork requirements can be daunting. A list of topics social services might be working on with a TGNC patient might include (but is not limited to) the following:

- *Gender marker changes*—Each state has different requirements, and the paperwork and court visits can be time consuming.
- *Name change*—Name changes are slightly easier than gender marker changes, but they can be a lengthy process involving legal proceedings.
- *Billing concerns*—Taking the time to review why claims may have been rejected and making phone calls to insurance companies can be time consuming.
- *Housing*—With the number of homeless TGNC patients, especially youth, finding a safe homeless shelter and housing options may be impossible depending on your location.
- *Advocating*—Working within the system will put a strain on time and emotions for individuals involved.
- *Benefits*—From disability applications to food stamps and other potential benefits, the paperwork involved is extensive and requires social services staff who are familiar with gender dysphoria and the challenges of the TGNC community.

GROUPS

One of the most helpful forms of treatment you can provide to a TGNC patient may not be your ability to provide gender-affirming therapy, medication management, or even social services. Rather, it might be group therapy. TGNC patients need to meet other TGNC patients to get social support. Unless you are part of the TGNC community—and even if you are—understanding all the complexities and challenges of TGNC people's day-to-day lives is beyond the scope of individual treatment alone. The TGNC community has, within its own framework, knowledge about the health care system, referrals, social hangouts, and the ins and outs of hormone and surgical options. There will be topics that will arise out of group sessions of which most cis-identified clinicians are unaware. The psychological support that one patient can provide to others within the framework of a safe and supportive group therapy is invaluable.

When thinking about group therapies offered, consider splitting up groups on the basis of gender identity. However, there are pros and cons to doing this, and different patient populations may have different needs. An easy and inclusive way to set up groups would be to have a transmasculine group and a transfeminine group. Ideally, there would also be a group dedicated to gender nonconforming individuals. Some clinics may have male- and female-identified groups that trans men and trans women, respectively, can join.

Do not expect all LGB patients to be supportive or trans-affirming in mixed groups. Within the LGB population, transphobia still exists. Expect there to be a lot of emotions and disagreements even within the TGNC community. Groups should focus on respecting both the similarities and differences among gender diverse people. Also, group leaders will need to be competent about individual TGNC patient needs and should understand the basics of medicinal and surgical treatments in order to facilitate discussion and provide accurate information when necessary.

CONNECTIONS WITH REFERRALS

Your list of resources and referrals should be just as extensive whether you are running an individual practice or are part of a larger system with social services available. However, finding other providers who are TGNC competent can be difficult. As many as 50% of TGNC patients have stated they had to teach their providers about TGNC care (Wichinski 2015), and most clinicians generally agree that their training in LGBTQ care is only fair or even poor (White et al. 2015). When speaking to other clinicians and organizations, be wary if you hear "We treat everyone the same." Understanding TGNC care is about knowing the challenges specific to the patient population; "...the goal of quality health care is for equity and not equality" (Quinn et al. 2015, p. 1162). TGNC-competent clinicians will know that gender diverse people need care that includes specific clinical knowledge and attention to areas that are not typical of the general population. At a minimum, your resource list should include the following:

- *Therapists*—Whether you plan to see the patient individually or not, a list of alternative TGNC-affirming therapists is needed for referral or for supplementing with alternative treatments.
- *Psychiatrists*—Just as with therapists, a list of TGNC-affirming psychiatrists is needed. These clinicians should not only be aware of the basics of TGNC care but should be an ally in advocating for surgical treatments should a patient desire them.
- *Primary care clinicians*—It is important to maintain a list of primary care clinicians who offer hormone therapy and who understand individual physical exam specifics.
- *Endocrinologists*—Although hormone therapy has largely moved to primary care clinicians, an endocrinology specialist referral may be re-

quired if there is no local access to a hormone prescriber or if complex issues arise.

- *Gynecologists*—Trans men who still have a uterus, cervix, and vagina will need regular screenings just as any cis female would. Currently, there are few gynecologists who are sensitive and knowledgeable about treating trans men.
- *Surgeons*—You should maintain a list of trans-competent surgeons who are well trained in gender-affirming surgeries.
- *Support groups*—List any local agencies that might have additional supportive services for patients, including informal groups, information sessions, and family education.
- *Legal services*—Local lawyers are crucial for stabilizing the lives of trans individuals, especially lawyers focused on civil rights, public health insurance, name and gender marker changes, and housing and public benefits.
- *Shelters*—For TGNC patients who are currently homeless, having a list of trans-friendly shelters can be lifesaving. Staff at a trans-friendly shelter will understand the individual needs of TGNC persons and will place them in a room that is gender appropriate.

SUMMARY

The biggest barrier a TGNC patient has in getting treatment is having a safe and trans-affirming clinic to go to. The list of providers who are TGNC competent is growing but remains small. In some parts of the country, they are nonexistent. Alterations to most practices are needed in order to make a clinic safe and affirming. The changes needed to a practice are not extensive, and a little effort can go a long way in making a clinic TGNC friendly. How much change is needed depends on both your goals and the patient population. If you are an individual practitioner, having a list of referrals and connections is crucial. Small changes to your medical record, billing, forms, and waiting room can greatly change the experience of a patient for the better. Larger clinics will need to think more broadly about the environment, security, staffing, and program options available. Whatever the current state of the clinic or practice you are working in, consider the experience TGNC patients have as they move through your space. Think about who they encounter and what they see on the walls and the registration clipboard. What services are available to them? As the world becomes safer for TGNC people to come out, there will be a growing need for services. All clinics should consider making changes in order to provide a safer environment and access to care for those who are gender diverse.

Key Points

- The number of TGNC patients is growing dramatically. There is vast room for improvement in the number of clinicians who can provide quality trans-affirming care.
- When considering how to make your clinic more trans friendly, think about the patients moving through your clinic and how they might interact with the facility and staff. This will give you a starting point in understanding what changes need to be made.
- A large portion of TGNC care is social in nature. Having referrals for housing, shelters, legal services, and organizations will provide basic needs for all TGNC patients.
- Try to create or alter the electronic health record to clearly state the patient's chosen name, gender identity, and legal gender. The more patient-specific you can make the record, the better.
- Consider mandating that all staff attend TGNC cultural competence training. A little staff education can make a big difference in the lives of patients.

QUESTIONS

1. Why does a clinic registration packet need a separate section that provides a patient's name and gender given at birth?

   A. You might need to contact the patient's birth family, and you would need to know what name to use.
   B. Insurance companies may reject a claim if the patient's name and gender marker are different from what appears on the insurance card.
   C. Clinicians need to know which of their patients are transgender so they can avoid having to ask about their gender identity during the session.
   D. It will alleviate staff curiosity.

2. What is the reason the number of TGNC patients is growing dramatically?

   A. The current youth culture is experimenting with trying out different gender identities.
   B. There are exponentially more people on the planet.
   C. TGNC growth may be due to genetic changes that are occurring because of the environment.
   D. TGNC patients are feeling safer when seeking health care.

3. In the unfortunate event that a TGNC patient needs to be hospitalized for psychiatric concerns, what steps can best help the patient feel safer?

   A. Step back and let the police and EMS take over the situation. They will likely know best.
   B. Get a colleague to stay with your patient while you go to get help.
   C. Stay with your patient while you have a colleague provide the patient's information, including gender identity, to EMS and police. Minimize the number of police in the room if possible.
   D. Treat the patient the same as you would any patient.

4. What part of a clinic might be the first area where a TGNC person encounters a problem?

   A. Registration paperwork.
   B. The clinician.
   C. The front desk staff.
   D. The restroom.

5. When designing a TGNC-friendly clinic, what is the best way to set up the restrooms?

   A. Design all the restrooms as single-stall restrooms.
   B. Label all the restrooms with a "gender-neutral" sign.
   C. Keep the restrooms as male or female.
   D. Have TGNC-specific restrooms.

ANSWERS

1. **The correct response is option B.**

   Claims may be rejected if the name and gender marker are not the same as what's on a patient's insurance card. Contacting the patient's family should be done only after discussing the parameters with the patient. Having a discussion about the patient's gender identity should be part of any gender-affirming evaluation. Staff need to know a billing and gender marker only when helping with administrative concerns.

2. **The correct response is option D.**

   As the world becomes safer for TGNC-identified individuals, more will feel comfortable seeking health care in gender-affirming practices.

3. **The correct response is option C.**

   In order to decrease the amount of stress on patients during a hospitalization, it is important that you stay with them so they feel safe. If possible, have a colleague intervene with EMS and the police to provide necessary information, including the patient's gender identity and pronouns. Too many police present in a small therapy office may traumatize the patient further, causing an increase in symptoms.

4. **The correct response is option C.**

   The front desk staff is likely to be the first place a TGNC person will encounter a problem in a non-TGNC-friendly clinic. Educating and training the front desk staff on how to work with TGNC people is crucial.

5. **The correct response is option B.**

   Although single-stall bathrooms are better than those labeled as male or female, gender-neutral signs will communicate to all patients and staff that people of all gender variants are welcome. Transgender-specific bathrooms can further create feelings of exclusion and force TGNC people to "out" themselves.

REFERENCES

Callahan EJ: Opening the door to transgender care. J Gen Intern Med 30(6):706–707, 2015 25743431

Deutsch MB, Buchholz D: Electronic health records and transgender patients—practical recommendations for the collection of gender identity data. J Gen Intern Med 30(6):843–847, 2015 25560316

James SE, Herman JL, Rankin S, et al: The Report of the 2015 U.S. Transgender Survey. Washington, DC, National Center for Transgender Equality, 2016

Pandya A: Mental health as an advocacy priority in the lesbian, gay, bisexual, and transgender communities. J Psychiatr Pract 20(3):225–227, 2014 24847996

Quinn GP, Schabath MB, Sanchez JA, et al: The importance of disclosure: lesbian, gay, bisexual, transgender/transsexual, queer/questioning, and intersex individuals and the cancer continuum. Cancer 121(8):1160–1163, 2015 25521303

Robinson A: The transgender patient and your practice: what physicians and staff need to know. J Med Pract Manage 25(6):364–367, 2010 20695249

Sevelius JM, Patouhas E, Keatley JG, Johnson MO: Barriers and facilitators to engagement and retention in care among transgender women living with human immunodeficiency virus. Ann Behav Med 47(1):5–16, 2014 24317955

Spack N: An endocrine perspective on the care of transgender adolescents. J Gay Lesbian Ment Health 13(4):309–319, 2009

Stone AL: Flexible queers, serious bodies: transgender inclusion in queer spaces. J Homosex 60(12):1647–1665, 2013 24175886

White W, Brenman S, Paradis E, et al: Lesbian, gay, bisexual, and transgender patient care: medical students' preparedness and comfort. Teach Learn Med 27(3):254–263, 2015 26158327

Wichinski KA: Providing culturally proficient care for transgender patients. Nursing 45(2):58–63, 2015 25585225

5

ADVOCACY

In all regards, practitioners should advocate for the rights of their transgender patients.

Allyson Robinson

ROBERT EADS WAS a man of trans experience who was diagnosed with ovarian cancer in 1996. Looking for treatment, he was turned away from more than two dozen doctors who didn't want to take him on as a patient. Only after a year of searching would anyone take his case, and by that time, the cancer had metastasized, and he ultimately died in 1999 (Robinson 2010).

All clinicians need to advocate for transgender and gender-nonconforming (TGNC) people. It's a necessary part of working with the population and may be the most crucial role we play. The inability to access competent care is the biggest problem facing the TGNC population, and discrimination and affordability seem to be the two main reasons for TGNC people not being able to access care (Cruz 2014). This deficiency in competent care exists in hospital settings, emergency departments, outpatient clinics, homeless shelters, and the prison system and is most noticeable outside the realm of mental health. The mental health care system also suffers from a lack of providers who are informed about the needs of the lesbian, gay, bisexual, transgender, and queer/questioning (LGBTQ) community, and wait times at some LGBTQ-affirming clinics can be as long as 2–3 years (Wise 2016). Because of these deficiencies, mental health professionals have a necessary and ongoing duty to advocate with other health care providers to help TGNC people get the most well-informed and compassionate care possible.

Advocating will take on a larger role for mental health professionals when working with TGNC people. Clinicians will find themselves advocating in new areas where they may not be comfortable because of lack of experience. One area that requires a great amount of time for advocating is with insurance companies. Not only do many insurance companies have policies regarding TGNC people that are vague and undefined, but some have policies that are discriminatory and potentially dangerous. Advocating with insurance providers for gender-affirming care on behalf of patients is a regular and necessary part of TGNC-affirming treatment.

Advocating can also be done through self-disclosure. Coming out is the self-acknowledgment and declaration to others that you are LGBTQ. For those clinicians who are LGBTQ themselves, coming out will have a significant impact on the attitudes and practices of those around them (Moll et al. 2014). Although LGBTQ persons should come out only when they feel comfortable doing so, mental health clinicians who out themselves will be in a place to educate other clinicians and help them to personify and even identify with those who have a diverse gender or sexuality.

Finally, the area where many clinicians should feel comfortable advocating for TGNC people is education. Both learning to improve your skill set and teaching less experienced clinicians will help propagate the growing literature of TGNC care and make health care and mental health treatment safer for individuals who are gender diverse. In this chapter I cover some clinical examples that are common to TGNC people in the health care system and give perspective on how to best advocate from the position of a mental health professional.

HOSPITALS

Hospitals can be very scary places for TGNC people. At best, hospitals have been described as invalidating and insensitive. At worst, they can be hostile and even unsafe. The vast majority of hospital staff, both medical and psychiatric, are uninformed about TGNC people. There are many hospital staff who hold negative views of the TGNC population and will sadly use their position to actively discriminate.

Case Example

Phillip is a 28-year-old man of trans experience. He has a history of bipolar I disorder with a number of past hospitalizations. He has been seen in a trans-affirming outpatient clinic for 5 years and has been mostly stable, although he remains symptomatic chronically. He has excellent insight into his symptoms and can identify when a manic episode is starting. Historically, when Phillip becomes manic, he becomes suicidal. He has always been a high risk for suicide because three of his family members completed suicide. Phillip tends to go to the hospital when he is manic because he and his treatment team are confident it keeps him safe from suicide until he stabilizes with supportive therapy and changes to his medication.

During past hospitalizations, hospital staff misgendered Phillip and put him in hospital rooms with cis female patients. He has been taking testoster-

> one for several years and has developed a somewhat masculine physique with facial hair and a deep voice. When staff attempt to put him in cis female rooms, the other patients become uncomfortable, wondering why a man has been put in the room with them. This situation usually forces Phillip to out himself to the other patients to provide an explanation, and before he is discharged, much of the unit knows he is a man of trans experience.
>
> On his most recent visit to an inpatient unit, Phillip had an exceptionally bad experience. The staff, despite knowing Phillip from previous hospitalizations, continued to put him in a cis female room. They also labeled his chart with his birth name instead of his chosen name. This caused all the staff interacting with him to use the name listed on the chart, so he was frequently misgendered and misnamed. In addition, the inpatient psychiatrist decided that testosterone was causing Phillip's manic symptoms and stopped the hormone even though Phillip and his outpatient psychiatrist were positive it was having no effect on his mood symptoms. Phillip was taking a low dose of testosterone and continued to have menstrual cycles. He happened to be having his period during the time of the hospital stay, but when he asked the nursing staff for feminine hygiene products, they told him he couldn't have them because he was a man and didn't need them.
>
> Phillip was rightfully upset. He was already very uncomfortable from having a manic episode, but the hospital staff were using the wrong name, misgendering him, blaming testosterone for his manic symptoms, and refusing to provide him with proper hygiene products. He called his outpatient psychiatrist to advocate for him. When the outpatient psychiatrist got in touch with the inpatient team, he told them that the hospital was treating Phillip differently because he was transgender. The lead psychiatrist asserted that this couldn't be true and went on to say, "We treat every patient the same."

Phillip's story is sadly not uncommon. An inpatient medical or psychiatric unit is already uncomfortable to most people. Patients are in a strange environment, in an uncomfortable bed, and usually unable to sleep because they are awakened for blood draws, vital checks, and examinations. For patients with bipolar disorder, this creates a difficult environment to recover from because the lack of sleep can exacerbate their symptoms.

Phillip's hospital stay highlights some of the major mistakes inpatient units make when working with TGNC people. First, despite what is written on their insurance card, patients should always be referred to by the name they want. It's not very difficult to make a chart notation that someone goes by a certain name. Staff tend to not have difficulty calling cis gender patients by their preferred name, so any name difficulties related to a person of trans experience is likely due to the patient's being transgender. Second, the room assignment for a person of trans experience should be in line with their gender identity. Phillip presented very masculine in his appearance. Only by outing himself as transgender could he explain to the other patients why he was in a cis female room. Staff should also not be outing anyone in order to calm the anxieties of other patients on the unit. Placing a person in a gender-appropriate room is the best possible treatment. If the staff feel a TGNC person may be at risk by being placed in a gender-appropriate room, then a single room is another option. This may raise questions among the other patients, however, and could lead to further isolation and feelings of being stigmatized. Talk to patients about their preferences.

Another mistake is the cessation of testosterone, a hormone that Phillip had been taking for several years and that was being monitored by him, his psychiatrist, and his primary care physician. Hormones causing psychiatric symptoms is exceptionally rare, and stopping the hormone will alienate the patient, invalidate their gender identity, damage the patient-staff alliance, and serve no therapeutic benefit (Dhillon et al. 2011). In the rare case that hormones are playing some factor in a patient's instability, the answer is not to stop them but rather to find a treatment that works with the patient's symptoms, allowing the continuation of hormone therapy. If patients want to take hormones, they do not need to get them from a medical professional. Given the dangers of unsupervised hormones, we should advocate for patients to continue to get prescribed hormones on both an inpatient and an outpatient basis.

A red flag when talking to any clinician is the statement "I treat all my patients the same." Clearly, TGNC people need individualized treatment, and using the exact same policies with them that you would with a cis person will create many of the problems noted above. Although TGNC people deserve the same level of expertise and standards of care that cis people do, they also require some individualized attention and protection given their history of being marginalized (Quinn et al. 2015).

EMERGENCY DEPARTMENTS

The emergency department is a place where decisions are made quickly. Moments spent in making a decision about patient care can literally be a matter of life or death. Although the majority of emergency room (ER) visits are not at such a high level of acuity, the intensity and energy that comes from an ER visit can be anxiety provoking and even terrifying for patients.

Many TGNC people are afraid of ERs, and they have reason to be afraid. Up to 21% of TGNC people may avoid the ER out of fear of discrimination because of their status (Brown and Jones 2016). Some postpone acute care because of this same fear (Vogel 2014). In no other place besides the surgical suite is the body objectified so much. TGNC people, in particular, might find their bodies being treated as a "special case" or "objects of curiosity" (Levitt and Ippolito 2014). There is no time for trust to develop in a doctor-patient relationship in the ER. Doctors review vital signs and lab work and perform a physical exam to make quick diagnoses and triage patients for further care. There is little space to talk about one's gender or sexual orientation unless the problem that brought the patient to the ER is directly associated with gender or sexuality.

TGNC people can expect to be misnamed and misgendered when going to the ER unless their identification and insurance card are identical to their gender identity and name. There is little to no privacy in most ER exam rooms, and a vulnerable conversation about one's gender identity will be overheard by other patients and frequently invalidated by the ER staff. This exposure to such an anxiety-producing environment probably explains why close to a quarter of TGNC people avoid getting care when they are sick out of fear of what will happen in the ER.

Advocating for TGNC people in an ER setting can be done in two major ways. First, if you speak to a clinician who is evaluating a TGNC patient you know, encourage that clinician to focus on the problem that brought the patient to the ER in the first place. The patient may be in the ER because of such emergencies as a heart attack, a stroke, substance withdrawal, or suicidal ideation. There is a tendency for the staff to focus on the fact that their patient is TGNC and not on the medical emergency. This can definitely happen in a psychiatric ER, where the fact that a person is TGNC is blamed for the psychiatric symptoms. A gender diverse patient might be experiencing suicidal ideation due to an untreated depression, but the ER staff explain away the symptoms by saying that many TGNC people have suicidal ideation and in this case, it's probably due to societal stressors. However, although societal stressors likely play a role in a TGNC person's depressive symptoms, a major depressive episode should not be minimized, and appropriate treatment should always be offered.

The second way to advocate for TGNC people in the ER is with regard to personal safety. TGNC people can be at risk of being physically assaulted just by being out in public. This is a population that is already in a vulnerable position with their bodies, and being exposed to strange clinicians in the ER can be traumatizing. Having an advocate present, be it a family member, a friend, a case worker, or a patient advocate, will significantly help reduce the stress TGNC people feel going to the ER and likely will make it easier for them to go when they need to. The presence of an advocate can provide safety, and the advocate can help explain to clinicians and staff a person's gender identity when the patient is too medically and/or psychologically stressed to do so.

Case Example

Martha is a 25-year-old woman of trans experience. She has identified as female since the age of 4. Her psychiatric history is significant in that she experienced many years of sexual abuse by an uncle who lived in her parents' home. She suffers from symptoms of posttraumatic stress disorder and has been seeing both a psychiatrist and a therapist for treatment. Her only medical problem is asthma, which is largely well controlled by her primary care doctor.

While Martha was walking on the street to her therapy appointment, local teenagers harassed her, as they had done before. In the past, they had called her names and made physical threats that turned into physical attacks. On this occasion, one of the younger neighborhood boys started calling her names and pulled out a knife, saying to her, "I'm going to cut off your penis for you." Martha was rightfully terrified and attempted to walk faster, but the boy caught up to her and tried to grab her arm. She pushed him away, but in the struggle his knife cut open her hand. She ran to the nearest train station and headed for the hospital, trying to apply pressure to her bleeding cut.

Once Martha was in the ER, she was taken in for treatment quickly given the severity of her cut. The registration staff asked for her identification and insurance card, calling her Mark and addressing her by male pronouns despite the fact that Martha presented as very feminine. Martha attempted to correct the staff, but they said they needed to use whatever name is on the identification card.

The ER doctor came in to examine Martha's cut. He asked her questions about her medical history and discovered she was taking estrogen. The doctor's questions were pointed, and he asked details about Martha's physical anatomy and genitals despite her hand being the acute medical problem. Martha couldn't believe the way she was being treated and started to feel anxious. When the ER doctor asked her if she was cut because she is a sex worker, Martha became overwhelmed and started to have a panic attack. The panic exacerbated her asthma, and she started to have an asthma attack as well.

The treating doctor immediately concluded that Martha might be suffering from a clot because of the estrogen she was taking and ordered an emergent magnetic resonance imaging (MRI) scan of her chest. Martha protested, saying she was having an asthma attack and just needed some time to relax. Despite Martha's protest, the doctor had security and a technician force Martha into a wheelchair and took her to get the MRI. They placed Martha on the MRI table and told her if she didn't get the MRI scan she could die. She fought with them, and they attempted to hold her down on the scanning table. Being held down gave her flashbacks to the sexual trauma she experienced as a child, and she started to dissociate. Thinking the patient had passed out from anxiety, the doctor, technician, and security decided to let Martha rest on the exam table until she could hold still enough to go into the MRI scanner. While the staff were distracted, Martha awoke and ran out of the room and out of the hospital. She vowed never to return to the ER and never received the stitches she needed for her hand.

Martha's case is a scary one. Several horrible events happened to Martha that day, and the health care system failed her in numerous ways. TGNC people frequently experience harassment. Martha experiences harassment just by leaving her home, and being physically attacked is not uncommon. It is lucky that Martha got away from the local teenagers before any more harm was done to her. However, once Martha was in the ER, the registration staff ignored her name and pronoun requests. She was already suffering from a deep wound in her hand, and now she was having to handle her feelings around being misgendered. Although the ER physician was correct in suspecting a blood clot as a potential cause of shortness of breath, Martha was clear about knowing it was an asthma attack, and her breathing was clearly brought on by the stress of the inappropriate conversation her doctor was having with her. Physicians do not need to ask detailed questions about a person's genitals when an injury has occurred on the hand. Furthermore, forcing Martha to have an MRI and holding her down in the process retraumatized her and caused flashbacks from the history of sexual abuse.

What Martha learned from this experience was that she cannot trust the ER as a place to seek help in times of need. Although there are many ER staff who are trans affirming, trans competent, and even TGNC themselves, the majority of ERs remain a scary place for individuals who are gender diverse.

CASE MANAGEMENT

The majority of advocacy that can occur in an outpatient clinic is covered in Chapter 4, "Establishing a TGNC-Friendly Clinic." One additional way that many outpatient clinics can begin to excel in advocacy is the addition of a case manager to their services. Case managers offer help in numerous ways, from providing social support to understanding the system and how to connect patients to the right services.

Case managers understand the laws around name and gender marker changes. They will sometimes go with patients to apply for housing, disability, or other social services. When it comes time for gender-affirming procedures, they can go with patients to surgery visits and help make sure enough time is taken to answer all the questions that patients might have.

Good case managers act, in some form, like a family member. The safety they provide is irreplaceable, and many TGNC people are able to get the care and services they need because they have a case manager in their life. Depending on the state where you practice, case management services may or may not be paid for by insurance providers. Regardless of the finances involved in staffing, case managers' advocacy with patient care is essential to any clinic that hopes to specialize in TGNC care.

HOMELESS SHELTERS

Case Example

Yolanda is a 40-year-old woman of trans experience who has identified as female since childhood. She has suffered from severe symptoms of disorganized schizophrenia for the past 15 years. She grew up in the rural South

> and moved to a larger city to find a more supportive environment. She started to develop symptoms of schizophrenia after she moved and slowly began to deteriorate without access to psychiatric or medical services. She purchased hormones off the street and contracted hepatitis from sharing needles.
>
> Yolanda eventually found care. She showed up at a local trans-affirming health clinic looking for treatment of minor medical concerns and was connected with a primary care doctor and a therapist. Because she was very disorganized, she was unable to make scheduled appointments, and her providers attempted to see her whenever she showed up at the clinic. In this way, they got her connected with appropriate treatment, including prescribed estradiol and an injectable antipsychotic for her disorganized symptoms. Yolanda was also connected to case management services.
>
> Case management helped Yolanda get into the shelter system. Because her name and gender marker did not match her gender identity, she was placed in an all-male shelter despite the fact that she was female identified and appeared very feminine. Shelter staff said their hands were tied and they were unable to place Yolanda in a female shelter without the appropriate documentation. Yolanda and her case manager filled out paperwork to have her name and gender marker changed in the state where she was born. The process was frustrating, and it took more than 1 year to get the changes made. The state Yolanda was from wanted her to have gender-affirming surgery before they would approve a gender marker change, but Yolanda wasn't in a psychologically fit place to have gender-affirming surgery. She was still recovering from symptoms of schizophrenia that was somewhat treatment resistant. She continued to stay in the all-male shelter, where she was harassed by the other clients, who knew she was a woman of trans experience. Yolanda was physically and sexually assaulted in the shelter. She eventually left the shelter because the process was too frustrating, and living on the street seemed better than dealing with the dangers of the shelter environment in which she had been placed.

A safe place in which to live is a basic necessity. Medical and psychiatric treatment will be futile if the patient does not have a place to sleep at night. The system failed Yolanda in providing her with basic supports. Yolanda had multiple problems, including homelessness, hepatitis, and schizophrenia. She was put in a bind because her state required her to have gender-affirming surgery before a gender marker change could occur on her identification card. The shelter wouldn't place her in an all-female facility without the gender marker change, and Yolanda couldn't begin the process because of her severe disorganized symptoms.

States and facilities will have rules that they follow. Even though these rules may be legislative in nature, accepting them as being set in stone would be a mistake. Working with TGNC people means constant advocacy, especially in situations such as this. The TGNC population is one that is historically marginalized, and state-run facilities and procedures often don't take into account their particular situations. Although cis people may be able to follow the necessary steps to receive services, TGNC people may not be able to do so and can require individualized treatment.

PRISON

Similar to shelters, prison systems follow rigid rules about where people are placed based not only on their gender markers but also their genitals. A woman of trans experience may have had her gender marker changed and may be receiving hormone treatment, but if she has a penis, she can be placed in an all-male prison. Frequently, the prison system will not provide appropriate care, including access to hormones. The dangers of having female-presenting TGNC persons in an all-male prison are serious. They will be harassed by prison staff and be in danger of physical and sexual assault from other inmates. Unlike Yolanda in the previous case example, TGNC persons in a prison system obviously can't leave the facility. They are confined to the circumstances that are given to them. Many people of trans experience come out of the prison system traumatized by what happened to them there. In addition to the usual psychological effects of long-term imprisonment, a TGNC person might have years of repeated trauma that can have lifelong effects.

INSURANCE

Insurance companies are a double-edged sword with regard to the care of a TGNC person. Although insurance companies may provide access to medicinal and surgical treatments for some, there is an ongoing redefining of policies and positions about what is "medically necessary" in the treatment of a TGNC person. Some companies will pay for hormone treatment and gender-affirming procedures, but only to a point. Breast augmentation and facial feminization for women of trans experience are, by many insurance providers, considered to be not medically necessary. Insurance companies are more likely to pay for top surgery for a man of trans experience than a woman of trans experience (see Chapter 17, "Transfeminine Top Surgery"). Gender politics still apply to the TGNC world, and these surgical options will be covered in the concluding chapters of the book.

Many insurance companies do not have medical professionals who are trans affirming or trans competent. The policies they put in place might be based on older suggestions regarding transgender care. The World Professional Association for Transgender Health (WPATH) has several versions of their standards of care that have been updated over the last 40 years as research and treatment understanding have improved. However, older versions of these standards exist online, and insurance companies may pick these versions on which to base their policies. It is up to clinicians to educate insurance companies on the most up-to-date recommendations and treatment guidelines. Patients also might frequently find themselves in situations where their insurance company isn't providing the access to care it should. TGNC people are well aware of the need to find "loopholes" in the system that will allow their health care provider to meet their particular needs (Roller et al. 2015).

TEACHING AND LEARNING

The only way for the mental health community to become more trans affirming and trans competent is for those who know TGNC care to teach those who don't. One study reported that as many as 50% of TGNC people had to teach their clinician about TGNC care (Wichinski 2015). The community of TGNC-affirming mental health professionals is growing, but it remains small and is not sufficient to meet the demands required by the TGNC population overall.

For most clinicians, only 1–2 hours of their professional training are dedicated to cover all LGBTQ topics (Callahan 2015). It is necessary for us to make time to teach those in training and educate others already in the field (Ettner 2013). Clinicians should be encouraged to treat TGNC patients with the help of consultation and supervision. One study found that simply educating clinicians about hormone treatment raised their willingness to prescribe hormones from 5% to 76% (Thomas and Safer 2015). With the help of a supervisor, inexperienced clinicians can become more comfortable understanding basic treatment needs and can identify their own professional areas that need improvement.

There are many organizations that can help foster a better understanding of working with TGNC people. WPATH continues to be the benchmark by which standards are set and includes some of the top thinkers and most experienced clinicians in the field. They have several branches, including the United States branch, USPATH, and hold a major conference every 2 years. The Association of LGBTQ Psychiatrists (AGLP) is a group of professionals who work to educate and advocate for LGBTQ mental health concerns. Their members meet at every conference of the American Psychiatric Association and have social events as well as educational seminars. Similarly, GLMA (formerly the Gay and Lesbian Medical Association) advocates for LGBTQ mental and physical health. They also have annual meetings made up of a variety of professionals. LGBTQ associations are present in most fields, and being a part of those organizations is necessary not only for teaching others but also for our own continued education and development. Given the lack of access to care and the history of marginalization, the American Psychiatric Association made a public statement about the discrimination of TGNC people (American Psychiatric Association 2012):

> **Therefore, the American Psychiatric Association:**
>
> 1. Supports laws that protect the civil rights of transgender and gender variant individuals
> 2. Urges the repeal of laws and policies that discriminate against transgender and gender variant individuals.
> 3. Opposes all public and private discrimination against transgender and gender variant individuals in such areas as health care, employment, housing, public accommodation, education, and licensing.
> 4. Declares that no burden of proof of such judgment, capacity, or reliability shall be placed upon these individuals greater than that imposed on any other persons.

For those of us who are already competent working with TGNC people, we must remember that the evolution of gender and sexuality will continue and is not finite. Going to conferences and learning from each other and our patients can help us to expand our collective knowledge and to provide better care. Culture will continue to expand, and more gender diverse people will express themselves in more diverse ways. The more open-minded and unattached to historical dogma you are as a clinician, the better you will be at working with those who are in different places on the gender spectrum.

SUMMARY

The TGNC population needs advocates as much as it needs access to care. Advocating for those who are TGNC is a necessary and crucial part of the work of a mental health professional. Having all clinicians provide trans-affirming care is a goal, but the first step is having all clinicians provide some level of appropriate care at all. Maintaining frequent communication between providers about individual patient needs and educating staff of inpatient units and in ERs will create a safer environment for TGNC people to get acute care when needed. TGNC people in shelters and the prison population need to have access to gender-appropriate placement and access to care such as hormones. Continued education and training of all clinicians are necessary regardless of their level of understanding and experience. Mental health professionals should join professional organizations to maintain their learning and provide education to those who are just starting their work with gender diverse people.

Key Points

- All mental health professionals should be prepared to serve as advocates for TGNC people.
- Places such as inpatient units and ERs, which usually provide safety and high-level care, can be invalidating and even dangerous for some TGNC individuals.
- Mental health professionals should take it on themselves to educate other clinicians who seem to lack an understanding of individuals who are TGNC.
- Rules that exist in shelters or prisons should not be accepted as static and need to be challenged for the sake of gender diverse patients.
- Professional organizations provide a place for clinicians to cultivate their skills and educate each other on TGNC care.

QUESTIONS

1. Samuel is a 25-year-old man of trans experience. He has been seen in your outpatient clinic for the past 4 years and has been in therapy during that time for treatment of posttraumatic stress disorder. Lately, he has been getting more depressed because his parents are refusing to speak to him as he transitions. He has become more suicidal with a plan, and both you and Samuel think it is important for him to be admitted for observation and medication changes. Once Samuel has been admitted to the inpatient unit, the attending psychiatrist calls to consult on the case. He says that Samuel's mood problems are due to testosterone, so he will be stopping the testosterone and starting an antidepressant. What should be your response?

   A. The attending psychiatrist probably is making a sound clinical decision. Tell him to do what he thinks is appropriate.
   B. Advise the attending psychiatrist to discharge the patient. Samuel is probably safer away from those who don't understand trans-affirming care.
   C. Explain to the attending psychiatrist the common risks and benefits of testosterone use and how it is likely not contributing to

Samuel's depression. Explain how stopping testosterone may make Samuel worse.

D. Connect Samuel with a legal advocate. This is malpractice.

2. Barika is a 33-year-old woman of trans experience. She has been suffering from bipolar disorder and is now homeless in a large city. She is an immigrant and has been applying for asylum because she is at risk of going to prison or being killed in her native country. She hasn't applied to change her identification gender marker. She is assigned to a male shelter despite having an external feminine appearance and identifying as female. Despite your protests, the head of the shelter says they must follow protocol. Barika's symptoms of depression start to worsen because of the harassment she receives from the other shelter clients. What should you do?

   A. Support Barika but let her know there is nothing that can really be done.
   B. Tell Barika it is safer for her to be on the street instead of in a male shelter.
   C. Help connect Barika with an inpatient unit that would be safer than where she is staying.
   D. Get legal services involved. You may need to speak with the agency that oversees the shelter facility.

3. How many hours of LGBTQ mental health training does the typical clinician receive?

   A. None
   B. 1–2
   C. 5
   D. 10

4. You are working in an ER and are consulted on the case of a 66-year-old woman who presents with symptoms of delirium and potentially a stroke. The ER clinician continues to refer to her as "he" and seems focused on the fact she is taking estrogen as the cause of these symptoms. The ER clinician wants your opinion. You notice no major work-up has been done. What would you suggest?

   A. Advise the ER clinician to evaluate for a stroke or identify the cause of the delirium as soon as possible.
   B. Ask to speak to the clinician's supervisor. This behavior is unethical.

C. It's likely to be something psychiatric, so suggest that the patient be transferred to inpatient psychiatry.
D. Spend time talking about trans care and educate the clinician about appropriate next steps.

5. You work in an outpatient clinic and are working on a case with another clinician who doesn't seem to understand the basics of trans care. She isn't hostile toward TGNC people but is definitely not skilled in trans-affirming care. What action should you take?

   A. Speak to the director and have the case transferred to someone else.
   B. Advise your colleague that she should educate herself before attempting to work with a TGNC person.
   C. The patient is probably going to receive good care because you know your colleague is a good clinician.
   D. Talk to your colleague and ask if you can provide her with some guidance and resources in working with TGNC patients.

ANSWERS

1. **The correct response is option C.**

   The attending psychiatrist needs to understand that the testosterone is likely not affecting Samuel's mood or causing depression. This is an opportunity to provide education about hormones to the clinician and turn him into an advocate for TGNC people. Samuel is safe in the hospital, but this learning example might improve the treatment of other TGNC people who come to that inpatient unit in the future. Building bridges instead of burning them is the best way to advocate.

2. **The correct response is option D.**

   Barika is not safe on the street or in the shelter. You have attempted to change the shelter director's mind regarding Barika, but shelter staff are not budging. Rules are in place, but they can be changed or broken. It's time to get legal help and go up the chain of authority until Barika is in a safe space. You might not be successful, but advocating for her in this moment is the best care you can provide.

3. **The correct response is option B.**

   Most clinicians receive approximately 1 hour of training in LGBTQ mental health.

4. **The correct response is option A.**

   This case is an emergency, and time is an important factor. The doctor's behavior can be discussed later. Right now, the patient needs to be evaluated for the cause of the delirium. Advise the doctor you can explain the risks and benefits of estrogen later.

5. **The correct response is option D.**

   You have an open-minded colleague who doesn't seem to understand the basics of TGNC care. With the right encouragement and support, she may become a trans-affirming specialist down the road. As long as the patient is safe, provide guidance and education to other colleagues. That is the only way that more trans-affirming providers will be around to provide care.

REFERENCES

American Psychiatric Association: Position Statement on Discrimination Against Transgender and Gender Variant Individuals. Arlington, VA, American Psychiatric Association, 2012

Brown GR, Jones KT: Mental health and medical health disparities in 5135 transgender veterans receiving healthcare in the Veterans Health Administration: a case-control study. LGBT Health 3(2):122–131, 2016 26674598

Callahan EJ: Opening the door to transgender care. J Gen Intern Med 30(6):706–707, 2015 25743431

Cruz TM: Assessing access to care for transgender and gender nonconforming people: a consideration of diversity in combating discrimination. Soc Sci Med 110:65–73, 2014 24727533

Dhillon R, Bastiampillai T, Krishnan S, et al: Transgender late onset psychosis: the role of sex hormones. Aust N Z J Psychiatry 45(7):603, 2011 21542781

Ettner R: Care of the elderly transgender patient. Curr Opin Endocrinol Diabetes Obes 20(6):580–584, 2013 24468762

Levitt HM, Ippolito MR: Being transgender: the experience of transgender identity development. J Homosex 61(12):1727–1758, 2014 25089681

Moll J, Krieger P, Moreno-Walton L, et al: The prevalence of lesbian, gay, bisexual, and transgender health education and training in emergency medicine residency programs: what do we know? Acad Emerg Med 21(5):608–611, 2014 24842513

Quinn GP, Schabath MB, Sanchez JA, et al: The importance of disclosure: lesbian, gay, bisexual, transgender/transsexual, queer/questioning, and intersex individuals and the cancer continuum. Cancer 121(8):1160–1163, 2015 25521303

Robinson A: The transgender patient and your practice: what physicians and staff need to know. J Med Pract Manage 25(6):364–367, 2010 20695249

Roller CG, Sedlak C, Draucker CB: Navigating the system: how transgender individuals engage in health care services. J Nurs Scholarsh 47(5):417–424, 2015 26243380

Thomas DD, Safer JD: A simple intervention raised resident-physician willingness to assist transgender patients seeking hormone therapy. Endocr Pract 21(10):1134–1142, 2015 26151424

Vogel L: Screening programs overlook transgender people. CMAJ 186(11):823, 2014 24982296

Wichinski KA: Providing culturally proficient care for transgender patients. Nursing 45(2):58–63, 2015 25585225

Wise J: Doctors are prejudiced against transgender patients, MPs say. BMJ 352:i252, 2016 26767717

6

LETTER WRITING

> How the gatekeeping role is performed has contributed to considerable tension between mental health professionals and transgender advocacy groups....
>
> *Jack Drescher*

IN WORKING WITH transgender and gender-nonconforming (TGNC) individuals, regardless of your practice location, you will likely be asked to write a letter attesting to a person's gender identity or readiness for surgery. In some circumstances, you may be asked to provide a letter stating someone can take hormones. There are laws and policies in place that will dictate these requirements. With the diversity of laws from state to state and the continued struggle for civil rights in the TGNC community, it is impossible to compose a comprehensive list of requirements. Having a connection to legal and case management services is crucial for both the provider and the patient. The confusion around changing laws continues to be one of the major barriers to accessing gender-affirming procedures for the TGNC population.

The World Professional Association for Transgender Health (WPATH) is a group of academic professionals who have been writing guidelines on necessary steps one should take before receiving hormone treatment or gender-affirming surgery. These guidelines are available for free through their Web site (WPATH 2017). They remain the most comprehensive standard for TGNC care and should be referenced as the ultimate source in current and up-to-date practices regarding TGNC treatment.

In addition to state laws that dictate the letter-writing requirements for mental health clinicians, there are also the arbitrary policies put forth by insurance companies and surgeons. Insurance companies sometimes take their requirements from older versions of the WPATH Standards of Care, and as a result, they may require inappropriate interventions and statements from clinicians. This problem will be highlighted in a case example later in the chapter. The policy makers involved with these insurance providers typically have very little to no experience working with the TGNC population. One of our most important interventions as mental health clinicians is to advocate for our patients when they are facing these types of barriers to care.

Surgeons will also have their own requirements. Although some of the surgeons involved in TGNC care are quite knowledgeable and set policies in place to protect both themselves and the patient, the majority of board-certified surgeons are not trained in gender-affirming procedures, and they may not have a firm understanding of the complexities involved in TGNC care. TGNC-affirming surgeons will have their own specific requirements depending on the procedure and the insurance company involved. As the relationship between mental health clinician and surgeon continues to grow around this topic, frequent communication is necessary to establish best practices and deliver safe and effective care in an efficient way.

For better or worse, the early WPATH Standards of Care recommended that TGNC people be involved in individual psychotherapy before receiving both hormones and surgical procedures. The most recent version removed these requirements and made mental health care an optional treatment to provide supportive interventions around transition (WPATH 2017). However, although mental health care treatment is not a requirement for medicinal or surgical interventions, both insurance companies and surgeons frequently require both long-term individual therapy and psychiatric involvement.

In the past, mental health clinicians have been noted to pathologize TGNC people simply for being gender diverse. Historically speaking, misguided efforts to convert or treat gender diversity have led to further trauma and bad outcomes, including suicide. Only in recent history have more gender-affirming standards been adopted by some major health organizations. Given the historical relationship between mental health and the TGNC population, mandating treatment prior to getting affirming interventions understandably leads to further negative feelings and mistrust of the general medical field (Drescher et al. 2012).

LETTERS FOR GENDER MARKER CHANGE

Everyone is assigned a documented biological sex at birth. Only recently has *intersex* become a possible choice (Segal 2017). People of trans experience will need medical professionals to attest to their gender identity in order to change legal documents such as government-issued identification, birth certificates, and passports. Laws are different depending on the state, with some asking for documentation of gender-affirming surgeries or hormones prior to making the gender marker change. Given that hormones and surgical procedures are voluntary options for TGNC people, these laws need to be changed. Depending on your location, these laws can greatly affect your ability to advocate for a gender marker change on a patient's identification or birth certificate.

Technically speaking, you can write a letter to change the gender marker of one of your patients if the patient meets the DSM-5 (American Psychiatric Association 2013) criteria for gender dysphoria. Six months of symptoms is enough to meet the criteria of gender dysphoria, although most of your patients will likely have years of symptoms prior to asking you for this type of letter. Details about the diagnosis of gender dysphoria will be covered in Chapter 7.

Consider all the times in which people use their identifications, and you'll quickly understand why a gender marker change is such an important event for those who are TGNC. How often are you asked to present your identification? This becomes particularly important and complicated when dealing with insurance companies. The gender marker on the insurance card needs to match what is on a person's government identification. For most hospitals and clinics, these gender markers are uploaded into their systems, and clinicians will see a gender marker on an electronic chart that matches the one on the insurance card. For mental health clinicians who are familiar with their patients, this won't create an issue because you'll already be well aware of your patient's gender identity and pronouns. For a first-time patient or for hospital and clinic staff, the gender marker documentation in the electronic record serves as a cue to the gender identity of the individual with whom they are interacting. The difference between being called Mister or Miss, male or female, he or she, rests on the letters M or F.

If you are placed in the fortunate position to be able to advocate for your patients to change their gender marker, a simple form letter can be used. Patients will need to have this letter notarized and take individual original copies to places such as the Department of Motor Vehicles or the office of Social Security. The letter will need to identify the person's gender specifically. A standard gender marker change letter might appear as follows (Callen-Lorde Community Health Center 2017a):

Date
RE: [patient name]
Birth date:
SS#:

To Whom It May Concern:

I, [your name], am the provider of [patient name], with whom I have a doctor-patient relationship and whom I have treated.

In my medical opinion, Mr. [patient name] is a man. Mr. [patient name] has had appropriate clinical treatment and has successfully completed his transition from female to male.

Mr. [patient name] should be considered male for all legal and documentation purposes, including on his passport, driver's license, and social security records. Indicating his gender as male will eliminate the considerable confusion and bias Mr. [patient name] encounters when using identification that does not accurately reflect his gender.

I declare under penalty of perjury under the laws of the United States that the foregoing is true and correct.

Sincerely,
[Your name]
[License and professional degree]

A TGNC person may wish to change their name as well, but this is done through the court system like any other name change. A licensed medical provider isn't needed.

Case Example

Alba is a 28-year-old woman of trans experience. She has a long history of gender dysphoric symptoms going back to childhood. Given the rural Midwest town where she grew up, she hid her symptoms most of her life out of fear that her family would disown her. Around the age of 22, she graduated from college and was accepted into medical school. She felt uncomfortable transitioning in medical school because she was living in a place where many of the doctors thought LGBTQ people were abnormal. She feared coming out, thinking she would fail out of medical school if her supervisors disapproved. After she graduated medical school, she went to residency in a more progressive urban environment to train as a family practitioner. She had spent her life dedicated to her studies and had sacrificed being comfortable with who she was in order to secure life in a career she loved.

Around her second year of residency, Alba decided it was time for her to come out and transition into a body she was more comfortable with. She was able to find a primary care doctor who prescribed her estrogen, and she continued her residency while taking on her new name, Alba, and presenting in feminine attire. She legally changed her name and got her gender marker changed with the help of her primary care doctor, all the while remaining one of the most beloved residents to both staff, fellow residents, and patients.

Alba had felt dysphoric most of her life from feelings of being in the wrong body, but being incredibly resilient, she suppressed those feelings for the sake of her education. Although she was very bothered by not having the gender in her mind and her body be aligned, she did not suffer from other psychiatric symptoms. She was incredibly healthy and, to her colleagues' amazement, made her transition from male to female in front of them without any major bumps in the road. Although not everyone goes through such a unilateral and one-directional transition, this was what felt right for Alba.

Alba sought support from other women of trans experience and her supervisors. She had met other professional colleagues who identified as TGNC, and she depended on their friendship and guidance in times when she needed support. Her friendship network was very solid. She had not had any romantic involvements as of yet because she was not comfortable in her current body. She was attracted to cis men and identified as a straight female. After taking hormones for more than 2 years, she was ready to have a vaginoplasty.

Alba saw her primary care doctor and asked for a letter of support. She had already located a surgeon who had experience performing vaginoplasty procedures, and, being a doctor herself, she was well aware of the potential risks and benefits. Alba was shocked, however, to find that her insurance company rejected her request for vaginoplasty because she had not been involved in psychiatric care and therapy for at least 18 months. Alba appealed, saying that she suffered from no mental illness and had no reason to see a mental health professional, but her insurance company claimed it was their policy and it could not be changed. Unable to negotiate anymore, Alba found a trans-affirming psychiatrist who agreed to meet with her weekly.

Alba found that she and the psychiatrist bonded well. She used the psychiatrist mainly for supervision to help her with her more difficult family practice cases. The psychiatrist offered supportive treatments but frequently documented that Alba was not in need of mental health treatment and the only reason they were seeing each other was to meet the requirements of Alba's insurance regarding vaginoplasty.

After 18 months of "treatment," Alba was finally able to get her psychiatrist to write a letter of support. She was about to graduate from residency and had been waiting for gender-affirming surgery for many years at this point. The psychiatrist supplied a basic letter of support for vaginoplasty, but Alba and her treatment team were shocked to find that this letter was also rejected. The insurance company provided Alba and her psychiatrist with a list of requirements that needed to be put in the letter. Some of those requirements included documentation that Alba was not a transvestite or "turned on" by wearing women's clothing, confirmation that Alba was not intersex, and also documentation that her gender identity was not due to a psychotic illness or mood disorder.

Both Alba and her psychiatrist were mortified that this had to be put in a document. Multiple phone calls and appeals yielded no results, and Alba's only choice was to follow the insurance company's rules regarding what had to be in the letter of support. She discussed this at length with her psychiatrist, and they both agreed that working within the system, for the present time, was the only way for Alba to get the surgical procedure she had so long desired.

Alba's story is not an uncommon one. Many TGNC people have identified as such for many years prior to asking for gender-affirming procedures. Only recently have public insurance companies started to pay for the procedures. Even when a patient has a long history of gender dysphoric symptoms, many insurance companies will require that the patient be involved with psychiatry, therapy, or both. However, according to WPATH Standards of Care (WPATH 2017), mental health treatment is not a requirement for surgical intervention. Although many TGNC people have a history of psychiatric symptoms and a need for mental health treatment, many do not.

Writing a letter of support for a gender-affirming procedure is a bit more complicated than writing a letter for a gender marker change. It's more complicated mainly because there are many different surgical procedures, and these procedures all have different requirements depending on the state in which the person lives, the insurance provider, and the surgeon who will be providing the treatment. WPATH has documented recommendations regarding letters of support for each of these surgical procedures. There is not yet an alignment between insurance companies and TGNC experts regarding the amount of evaluation and observation that goes into a letter of support for gender-affirming surgery. The system will likely remain complicated for years to come, but there are some basic components that are necessary in all letters of support. These include specifics about the patient, how long they have been on hormones (if applicable), the specific surgical procedure they are seeking, a brief history of their mental health, and their capacity to understand the risks and benefits of the procedure. These letters are *not* intended for the mental health clinician or the primary care clinician to identify someone as TGNC. Gender identity remains in the hands of the individual. Although gender identity remains in DSM-5 as an avenue to care, the goal of evaluation for surgery is not to diagnose but to assess for safety.

CAPACITY EVALUATIONS

Most psychiatrists are familiar with capacity evaluations, but other mental health clinicians may not be because these evaluations are not a regular part of their training. The words capacity and competency frequently get mixed up. *Competency* is a legal term used by a judge to decide a person's ability to make decisions. *Capacity* is more a medical term that identifies patients' ability to make an informed decision about their care. Capacity evaluations are typically not done because most patients, even those with serious mental illness, can understand and make decisions for themselves. TGNC people also have capacity to make decisions about their bodies and treatments. However, insurance companies and many surgeons require a mental health clinician to attest to a patient's capacity and readiness for surgery. When assessing someone for capacity, consider these four major elements (K. Donnelly-Boylen, personal communication, February 15, 2017):

1. Can the person express a clear and consistent choice?
2. Do they understand the proposed treatment?
3. Can they appreciate how the treatment will apply to them in particular?
4. Do they demonstrate reason around making their decision?

The concept of capacity does not have to be a complicated one. The clinician writing the letter should have a basic familiarity with the risks and benefits involved. (For details about hormones and surgical procedures, see the chapters in Part III, "Primary Care and Hormone Treatment," and Part IV, "Surgical and Nonsurgical Gender-Affirming Procedures.") Generally, a mental status exam with some basic open-ended questions about the person's history and understanding of the surgical procedure will provide the necessary information for you to feel comfortable writing a letter of support. Some of the questions you might include in your evaluation are the following:

- Please explain to me your understanding of the risks around the surgical procedure you are seeking.
- How do you see the surgery affecting your life?
- What are the alternative treatments available to you and why are you choosing this procedure over the alternatives?
- Do you see any potential drawbacks to having the procedure?
- What is your plan for recovery, and do you know the recommendations after surgery?

These basic questions will likely give you insight into your patient's understanding of the surgery. Most TGNC people will have done plenty of research on the procedures and know much more than you do about the potential risks and recovery. This may also be a time to clarify any misunderstandings and misinformation your patient may have gotten from Internet sources or word of mouth.

LETTERS FOR SURGERY

The letter of support for surgery should include all the basic elements, specifically addressing the name of the procedure, the patient's capacity, and their history of gender-affirming treatments. A recovery plan would likely help both the patient and the surgeon make sure they understand what to do after the procedure. A template to start from would be as follows (Callen-Lorde Community Health Center 2017b):

Date
Patient Name:
Patient DOB:
Dear Dr. [surgeon's name],

[Patient name] has been a patient of mine since [date of first visit]. I am writing this letter in support of [patient name] undergoing [choose one: metoidioplasty/vaginoplasty/phalloplasty/hysterectomy/oophorectomy/orchiectomy/bilateral reduction mammoplasty with chest reconstruction/breast augmentation]. [Patient name] experiences persistent gender dysphoria, and I am in support of this gender-confirming surgery as the next step in their transition process. [Patient name] was determined to have capacity to make informed consent around this procedure. This procedure is medically necessary to treat their gender dysphoric symptoms.

[Provide relevant psychiatric history here, including diagnosis, recent hospitalizations or suicide attempts, whether the symptoms are well controlled, and why the patient is ready for surgery at this time, in your opinion.]

[Patient's name]'s current medical hormone regimen includes [insert currently prescribed hormone], which they have been taking since [insert hormone start date].

or

[Patient name] is currently not taking hormones because [fill in the reason].

Please call me at XXX-XXX-XXX with any questions or to arrange follow-up care.

Sincerely,
[Your name]
[License and professional degree]

The specific components of this letter will likely be different from state to state and from surgeon to surgeon. Insurance companies may change the letter requirements from patient to patient and give no detailed guidelines about how to write a letter of support. Sometimes, a formatted template letter will meet the requirements, and other times a more detailed biography of the patient's gender history is needed. If your state has laws specifically protecting TGNC people, it might help to include reference to those laws specifically highlighted in your letter of support. Unfortunately, as more people ask for gender-affirming procedures, more requirements may be put in place to limit the number of those who have access to care. This may be largely due to monetary reasons as decided by insurance providers, or surgeons may require more information related to their comfort level and for medical-legal reasons.

SUMMARY

The thing to keep in mind is that letters of support are being asked for more often than experts and guidelines such as those of WPATH recommend. Having TGNC people go through a process to certify that they meet the arbitrary requirements necessary to get a gender-affirming procedure is paternalistic and does not honor patient autonomy.

With gender dysphoria being listed as a mental health diagnosis, letters of support written by mental health clinicians remain a necessary step for TGNC people who are looking to have gender-affirming surgical procedures. Although requiring TGNC people to see mental health professionals is stigmatizing and creates further barriers to gender-affirming treatments, clinicians are in a unique position to use these requirements in a positive way and to advocate for their patients. Mental health professionals have more time to meet with their individual patients than a surgeon does, and letter-writing appointments can serve as a time to cover what will happen before, during, and after surgery. As the mental health clinician involved, you can help make sure that all your patient's questions have been answered and that the patient is fully aware of what will be taking place. It's unclear if the policies around TGNC people being evaluated by a mental health clinician will ever change, but in the meantime, mental health providers can easily become comfortable with writing letters of support for surgery and should become familiar with the basic ideas of capacity in an evaluation.

Key Points

- State laws regarding gender marker changes vary widely and can shift over time.
- Having access to both legal consults and case managers will help with understanding requirements in your specific state.
- Letters of support from a mental health clinician are still required for gender marker changes and gender-affirming surgical procedures.
- The main goal of a letter of support for surgery is to evaluate for capacity around the surgical procedure.
- *Capacity* is a clinical term used to describe a patient's ability to understand and make decisions about treatment options.

- There is a lack of mental health professionals who are familiar with and know how to write letters of support.
- Most clinicians can quickly become comfortable with writing letters of support once they understand the basic concepts.

QUESTIONS

1. A TGNC patient comes to your clinic and asks for a letter of support to change their legal name. What is your response?

    A. Evaluate the patient for capacity to make sure they understand all the ramifications of changing their name.
    B. Tell them that they shouldn't change their name without at least a year of therapy.
    C. Changing their name would be the same process as anyone else changing their name. It is done through the court system.
    D. Refer them for hormones first.

2. A patient has been coming to your clinic for the past few weeks and tells you he was told he is labeled as female in his chart, but he identifies as male. He has changed his government-issued identification and wants to change the label in his chart. How should you respond?

    A. Tell the patient that the sex identifier in the chart needs to match the insurance card for billing purposes. The patient should update the gender identity on the insurance card first, and then the electronic record can be updated as well.
    B. Tell the patient that it's important to document the patient's gender assigned at birth for medical reasons.
    C. Tell the patient that it's impossible to change that label, even if the patient has the government identification changed.
    D. Have the record updated immediately with the appropriate gender marker.

3. What is the main purpose for writing a letter of support?

    A. To affirm that your patient is transgender.
    B. To meet the requirements of an insurance company.

C. To affirm the patient has capacity to make decisions around gender-affirming procedures.
D. To encourage a surgeon to perform the gender-affirming procedure.

4. Which of the following is not a core part of a capacity evaluation?

A. Seeing if the patient communicates a clear and consistent message.
B. Asking about how the procedure will affect the patient personally.
C. Seeing if the patient's reasoning around choosing the procedure makes sense.
D. Testing the patient to see if they understand all the details of the surgical procedure.

5. Which of the following should be included in a letter of support?

A. Whether or not the patient is on hormone treatment.
B. Whether there are any mental health concerns.
C. That the procedure is medically necessary.
D. A statement about capacity.
E. All of the above.

ANSWERS

1. **The correct response is option C.**

Name changes are done through the courts. A letter of support is not needed.

2. **The correct response is option A.**

Although you want to remain gender affirming, if a billing department uses M or F for someone and it doesn't match what is on the insurance card, the claim could be denied. The patient needs to have the insurance card updated so the electronic record can reflect what's on the insurance card.

3. **The correct response is option C.**

Letters of support are all about capacity, not diagnosis.

4. **The correct response is option D.**

   Although a patient needs to understand the risks, benefits, recovery, and follow-up around gender-affirming procedures, the vast majority of people, including the mental health professional involved, will not know all the details. That level of expertise is left to the surgeon.

5. **The correct response is option E.**

   Technically, the only thing really needed in a letter of support is the patient's capacity to make a decision around gender-affirming treatment; however, most insurance companies and surgeons will want you to include basics about the patient's mental health history and history of hormone treatment, if any.

REFERENCES

American Psychiatric Association: Diagnostic and Statistical Manual of Mental Disorders, 5th Edition. Arlington, VA, American Psychiatric Association, 2013

Callen-Lorde Community Health Center: Gender Marker Change. New York, Callen-Lorde Community Health Center, 2017a

Callen-Lorde Community Health Center: Mental Health Surgery Letter. New York, Callen-Lorde Community Health Center, 2017b

Drescher J, Cohen-Kettenis P, Winter S: Minding the body: situating gender identity diagnoses in the ICD-11. Int Rev Psychiatry 24(6):568–577, 2012 23244612

Segal C: Nation's first known 'intersex' birth certificate issued in New York City. PBS NewsHour, January 5, 2017. Available at: www.pbs.org/newshour/rundown/new-york-city-issues-nations-first-birth-certificate-marked-intersex/. Accessed May 6, 2017.

WPATH: The Standards of Care. World Professional Association for Transgender Health, 2017. Available at: www.wpath.org/site_page.cfm?pk_association_webpage_menu=1351&pk_association_webpage=4655. Accessed May 6, 2017.

Part II

Mental Health–Related Topics

7

THE GENDER DYSPHORIA DIAGNOSIS

> My problem isn't that I was born transgender. My problem is that I wasn't born female.
>
> *A woman of trans experience*

THE QUOTATION ABOVE was spoken to me by a long-term patient who is a woman of trans experience. It sums up the arguments that go into having or not having a psychiatric diagnosis of gender dysphoria. The presence of gender dysphoria in the fifth edition of the *Diagnostic and Statistical Manual of Mental Disorders* (DSM-5; American Psychiatric Association 2013) is a controversial one (Drescher et al. 2012). There are proponents who would like to see the diagnosis removed altogether, and there are many who would like to see some form of diagnosis remain. Even trying to understand what gender dysphoria means is complicated. Understanding the diagnosis of gender dysphoria and how to apply it to patient care means knowing it from a historical, cultural, and scientific perspective.

GENDER VARIANCE IS NOT A MENTAL ILLNESS

A diagnosis of gender dysphoria can and should be used in cases where treatment is necessary. However, the presence of gender variance in itself does not imply the presence of a mental disorder. Further, although gender dysphoria is found in psychiatry's diagnostic manual, DSM, the World Health Organization is preparing to move its gender diagnoses (referred to as *gender incongruence*) out of the mental disorders section of the *International Classification of Diseases* (ICD) and into a new chapter provisionally called

"Conditions Related to Sexual Health" (Drescher et al. 2012; Reed et al. 2016). However, many people still associate the word *transgender* with some sort of pathology, viewing individuals who fall outside the binary view of gender—male or female—as abnormal. Mental health professionals should continue to educate those who believe this and teach the larger community about varied gender expressions in the range of human development.

Regarding the diagnosis of gender dysphoria, there are those who are against having the diagnosis in DSM-5 and those who would like the diagnosis to remain (Drescher 2010). Of those who are against having a diagnosis, many cite the removal of homosexuality from DSM-II as an example of why the presence of gender dysphoria in DSM-5 is stigmatizing. This removal was based on scientific research but also in part on political advocacy (Drescher 2010). Homosexuality remained in DSM until 1973, when it was removed for several reasons. Some of those reasons included the emerging belief within psychiatry that a psychiatric diagnosis should involve some degree of distress and/or impairment or "dysfunction" in the affected individual. If gay people were neither distressed nor disabled by their homosexuality, then there was no need to give them a diagnosis (Drescher 2003; Spitzer 1981). However, the research of Evelyn Hooker (1957) first showed that people who are homosexual don't necessarily experience impairment or distress. Although the evolution of DSM in regard to homosexuality took many years, the removal of homosexuality from DSM signified that the American Psychiatric Association was evolving as society did.

The diagnosis of homosexuality as a mental illness was stigmatizing and damaging and continues to have lingering effects on the lesbian, gay, bisexual, transgender, and queer/questioning (LGBTQ) community. Some people still believe that people with a diverse sexual orientation are mentally ill and need reparative therapies in order to correct their "deviance." DSM represented these beliefs, and, by listing homosexuality as mental illness, communicated to gay and lesbian people that they were abnormal and needed treatment for their personal sexual feelings and identity. Many people believe that the presence of gender dysphoria in DSM-5 has similar effects. It communicates to those who are gender diverse that something is wrong with them that needs treatment. Furthermore, it provides written evidence to those who see gender diversity as a sin or abnormality in need of repair. Only by removing gender dysphoria from the list of mental illnesses can the wounds between mental health professionals and the TGNC community begin to heal. Table 7–1 compares sexual orientation and gender identity and how they have been pathologized in DSM. It has been altered from its original form (Drescher 2010) to include updates.

On the other side of the debate are those who advocate for gender dysphoria to remain in DSM as an avenue to treatment. Much of the modern

TABLE 7–1. Pathologization of homosexuality and gender variance in DSM

	Homosexuality	Gender variance
Year of first appearance in DSM	1952	1980
Current status in DSM	Not present	Gender dysphoria diagnosis
Year removed from DSM	1973	NA
Scientific rationale for category	Alternative model to religious views of homosexuality as a sin	Alternative model to transsexualism being due to psychosis or neurosis
Medical rationale for category	Justified conversion therapy	Justified hormone and surgical interventions
Did diagnosis lead to increase in access to care?	NA	Yes, with insurance providers paying for gender-affirming procedures
Role of activism	Removal occurred because of APA debates from 1970 to 1973	Led to change of name from gender identity disorder to gender dysphoria
Medical consequences of removing the diagnosis	None noted	NA
Relationship to civil rights	Civil rights followed removal from DSM	Civil rights preceded removal of gender identity disorder from DSM
APA Practice Guidelines	NA	APA Toolkit published in 2017
APA position statement of support	Opposed discrimination (1974)	Opposed discrimination (2012)

Note. APA = American Psychiatric Association; DSM = Diagnostic and Statistical Manual of Mental Disorders; NA = not applicable.
Source. Adapted from Drescher 2010.

controversy around the presence of gender dysphoria in DSM-5 is not over whether or not being gender diverse makes one mentally ill but in how various optional treatments will be provided to people who wish to change their body to reflect their mind. Psychotherapy is needed for many who are gender diverse not because gender diversity inherently causes mental health symptoms but because the treatment by the larger cis society of TGNC individuals reinforces transphobic beliefs and creates a minority stress (the general stress caused by being part of a minority group that is not accepted or is marginalized in mainstream culture) that impacts the mental health of every TGNC person. Symptoms of depression, anxiety, panic, and trauma can manifest from these stressors. In addition, because of the cost of hormone therapy and gender-affirming surgeries, these treatments are not possible without insurance coverage unless the seeker is independently wealthy. Very few people, regardless of their gender status, can afford these therapies. Therefore, keeping the gender dysphoria diagnosis in DSM makes it possible for individuals most in need of services to access them.

The majority of mental health professionals who work with the TGNC population fall on both sides of the debate. Although we would like to see the diagnosis of gender dysphoria removed from the list of mental illnesses, there is an understanding that TGNC people need treatment because of societal transphobia and the cost of gender-affirming treatments. Until a time when there is a better understanding of TGNC people and a less stigmatizing route to therapies exists, gender dysphoria will remain a double-edged sword that will continue to both help advocate for the TGNC population and hinder healing.

WHAT IS GENDER DYSPHORIA?

The DSM-5 criteria for gender dysphoria in adolescents and adults are shown in Box 7–1.

Box 7–1. DSM-5 Diagnostic Criteria for Gender Dysphoria

Gender Dysphoria in Adolescents and Adults **302.85** (F64.0)

A. A marked incongruence between one's experienced/expressed gender and assigned gender, of at least 6 months' duration, as manifested by at least two of the following:

1. A marked incongruence between one's experienced/expressed gender and primary and/or secondary sex characteristics (or in young adolescents, the anticipated secondary sex characteristics).

2. A strong desire to be rid of one's primary and/or secondary sex characteristics because of a marked incongruence with one's experienced/expressed gender (or in young adolescents, a desire to prevent the development of the anticipated secondary sex characteristics).
3. A strong desire for the primary and/or secondary sex characteristics of the other gender.
4. A strong desire to be of the other gender (or some alternative gender different from one's assigned gender).
5. A strong desire to be treated as the other gender (or some alternative gender different from one's assigned gender).
6. A strong conviction that one has the typical feelings and reactions of the other gender (or some alternative gender different from one's assigned gender).

B. The condition is associated with clinically significant distress or impairment in social, occupational, or other important areas of functioning.

Specify if:

With a disorder of sex development (e.g., a congenital adrenogenital disorder such as 255.2 [E25.0] congenital adrenal hyperplasia or 259.50 [E34.50] androgen insensitivity syndrome).

Coding note: Code the disorder of sex development as well as gender dysphoria.

Specify if:

Posttransition: The individual has transitioned to full-time living in the desired gender (with or without legalization of gender change) and has undergone (or is preparing to have) at least one cross-sex medical procedure or treatment regimen—namely, regular cross-sex hormone treatment or gender reassignment surgery confirming the desired gender (e.g., penectomy, vaginoplasty in a natal male; mastectomy or phalloplasty in a natal female).

Notice that the focus of the diagnosis is not the presence of gender variance but the person's reaction to both their physical anatomy and their societal prescribed gender role. The diagnosis on the surface appears rather simple. If a person meets one of the criteria for gender dysphoria, they likely meet criteria for many, if not all, of the others. When the diagnostic process is examined more closely, however, the complexity of diagnosing gender dysphoric symptoms will become more evident and it will become more obvious why research and academic understanding of these symptoms can be difficult.

Gender dysphoric symptoms related to the anatomy of an individual are objective. A man of trans experience who has breast tissue and a vagina can experience dysphoric symptoms around the presence of these body parts and can seek to have them removed or altered. For many clinicians, a thought experiment in which the person considers waking up in the body of a different gender will facilitate empathy as to why certain body parts might lead to uncomfortable or dysphoric symptoms. It is easy for many clinicians to imagine, and symptoms related to anatomy are also easy to document when making a formal diagnosis of gender dysphoria.

Regarding gender roles, the idea of what is male or female is part genetic, part hormonal, and part societal. Cis men and cis women in society have general roles that are traditionally followed and socially accepted. Although there is some variance in these roles (see section "Is Gender Dysphoria Societal?"), most people have ingrained stereotypes about what makes a person masculine or feminine. Until there is a better understanding of what is genetic or hormonal in origin versus what is societal, dysphoric symptoms around gender roles will be somewhat subjective and will be contextual only in the narrative of the individual. Although some of these dysphoric feelings around gender roles may seem obvious to most clinicians, considering the societal assumptions being made will highlight why gender diversity is intrinsically not a mental illness. Many TGNC people are having dysphoric "symptoms" in part because society shuns those who break gender stereotypes and we collectively as a society are asking individuals born with a certain anatomy to behave in a certain way.

HISTORY OF GENDER DYSPHORIA

The history of a transgender diagnosis, as stated in Chapter 3, "Historical Background," goes back to Karl Heinrich Ulrichs identifying "a female psyche existing in a male body" (Group for the Advancement of Psychiatry, LGBT Issues Committee 2015). Although Ulrichs may have been talking about homosexuals and not individuals who are TGNC, his statement still represents an initial academic understanding of how the gender of the mind and the sex of the body may not correlate.

A diagnosis related to gender was not present in either DSM-I or DSM-II (Drescher et al. 2012). Early on, academics and clinicians confounded the concepts of sexual orientation and gender identity. A person assigned male sex at birth who identified as female might have been defined by the medical community as homosexual. It was argued that the presence of gender variance related to the individual's wish to sexually identify with the opposite gender or because that person was attracted to individuals of the same gender. Blanchard (1989) described these concepts as *autogynephilia*. These ideas don't apply to the large gender diverse community, with the understanding that sexual orientation and gender identity are two separate phenomena. This early thinking, however, convoluted the understanding of what is gender diversity and what is sexual orientation diversity. Although different, these two groups make up the LGBTQ community and continue to be intertwined today, for better or worse.

Throughout the twentieth century, psychoanalytic thought stigmatized those who are gender variant and sought to repair them. Mental health providers considered the basis of gender diversity to be neurotic in nature, and many in the medical community opposed (and some still do) any hormonal or surgical interventions with TGNC people. Instead, they supported reparative treatments to help TGNC people comes to terms with their sex assigned at birth. These treatments did more harm than good, and it wasn't until the latter half of the twentieth century that gender diversity started to be seen as a normal variation in the human condition. In 1969, Virginia Prince, a transgender activist, was probably the first person to use the term *transgender*. With the opening of gender clinics around the country in the past decade, the larger mental health community started to focus on how to identify and work with people who were gender diverse and requesting gender-affirming treatment.

The diagnosis of *gender identity disorde*r (GID) first appeared in DSM-III (American Psychiatric Association 1980). The word choice around this diagnosis was problematic from the start. The name itself implies that the disorder or mental illness is due to a person's gender identity. A larger debate occurred around the presence of GID in children. Tables 7–2 and 7–3 summarize how disorders related to gender identity have evolved over time in DSM and ICD, respectively.

In DSM-IV, GID was retained as a diagnosis, specifying adolescence or adulthood. By this time, homosexuality had been removed from DSM, and arguments were building for the removal of GID as well. The presence of GID encouraged the stigmatization of gender diverse people and continued to focus on gender identity as a mental illness rather than a dysphoric reaction to the person's sex assigned at birth.

DSM-5 helped change this stigmatization. The terms *gender identity* and *disorder* have been removed from the new diagnosis, shifting the diagnosis to the body and not the mind. The diagnosis of gender dysphoria is related not to an individual's gender identity but to the person's gender. *Dysphoria* is a word commonly used among mental health professionals to refer to an emotional or affective state generally characterized by depressed mood, anxiety, or agitation. The dysphoria is related to a person's sex assigned at birth and assigned gender role; how patients view themselves to be in their minds has been removed from the diagnosis.

TABLE 7–2. Gender identity diagnoses in DSM

Edition	Parent category	Diagnosis name
DSM-I (1952)	NA	NA
DSM-II (1968)	Sexual deviations	Transvestitism
DSM-III (1980)	Psychosexual disorders	Transsexualism Gender identity disorder of childhood
DSM-III-R (1987)	Disorders usually first evident in infancy, childhood, or adolescence	Transsexualism Gender identity disorder of childhood Gender identity disorder of adolescence or adulthood, nontranssexual type
DSM-IV (1994)	Sexual and gender identity disorders	Gender identity disorder in adolescents or adults Gender identity disorder in children Gender identity disorder not otherwise specified
DSM-IV-TR (2000)	Sexual and gender identity disorders	Gender identity disorder in adolescents or adults Gender identity disorder in children Gender identity disorder not otherwise specified
DSM-5 (2013)	Gender dysphoria	Gender dysphoria in adolescents or adults Gender dysphoria in children Other specified gender dysphoria Unspecified gender dysphoria

Note. NA = not applicable.
Source. Drescher et al. 2012.

TABLE 7–3. Gender identity diagnoses in ICD

Edition	Parent category	Diagnosis name
ICD-6 (1948)	NA	NA
ICD-7 (1955)	NA	NA
ICD-8 (1965)	Sexual deviations	Transvestitism
ICD-9 (1975)	Sexual deviations	Transvestism Trans-sexualism
ICD-10 (1990)	Gender identity disorder	Transsexualism Dual role transvestism Gender identity disorder of childhood Other gender identity disorders Gender identity disorder, unspecified
ICD-11 (2015)	Remains to be seen	Remains to be seen

Note. NA=not applicable.
Source. Drescher et al. 2012.

WHAT GENDER DYSPHORIA IS NOT

Many clinicians are afraid to give the diagnosis of gender dysphoria because they feel they don't have a comfortable understanding of the patient's history and don't want to incorrectly assign a diagnosis. I would argue that the diagnosis of gender dysphoria is largely a simple one to make. Our patients typically come in to an evaluation already expressing many of the criteria called for in DSM-5. A review of the patient's gender identity and gender expression history will provide key evidence for the diagnosis, thus leading to avenues of care such as hormonal therapy or gender-affirming surgeries.

To ease the fears of clinicians new to working with TGNC people, it might be helpful to briefly explore the rare instances that would not lead to a diagnosis of gender dysphoria. *Intersex* (formerly referred to as *hermaphrodite*) is one of these rule-out diagnoses. Intersex people are those who are born with ambiguous genitalia due to a genetic or hormonal diversity in utero. It would be unusual for those who are intersex to see a mental health provider expressing new gender dysphoric symptoms. This is because most intersex children are identified early on and get supportive treatments along with family interventions. Modern guidelines encourage parents to let children with ambiguous genitalia age enough to identify their gender themselves. This will prevent the need for gender-affirming procedures later in life. Although many of the hormone therapies and gender-affirming procedures are available to intersex people, their diagnosis is more pediatric in nature, and they are not usually diagnosed by a mental health professional. Intersex people are more common in society than one might think, making up about 1.7% of births (Blackless et al. 2000).

Another rule-out diagnosis is transvestism (Box 7–2). A common source of confusion in the general population is thinking that transgender people and transvestites are the same. Although transvestites cross-dress, they are typically heterosexual cis male identified and wear traditional female clothing for sexual pleasure. A transvestite wears female clothing but does not identify as female (American Psychiatric Association 2013).

Box 7–2. DSM-5 Diagnostic Criteria for Transvestic Disorder

Transvestic Disorder 302.3 (F65.1)

A. Over a period of at least 6 months, recurrent and intense sexual arousal from cross-dressing, as manifested by fantasies, urges, or behaviors.

B. The fantasies, sexual urges, or behaviors cause clinically significant distress or impairment in social, occupational, or other important areas of functioning.

Specify if:

With fetishism: If sexually aroused by fabrics, materials, or garments.

With autogynephilia: If sexually aroused by thoughts or images of self as female.

Specify if:

In a controlled environment: This specifier is primarily applicable to individuals living in institutional or other settings where opportunities to cross-dress are restricted.

In full remission: There has been no distress or impairment in social, occupational, or other areas of functioning for at least 5 years while in an uncontrolled environment.

Case Example

James is a 45-year-old cis gender heterosexual man. He identifies as male and has since he was a child. He works during the day as a banker but likes to spend some of his evenings dressed in women's clothing. He likes the feel of the clothing and has erotic feelings when he wears dresses and pantyhose. James has been married for 20 years to a cis woman. She knows about James's proclivities and enjoys taking part in role play with him while he is dressed in female clothing. James sometimes likes to go to gay bars dressed in female clothing but does not identify as gay or as female; he enjoys the chance to be around people who won't judge him for his clothing choices.

Although wearing the clothing associated with a specific gender is one part of the gender dysphoria diagnosis, it is not the entire picture. When clinicians come across someone who is gender atypical, they may be quick to diagnose that person as having gender dysphoria. However, there are many men like James who like to dress up in female clothing for erotic reasons. James even likes to go to gay bars so that he can dress up in female clothing in public. This alone does not make James transgender, although he might self-identify at any point on the gender spectrum. The important difference is his identity and the lack of other gender dysphoric symptoms. Mental health professionals who meet patients who fall outside the norm of their usual cis gender patients may be impetuous in their diagnosis. It is also possible that someone like James would go on to express gender dysphoric symptoms. It is necessary to look at the whole person, taking into account the patient's gender identity and gender history over time.

People may also confuse those who are known as drag queens as people who are TGNC. Remember that gender identity and gender expression are on a continuum. Drag queens and drag kings are people who dress up in the opposite gender's clothing for entertainment purposes. They are generally performers who take on opposite gender identities to provide entertainment and make an income. Although they may not be the same as TGNC, there might be circumstances where drag queens or kings come to identify as TGNC, and some may decide to transition at some point in their life. Because TGNC people have been stigmatized and marginalized for so long, coming out and identifying as TGNC may take time for some people. A person will report their gender identity to you, and if someone who previously dressed in drag for entertainment purposes now identifies with that gender, it will be clear in the patient's history from the psychiatric evaluation.

Case Example

Nicki is a 26-year-old woman of trans experience. She was raised in a somewhat isolated environment, was provided with home schooling, and didn't come across anyone she knew of as non cis or non straight until college. She was an only child and knew that she was different because her parents got angry with her about the clothing she wanted to wear and the toys she wanted to play with. Although her parents viewed her as a boy, she felt very feminine inside.

Once she got to college, Nicki met young men who identified as gay. In sharing her experiences with them, she started to understand herself to be a gay man. At this point, she still had not been exposed to anyone who was transgender and thought of herself as a gay man. During college, Nicki went to gay bars and started to identify with the drag scene. She enjoyed putting on dresses and makeup and having crowds cheer for her while she sang and performed. The experience was very validating for her, and she looked forward to performance nights, mainly because they gave her a chance to dress and present in a way that was more comfortable for her and more in line with how she saw herself.

Toward the end of her college years, Nicki learned about TGNC people and discovered what it meant to be gender diverse. For the first time, she was able to see that someone could be assigned a sex at birth but identify with the other gender, and her past and how she had felt most of her life started to make more sense. In meeting other TGNC people, she was given the mental freedom to identify as female and didn't need a reason, such as performing in drag, to dress and express herself in the way she had always wanted. However, she continued to perform because she enjoyed singing and entertaining people.

Many people in the drag community do not have the same experience as Nicki, but some do. The diagnosis of gender dysphoria is specific to a person's discomfort with their sex assigned at birth. The criteria for gender dysphoria consist of a list of symptoms related to a dysphoric state around a person's assigned sex and gender role. People who dress in drag for entertainment or financial reasons do not fit this diagnosis. What one does for entertainment is not the same as one's gender identity. There are some who dress in drag who might come to identify with that gender, but whether or not an individual eventually identifies as transgender is a personal decision. A circumstance such as what happened with Nicki would be discovered during an appropriate review of a patient's history and development.

Gender dysphoria can also be confused with other cultural phenomena. An astute mental health clinician will be mindful of people who present from other cultures. In Samoan culture, for instance, there are those who are called *fa'fafine* who don't fall into a neat binary gender (Adams et al. 2013). These are people assigned male at birth who identify in many ways with both the female and male genders. Individuals who are fa'fafine may have gender dysphoric symptoms around their body or assigned gender role, but their gender diversity is also accepted within Samoan culture. An in-depth history and review of symptoms would help distinguish what is culturally related and what is gender dysphoric in nature. There are other examples of gender diversity and atypical gender roles around the world, such as the Métis, Bakla, and Muxe. Be particularly careful when evaluating patients from cultures different from your own.

IS GENDER DYSPHORIA GENETIC?

If you ask most people, they would probably say that being transgender is due to genetic or hormonal diversity (Furnham and Sen 2013). There have been only a handful of studies looking for genetic explanations for gender diversity. Laura Erickson-Schroth has done an extensive review of the literature, looking at findings from studies of siblings, twins, and chromosomal abnormalities (Erickson-Schroth 2013). One might think that being TGNC would have a genetic basis, with some combination of chromosomes such as XXY, XXX, or XYY. What has been discovered so far is that individuals who are TGNC typically do not have chromosomal variance, and there is no genetic explanation for why they identify as TGNC. There is also no genetic explanation for why people identify as cis gender.

IS GENDER DYSPHORIA HORMONAL?

Researchers have also searched for hormonal explanations for gender diversity (Erickson-Schroth 2013). Postmortem studies of the brains of TGNC individuals do reveal similarities in the size of brain structures of TGNC individuals and individuals whose gender identity corresponds to the same sex or gender assigned at birth. These studies are problematic because there are so few of them and the number of subjects remains small. The jury is still out as to whether there are hormonal changes that happen in utero or whether people who are TGNC are born with brain structures that align with their ultimate gender identity rather than their assigned sex at birth. More research needs to be done to help identify why people become cis or trans. Understanding the human condition of gender is still a work in progress.

IS GENDER DYSPHORIA SOCIETAL?

There are obviously some inborn traits that are generally what we would refer to as male or female. The addition of testosterone or estrogen helps exemplify these traits and behaviors, which can largely be explained by the hormones themselves. For example, there seems to be a correlation between the addition of testosterone and an increase in sex drive. Conversely, there appears to be a correlation between the reduction of testosterone and a decrease in sex drive. Some might say that sex drive doesn't necessarily decrease, but the expression of the sex drive changes. Individuals with higher levels of testosterone may respond more to visual cues of sexuality, whereas those with more estrogen respond more to emotional cues. These are general statements but help point out that there are gender characteristics associated with hormones and being male or female.

The majority of other gender characteristics are probably more societal and culturally defined over time. The world has diverse views of what characterizes a traditional male or traditional female, expressed in the clothing people wear, how they act, and the work they value, for example. Thousands of years of human evolution, along with individual cultural evolutions, have helped shape these views. What it means to be a cis man in Italy can be quite different from what it means to be a cis man in Mongolia. Noticing these individual differences will help mental health clinicians and researchers to distinguish what is nature and what is culture.

DIAGNOSIS AND OUR PATIENTS

Although the focus in this chapter is on the diagnosis of gender dysphoria and being able to distinguish symptoms to make an appropriate clinical diagnosis, it should be pointed out that assigning the diagnosis of gender dysphoria will have an effect on the clinician-patient relationship. The TGNC community is well aware of the stigma assigned to them by mental health professionals over time, and individuals are justified in being cautious about receiving a stigmatizing diagnosis from their mental health clinician. Before assigning a gender dysphoria diagnosis, mental health clinicians should discuss with their patients the reasons for the diagnosis. Mental health providers will use the diagnosis of gender dysphoria largely when access to care is needed. It can help justify to insurance providers treatments such as psychotherapy, hormone therapy, and gender-affirming surgeries. Giving someone the diagnosis of gender dysphoria does not mean that person is mentally ill, but it does signify that the patient has symptoms related to their assigned gender. TGNC people need access to mental health care not because gender diversity is a mental illness but because the stress of being gender diverse in a larger gender dichotomous world can be taxing and stressful over time. Because of this, people with gender dysphoria may exhibit a range of symptoms leading to misdiagnoses such as borderline personality disorder, bipolar disorder, or even schizophrenia. This information will be covered in more detail in Chapter 8, "Gender-Affirming Mental Health."

There are people who are gender diverse and identify as TGNC but do not meet the criteria for gender dysphoria. It is possible to be on the TGNC spectrum and not have symptoms related to one's gender identity or gender expression. Being gender diverse is not the same as having gender dysphoria.

GENERAL INTERVIEW QUESTIONS

Gender identity development is not typically taught in mental health training programs, and many clinicians don't know the basic questions to ask to inform a diagnosis of gender dysphoria. A first-time mental health evaluation may or may not be the time to discuss gender. It is important to ask all patients about their gender identity, but a person's comfort level and connection with the mental health clinician is more important than reviewing a gender history. Asking permission to discuss gender-specific topics is the most sensitive and respectful way to approach your patient's gender history. Although the majority of TGNC people in treatment will provide the details needed to understand the basics of their identity, clinicians should be aware of certain open-ended questions to start a dialogue around gender identity. Some of these questions could include the following:

- Gender and sexuality are unique and personal. Help me understand how you identify with regard to both your gender and sexual orientation.
- Would you say the gender you were assigned at birth is the same as or different from how you identify now?
- Do you remember feeling different when you were younger? As if you didn't fit in?
- Were you ever uncomfortable with the clothing you were asked to wear early on?
- What type of toys did you play with growing up?

- Do you remember who you pretended to be in your childhood fantasies?
- What was puberty like for you? How did you respond to the changes in your body?
- How do you feel with regard to your body now? What do you like and not like about your physical self?
- What gender do most people see you as? What is that experience like for you?
- How do you imagine yourself to be?

SUMMARY

The diagnosis of gender dysphoria has evolved over time. Currently, mental health providers are attempting to limit stigmatization and provide access to care. Mental health professionals have traditionally overdiagnosed gender variant patients and have confused gender identity and sexual orientation. The diagnosis of gender dysphoria in DSM-5 focuses on patients and their feelings around their physical self and their assigned gender role. Mental health providers will need to discuss the diagnosis of gender dysphoria with their patients in order to decrease the feelings of being stigmatized and help heal the relationship between the TGNC community and the larger mental health world.

Key Points

- Gender variance, once categorized as a psychiatric problem, is increasingly being viewed in many societies and cultures as a normal expression of the human condition.
- Gender dysphoria focuses on a person's relationship with their body and assigned gender role.
- The diagnosis of gender dysphoria remains controversial because although it provides avenues to treatment, it also labels TGNC people as mentally ill.
- There is no clear genetic explanation for gender diversity. There is also no clear genetic explanation for people who are cis gender.
- There is no clear hormonal explanation for gender diversity, and the research remains limited by small sample sizes and few studies.

- Gender can be expressed in various ways across cultures, and a formal diagnosis should be applied only when a person is clearly having gender dysphoric symptoms.
- Providers should discuss the diagnosis of gender dysphoria with their patients and be prepared to explain why a diagnosis may be necessary.

QUESTIONS

1. In which edition of DSM did a diagnosis related to gender first appear?

    A. DSM-I.
    B. DSM-II.
    C. DSM-III.
    D. DSM-IV.
    E. DSM-5.

2. You are working in an emergency room and are asked to evaluate a patient named Aron. Aron came in with symptoms of depression, including anhedonia, decreased sleep, poor appetite, and depressed mood, and is having thoughts of suicide. There is a strong family history of depression, and Aron had a maternal aunt who completed suicide. Aron identifies as "they" and presents with both traditional masculine and feminine attire. When asked about their gender and symptoms, Aron reports they are happy with their gender expression. They were assigned male at birth and want to keep their body the way it is with no changes. Aron reports that people frequently harass them on the street, which makes their symptoms of depression worse. What would you say is Aron's diagnosis?

    A. Major depressive disorder.
    B. Both major depressive disorder and gender dysphoria.
    C. Gender dysphoria only.
    D. Borderline personality disorder.

3. Evan is a 30-year-old gay-identified cis male. He has been seeing you in an outpatient clinic for treatment of panic disorder with agoraphobia. He finds it difficult to leave the house and be around other people. Evan also performs drag on the weekends to support himself. He says that

when he dresses up in drag he feels protected and is free to be a different person. His persona, Dragonysis, is funny and more extroverted than he is, and he enjoys the reactions he gets from an audience when he is performing. How should you focus your treatment with Evan?

A. Evan is clearly suffering from gender dysphoria, and he should be confronted about his true gender identity.
B. Evan is seeking treatment of panic attacks. His persona as a drag queen may offer valuable insight into steps that Evan can take to help overcome his anxiety.
C. Evan probably has dissociative identity disorder. Having two personas is probably from a history of trauma.
D. Evan should just live in drag all the time. He wouldn't have panic attacks then.

4. Sue is a 19-year-old woman of trans experience. She recently came out and has been seeing you for supportive psychotherapy. Her family is largely unaccepting of her gender identity, and strangers frequently call her names and yell at her on the street because of her appearance. She would like to take estrogen and ultimately wants breast augmentation and vaginoplasty. She comes to you in tears one day with a bill she received from your clinic. She says you diagnosed her with gender dysphoria and she thought you were different in understanding that she was truly born female. How should you respond?

   A. Tell her that people assigned one sex at birth who identify as a different gender have gender dysphoria.
   B. Apologize and agree to change her diagnosis to adjustment disorder.
   C. Tell her she needs that diagnosis if she wants to receive hormones.
   D. Discuss the diagnosis with the patient and explain the meaning of gender dysphoria as a reaction to physical self and assigned gender role.

5. What is the genetic explanation for gender diversity?

   A. Gene diversity such as XXY and XYY creates gender diversity.
   B. There is no clear genetic reason for the existence of cis or trans people.
   C. Hormonal changes in utero explain gender diversity.
   D. The brains of gender diverse people are different.

ANSWERS

1. **The correct response is option C.**

   Diagnoses corresponding to gender first appeared in DSM-III.

2. **The correct response is option A.**

   There is no evidence for gender dysphoria in Aron, but there is clear evidence of major depressive disorder. People who are suicidal and TGNC are typically overdiagnosed as having borderline personality disorder.

3. **The correct response is option B.**

   Evan has not expressed symptoms of gender dysphoria, but he does report clear symptoms of panic and would like treatment for his panic attacks. Having a drag persona is part of the diversity of gender expression and is not necessarily the same as gender dysphoria.

4. **The correct response is option D.**

   Sue needs to be provided psychoeducation about what gender dysphoria is. She might be thinking that your diagnosis means she is mentally ill because her gender identity and sex assigned at birth do not line up. Reassure her that you respect her gender identity and explain to her why the diagnosis is being used.

5. **The correct response is option B.**

   Although there are small findings, the research into why gender diversity exists, as well as why cis gender people exist, is limited, and much more study is needed.

REFERENCES

Adams J, Dickinson P, Asiasiga L: Mental health promotion for gay, lesbian, bisexual, transgender and intersex New Zealanders. J Prim Health Care 5(2):105–113, 2013 23748391

American Psychiatric Association: Diagnostic and Statistical Manual of Mental Disorders, 3rd Edition. Arlington, VA, American Psychiatric Association, 1980

American Psychiatric Association: Diagnostic and Statistical Manual of Mental Disorders, 5th Edition. Arlington, VA, American Psychiatric Association, 2013

Blackless M, Charuvastra A, Derryck A, et al: How sexually dimorphic are we? Review and synthesis. Am J Hum Biol 12(2):151–166, 2000 11534012

Blanchard R: The concept of autogynephilia and the typology of male gender dysphoria. J Nerv Ment Dis 177(10):616–623, 1989 2794988

Drescher J: An interview with Robert L. Spitzer, MD. J Gay Lesbian Psychother 7(3):97–111, 2003

Drescher J: Queer diagnoses: parallels and contrasts in the history of homosexuality, gender variance, and the diagnostic and statistical manual. Arch Sex Behav 39(2):427–460, 2010 19838785

Drescher J, Cohen-Kettenis P, Winter S: Minding the body: situating gender identity diagnoses in the ICD-11. Int Rev Psychiatry 24(6):568–577, 2012 23244612

Erickson-Schroth L: Update on the biology of transgender identity. J Gay Lesbian Ment Health 17(2):150–174, 2013

Furnham A, Sen R: Lay theories of gender identity disorder. J Homosex 60(10):1434–1449, 2013 24059967

Group for the Advancement of Psychiatry, LGBT Issues Committee: LGBT Mental Health Syllabus, 2015. Available at: www.aglp.org/gap/6_transgender. Accessed April 29, 2017.

Hooker E: The adjustment of the male overt homosexual. J Proj Tech 21(1):18–31, 1957 13417147

Reed GM, Drescher J, Krueger RB, et al: Disorders related to sexuality and gender identity in the ICD-11: revising the ICD-10 classification based on current scientific evidence, best clinical practices, and human rights considerations. World Psychiatry 15(3):205–221, 2016 27717275

Spitzer RL: The diagnostic status of homosexuality in DSM-III: a reformulation of the issues. Am J Psychiatry 138(2):210–215, 1981, 7457641

8

GENDER-AFFIRMING MENTAL HEALTH

Sometimes we get so focused on the body, we forget that health also encompasses the mind, our emotions, and our mental health.

Thomas Sasso

GENDER-AFFIRMING mental health care begins with therapists learning to be competent providers for transgender and gender-nonconforming (TGNC) patients. The sections in this chapter provide a basic overview of major topics within the realm of TGNC health care, and your familiarity with these topics will form the groundwork for providing TGNC-competent care. In general, therapists do not have insight into the lives of their patients before the first session starts, and the experience of therapist and patient processing the patient's life experience is what informs the therapist of the intimate details of who the patient is and what is important to them. Although the same can be applied to TGNC people, the majority of mental health professionals are in a disadvantaged starting place in processing patient experience because most of the population do not identify as gender diverse.

There is an accepted understanding among the general population about certain aspects of being male or female, and mental health professionals will use these cultural stereotypes to inform their treatment of TGNC patients. According to society, men and women are supposed to think a certain way, behave in certain patterns, and want certain things. Historically speaking, when the American Psychiatric Association removed homosexuality from the *Diagnostic and Statistical Manual of Mental Disorders* and acknowledged diverse sexual orientations, traditional male-female dichotomies, along with gender stereotypes, started to blur. Now that gender diverse people are better represented in the mainstream, all gender stereotypes are being brought into question. In the past, the mental health professional could make some basic assumptions based on the patient's gender identity describing ways in which he or she might view the world. A TGNC person largely removes these assumptions, and the situation leaves the mental health clinician in uncharted territory without direction.

Nancy McWilliams, arguably one of the world's preeminent psychoanalytic psychotherapists once said,

> One frequently heard analogy for the role of the analytic therapist, a role that claims authority about process, but uncertainty about content, is that of the trail blazer or travel guide. If one is walking through an alien jungle, one needs to be with someone who knows how to traverse that terrain without running into danger or going in circles. But the guide does not need to know where the two parties will emerge from the wilderness; he or she (or they) has only the means to make the journey safe. (McWilliams 2011, p. 31)

Although the majority of therapy done with patients who are TGNC is not psychoanalytic in nature, this quotation provides a good example of why a TGNC-competent therapist is needed when working with TGNC people. So many aspects of TGNC care are TGNC specific.

TGNC people have higher rates of depression, anxiety, substance abuse, HIV, trauma, and suicide (Bockting et al. 2013; Brown and Jones 2016; Budge et al. 2013; Mustanski et al. 2016). In my opinion, this is largely due to the effects of growing up gender diverse in a cisgender world. If the world were more open to gender diversity, rates of mental illness among the TGNC population would likely mimic those of cisgender people. The experience of being gender diverse creates thoughts, emotions, and experiences that are not familiar to most mental health professionals, and being familiar with gender diverse experiences is crucial if you plan to engage and work with TGNC patients (Sevelius et al. 2014; Zelle and Arms 2015).

Case Example

Marisol is a 44-year-old woman of trans experience. She came to an urban outpatient clinic for treatment of severe treatment-resistant schizophrenia, disorganized type. Previously, she had worked for a number of years with several residents and therapists in training who provided her with mental health treatment aimed at reducing her symptoms of schizophrenia. Her past was difficult to assess because she is a poor historian, but she had developed tardive dyskinesia (a movement disorder typically caused by antipsychotic medication), signaling a long history of medication management. She appeared in traditionally female attire with long hair and makeup and was very disorganized, with dirty, unkempt clothing and poor grooming, which led the clinicians to assess her as a low-functioning patient with treatment-resistant chronic and persistent mental illness. Marisol spent most of her time trying to organize her day, and getting from her home to the clinic or to her rehabilitation job required excessive mental energy.

Marisol's gender identity was never a main focus of treatment. She had already changed her identification cards to match her name and gender marker, and she was called by her appropriate name and pronoun throughout the clinic. Gender-related aspects of her treatment, such as availability of hormones or surgical options, were not brought up because clinicians were focused on treating her psychotic symptoms. She never brought up gender-affirming treatments, but over time it became clear that she didn't know they were options available to her.

Marisol was placed on a regimen of an injectable antipsychotic medication and was stabilized with continued medication treatment and supportive psychotherapy. She remained very symptomatic but largely stable. Eventually, one of the trainee clinicians, who had become informed about TGNC-affirming treatments, had a discussion with Marisol about her gender identity along with all the options available to her, such as hormone treatment and gender-affirming surgical procedures. Further psychotherapy would target her views of her gender and what steps she would like to take, if any, to align her body and mind.

It became evident that Marisol had been having continued symptoms of gender dysphoria, but they were being ignored because of her diagnosis of schizophrenia. One way that gender dysphoria manifested itself occurred during visits to her parents. They were not accepting of her gender identity, and when they saw her, they would convince her to cut her hair and wear male-identified clothing. The treatment team always knew when Marisol had visited her family because of the clothing and haircut. She would be severely depressed following these visits, which typically happened about two times per year.

Once Marisol was connected with gender-affirming care, she started receiving hormones and was given information about surgical procedures. She remained quite ill with regard to her psychotic symptoms, but she was stable overall and understood the risks and benefits of her medicinal treatment. With the help of her clinicians, she was able to understand what options were available to her and which options would be right for her and her body. Therapy also targeted her relationship with her family members, and she learned how she could best protect herself and prevent depressive symptoms when she decided to see her family in the future.

STARTING TREATMENT

For a clinic to be more TGNC friendly, trans-affirming treatment will need to continue during all mental health sessions. Whether you are a psychiatrist, psychologist, social worker, case manager, or other mental health professional, your initial evaluation will communicate to the TGNC patient your level of knowledge of and competence and comfort with TGNC concerns. In the case above, Marisol was lucky in some ways. She had already changed her name and her gender marker on her identification and insurance card. The staff referred to her as female and by her chosen name. Her going through the process of changing her name and identification without the help of case management was pretty extraordinary considering her level of disorganization.

Despite not being in a trans-affirming clinic, Marisol ultimately connected with trans-affirming clinicians. Although they didn't focus on medicinal and surgical treatments available to her, they respected her gender identity and name, which is the bedrock to starting TGNC care. It is crucial that all TGNC patients are addressed by their correct name and pronoun. The means necessary to document these items in a patient chart will depend on the type of record being used. Most medical records don't have the sophistication for gender diversity, and most clinicians will need to create work-arounds (see Chapter 4, "Establishing a TGNC-Friendly Clinic").

MIND OVER BODY?

TGNC people want both to be treated like other patients and to have their particular and unique needs met by their providers. As a general rule, the mental health clinician should start the evaluation process just as they would any other evaluation. Unless the patient starts with gender dysphoria as the chief complaint, a review of systems, gender identity, and sexual orientation can come later in the interview. These first moments of an interview are your opportunity to convey your comfort with and knowledge of TGNC care. The patient needs to feel at ease with you, and if you start asking questions about gender identity from the start, you could create a situation where the patient feels their gender is being tokenized.

Attend to the chief complaint and the general evaluation first. Focus on the patient's symptoms as well as past psychiatric history, family history, substance history, medical history, and social history. Once the social history is brought up, information about gender identity should naturally flow. Sadly, many TGNC people become estranged from their biological families early in life. They are exposed to violence, assault, and substances and experience suicidal ideation more than their cis counterparts. When taking a chronological history, document when gender dysphoric symptoms started to appear. Some patients may respond well to validating statements that convey both empathy and knowledge about TGNC concerns: "When did you discover your gender identity?" "At what point did you realize you were female?" For many who have grown up in places isolated from gender diversity, it may take years to put together all the pieces and to understand the basis of many of their symptoms. For this reason, people may come out as transgender or gender nonconforming at any point in their life.

The mistake many clinicians make when working with TGNC people is focusing on the body and not the mind. Gender is not present in the body; it rests within the mind. Starting off with questions about the body conveys the wrong intention and could make your patient uncomfortable. Conduct your evaluation as you would any other, but focus on gender and sexuality when they come up naturally during the interview. You'll find that getting in the habit of asking how people identify regarding their gender and sexual orientation will quickly become easy, and you might discover things about your patients—cis or transgender—you wouldn't have known otherwise. Remember that all types of medicinal and surgical treatments are available as options to patients, but some patients may not think or feel these treatments are right for their body.

INDIVIDUAL THERAPY AND IMPARTIALITY

How individual therapy is conducted with a TGNC person will largely depend on the patient's presenting problem. Gender will be the lens through which you view the symptoms. Whether the underlying condition is a mood disorder, psychosis, anxiety concerns, or a mild adjustment disorder, when those same symptoms arise from the evaluation of a person who is also TGNC, they should be treated just as symptoms that arise from any other evaluation.

You will find that the many TGNC patient histories laden with trauma, transphobia, and adversity will be paired with strength, resilience, and hope. Therapy should be particularly nonjudgmental, gender affirming, and empathic in nature. TGNC people don't have many others who are supportive of their gender diversity, and this is your chance to be that one person who hears them and understands them.

Maintain a stance that gender and sexual orientation remain on a spectrum and are also fluid. When discussing gender-affirming treatments, reassure patients who are ambivalent about change that this is a normal part of a transition process and there is no one way or right direction. Each individual should proceed at whatever pace is most comfortable for them. The mental health professional is there not to police the patient's gender but to increase understanding of it, by both the patient and the therapist (Drescher 2015; Silverman 2015).

Case Example

Justine is a 36-year-old woman of trans experience. She suffered for years from major depression and alcohol abuse secondary to having to hide her true identity. She got married and had children and spent years in therapy trying to treat symptoms of depression that were a response to her attempts to cover up her gender identity.

Justine works as a lawyer at a very conservative firm. The other partners would be very uncomfortable if she decided to transition at work, and she had concerns about what would happen to her job. Her family is somewhat supportive, but they don't understand what it means to be transgender. Justine's sons have had a hard time with the transition and have reacted with behavioral problems at school.

Justine is in individual therapy and is coming to terms with her own sense of self as well as her gender identity. Her therapist is providing an open space for her to explore ideas about herself that align with her true self. In addition to exploring her own sense of identity, Justine and her therapist are working on the outside social stressors in her life and how to manage them. Her wife and sons are part of that stress, asking Justine to explain gender identity and transition to them just as she is starting to discover their meaning for herself. Playing this role has created ambivalence and confusion for her. She wants to maintain a relationship with her wife and sons but needs to do so as Justine and not as the man she had appeared to be.

In addition to her family stress life, her work stress life causes her more anxiety. Although she is not tied to her job permanently, she has a good position and salary after having worked at her firm for many years. Coming out would almost certainly jeopardize that position. Although Justine has accrued some savings, she is worried about providing for her family and ultimately sending her sons to college.

Justine goes back and forth in her therapy sessions. Some days she is ready to move forward with outing herself at work. Other days she goes back in the closet and says that the decision to finally transition would be too damaging on her family and work life. She sometimes thinks she would rather suffer alone than cause pain to others. Reaching a point of being halfway out of the closet, presenting as female in her personal life and male in her work life, has been discussed as an option, but Justine feels the need to make an ultimate decision regarding her gender presentation.

The role of the therapist in Justine's case is not to encourage transition. The role is to help Justine identify what it is she wants out of life and understand the possible effects of her decisions. The therapist should remain nonpartial in moments like these and should not push Justine out of the transgender closet in any way. The patient needs to understand that there are risks and benefits to transitioning and risks and benefits to not transitioning, and the therapist's task is to help the patient tolerate the anxiety that unfolds as she struggles with these choices. No matter how long it takes. Justine's decisions going forward, whatever they may be, are going to be difficult decisions that are likely to have consequences. Although Justine may think it's easier for her to suppress her gender feelings and not go forward with any kind of transition, she should be reminded of the psychological toil it has taken on her in the past. She has every right to continue this path, but she should fully explore the implications of whatever choices she makes.

When working with patients who are TGNC, continue to filter your interventions through a gender diverse lens. You may be using psychodynamic, cognitive, behavioral, or other forms of therapy, but whatever the modality, patients' experience and recovery will be affected by their TGNC identity. There should always be room in the therapy session to discuss TGNC-specific concerns and how they are relating to treatment and recovery. It is up to the clinician to maintain support while remaining largely neutral. However, it is perfectly acceptable to bring up topics regarding TGNC culture of which the patient may not be aware. Some patients are not clear on what services are available to them and how their bodies can change as a result of these interventions. As a TGNC-competent mental health professional, you should provide both treatment options and acceptance of your patient simultaneously.

THE PRESCRIBER AND THE GATE KEEPER

Psychiatrists and other mental health prescribers still have a long way to go to repair the damage caused by our predecessors, who stigmatized and overmedicated TGNC people in order to "cure" them. The practice of conversion therapy, which uses various techniques to change an individual's sexual orientation, has been banned by multiple mental health organizations (including the American Psychiatric Association, the American Psychological Association, the Pan American Health Organization and World Health Organization, and the Royal College of Psychiatrists) and is largely believed to be dangerous and unethical. Similarly, there is advocacy to ban similar practices designed to change a person's gender identity.

Depending on insurance requirements, clinicians may need to diagnose patients with gender dysphoria in order for them to be eligible for insurance reimbursement for some treatments. A conversation with patients regarding why this diagnosis is necessary will be crucial when developing rapport. Patients should understand from the start of treatment that our goal will never be to convert them to being cis, but we will provide therapeutic and medicinal interventions that can help ease symptoms and clear a pathway for patients to discover their true selves as they envision them.

Prescribing psychoactive substances requires a basic knowledge of hormones and TGNC culture. Some medications may affect psychiatric treatments that use hormones. One clear example is that of spironolactone, which blocks testosterone but also functions as a diuretic. In addition, patients taking spironolactone and lithium might find a decreased need for lithium because of the potential of spironolactone to increase lithium levels in the body. Many of the psychiatric medications do not interact with hormones and taking them together is quite safe, so psychiatrists should not be afraid of treating psychiatric symptoms while a patient is receiving hormone treatment. However, it is important for prescribers who are new to the TGNC field to remain vigilant of potential interactions.

Case Example

Yvette is a 22-year-old woman of trans experience. She recently was connected to psychiatric care and is seeing a primary care doctor who is providing her with estrogen and spironolactone. She has been taking estrogen for only 3 months and is starting to report increased symptoms of mood lability. She reports that she is multitasking more than usual, but things seem to affect her more intensely than before. She is having some crying spells. Despite this, she has no other major symptoms of depression and denies lack of energy, anhedonia, or suicidal ideation. Her psychiatrist discusses the possibility of an antidepressant, but Yvette says that she would like to avoid additional medication and thinks her mood changes might be a reflection of the changes happening with estrogen. Yvette goes to a support group, where she hears about other people's experiences with estrogen over time, and some of the members of the support group note that her experience is rather common.

Mental health professionals who work with patients receiving hormone therapy will, over time, become comfortable with the typical changes that can take place. There are many anecdotal reports of changes to mood symptoms when patients take estrogen, progesterone, or testosterone. These mood changes are rarely dangerous. They are generally not pathological but rather are more stereotypical of what hormones do in cisgender people. Some studies report protective factors with initiating hormones, such as decreased psychotic symptoms (Dhillon et al. 2011). Yvette noticed a positive change in her mood after starting estrogen. She felt mere emotions, which seemed more natural to her. It would not be surprising for someone with previously cis male levels of estrogen in their system to start experiencing increased emotional range after months of estrogen treatment. Be careful not to overpathologize small behavioral and emotional changes. These may be normal results of the hormone treatment process. For details about hormones, see Chapter 14, "Transmasculine Hormones," and Chapter 15, "Transfeminine Hormones."

GROUP THERAPY

Group therapy can be crucial to the development of a patient's gender identity as a TGNC person. Participating in a support group that is specific to the experiences of a trans woman, trans man, or gender-nonconforming person accomplishes several things. First, the patient will be in a room with others who have had a similar, although definitely not the same, life experience.

This shared experience will provide fertile ground for facilitating delicate issues that might take longer to reach in individual psychotherapy. Knowing that other people in the group may have similar questions, fears, and shame can bond group members and encourage sharing of a collective narrative. A group leader will facilitate the cohesion of the group, allowing group members to process each of their experiences. Learning about others who may be like them will dissipate uncertainty and isolation, and hearing about different life perspectives will give each group member further options about the different ways TGNC persons can express themselves.

MENTAL HEALTH RESOURCES

When working with TGNC people, consider all community support options as avenues to care. In addition to providing individual or group treatment, part of TGNC-affirming therapy involves connecting patients to outside resources that may further support them. Most large urban settings have an LGBTQ center, and these centers typically have support groups. These support groups can be generally focused on all queer people or individually focused on subgroups such as trans men or trans women.

For patients dealing with substance abuse concerns, there are LGBTQ-specific Alcoholics Anonymous (AA), Crystal Meth Anonymous (CMA), and Narcotics Anonymous (NA) meetings. Many LGBTQ people might find it easier to attend meetings with others of a similar background and identity, although these meetings may not be completely free from harassment.

INTERNALIZED TRANSPHOBIA

Growing up gender diverse in a largely cisgender world is very difficult. From a young age, we are bombarded with gender stereotypes, and those who fall outside of a typical gender presentation are ridiculed, bullied, and even killed. Our culture has traditionally represented those who fall outside the classic gender dichotomy of male and female as odd, deviant, dangerous, or sometimes someone to be laughed at. TGNC people see these representations over time and internalize thoughts about themselves and the larger gender diverse community. Sometimes these thoughts are on the surface and are present in sessions and during treatment. Other times they can be buried, suppressed, or repressed, and echoes of them affect the person's work, relationships, and life. The internalizing of negative gender diverse views is called *internalized transphobia* (Levitt and Ippolito 2014). Internalized transphobia is present in any person who has been exposed to negative gender diverse views or stereotypes—which includes most people—and should always be talked about in therapy sessions. Psychoeducation should be provided that internalized transphobia is a universal experience to some degree. Most people are afraid to speak about these internalized views because they are ashamed that they are having them. However, these views should be normalized because it is impossible not to internalize some of those thoughts while being bombarded with negative representations. If not attended to, internalized transphobia can be serious and can even increase a person's risk of suicide (Perez-Brumer et al. 2015).

CIS COUNTERTRANSFERENCE

A pitfall many clinicians might run into when working with TGNC people is their countertransference toward gender diverse people. Cis and trans countertransference can occur with any mental health professional regardless of their gender identity. Clinicians should remain vigilant of their own feelings toward patients. Managing ambivalence, particularly around gender, can be difficult. Even the most well-meaning provider may be tempted to push patients who are more gender nonconforming toward the male or female poles of the gender spectrum. Whether or not TGNC patients are taking hormones or having a gender-affirming surgery says nothing about their progress and success in treatment. There is no "typical" TGNC case. Each person needs to be approached individually, and patients should be directing their treatment plan, informing the clinician on where they want to go in gender-affirming care.

For clinicians who are new to TGNC care, managing countertransference may mean that they are not the appropriate mental health professional for that particular patient. There are very skilled and experienced TGNC-competent clinicians who may not be appropriate fits for some patients. Knowing when a patient needs a form of treatment you can't provide and transferring the patient to another provider may be the best next step in care.

SPECIAL TOPICS

In this section, I discuss special topics that are pertinent to the TGNC population. It is reasonable to believe that topics generally arise not inherently because one is TGNC but from growing up and living gender diverse in a largely cisgender world. This list of topics is by no means exhaustive but suggests a general overview of themes that may present themselves during your work with TGNC individuals. Not all gender diverse people will have these experiences, but any TGNC patient you work with should be screened for the presence of them.

Suicide

Suicide attempts and completion are very common in the TGNC population. Some studies report that as many as 50% of TGNC people have attempted suicide in their lifetime (Hoshiai et al. 2010; Spicer 2010). Given the severity of this problem, all TGNC people should be screened for suicidal ideation. Those with suicidal thoughts need to be further screened for ways, means, and intent. Patients with a history of suicidal ideation or attempts in their past or their family's past should be screened regularly. A safety plan can be made with patients, identifying ways to decrease suicidal ideation as well as safe places for them to go when they feel in danger.

Substance Use

Substance use is present in larger numbers not only in the TGNC population but also the LGBTQ population in general. One reason for this, as mentioned previously, is the presence of internalized transphobia, which is common in our cisgender world. This internalized transphobia may lead to increased levels of anxiety and depression, which are commonly self-medicated by substances, particularly alcohol.

A second reason why substances may be present more often in the TGNC population is the presence of deep-rooted social traditions. Many LGBTQ people learn to socialize and meet others in their community through queer-oriented bars. These establishments provide a safe space for gender diverse people to meet others who are like them. It also provides an easy way for those who might be anxious about socializing or identifying with the TGNC community to have easy access to alcohol.

Whether someone might be self-medicating, socializing, or just having fun, substance use is intimately entwined in the queer community, and gender diverse people may frequently be in situations where substances are presented to them and given to them. For those in recovery, this can be particularly challenging because finding social outlets that also don't trigger a relapse can be difficult.

Violence

Violence is common within the TGNC community as well. Individuals who are TGNC are at risk of being the victim of hate crimes. As many as 10% of TGNC people have reported being attacked because of their gender status (James et al. 2016), and many TGNC-identified people die yearly simply because they are gender diverse. Given this knowledge, clinicians should be mindful of their patients and how they get to their sessions. Leaving their homes, depending on where gender diverse patients live, can mean risking their life. Taking public transportation can be dangerous if fellow commuters perceive a person as being transgender and are hostile toward them. Patients who miss frequent sessions should not necessarily be labeled as nonadherent and discharged from your services. Attempt to understand the barriers that are preventing them from reaching treatment. If those barriers include fears of being assaulted, these are realistic concerns, and social services should try to help facilitate safe ways for patients to get to treatment.

Domestic or intimate partner violence should not be ignored. Even TGNC patients who are in relationships with other TGNC people can experience intimate partner violence. Patients may feel ashamed or afraid to bring up this topic. Sometimes they are closely connected with the violent partner, and they are worried you will try to separate them. Making space in sessions to talk about violence, without threat of action on the part of the therapist, will help identify those patients who might be too afraid to broach the subject.

Shame

Shame is a common theme in the TGNC world. The gender diverse community is taught by society at large, including even some people within the LGBTQ community, that they are deviant and mentally unstable. TGNC people typically experience many symptoms of depression and anxiety, which only confirm their shame at being "crazy." It is the job of the clinician to provide accurate clinical information about the lives of those who are TGNC. It is common for TGNC people to experience symptoms of depression, anxiety, and other forms of mental illness, typically due to being in unsupportive environments. TGNC people are not inherently "crazy" any more than any other person. Although everyone's experience is unique, sometimes normalizing a person's narrative can help with feelings of shame and isolation.

Trauma

Trauma can be an underlying if not a major theme in the lives of many TGNC people. In addition to experiencing intimate partner violence and random attacks, as discussed in the previous subsections, many TGNC people come from families who don't understand them. These families can be more passive and show little or no interest in the gender identity of their child. They can also be outright hostile, subjecting any gender diverse young person to physical and even sexual abuse. TGNC people also deal with their families, friends, schools, churches, and other social institutions misgendering them and having a range of reactions from disconnecting with them to hostility because they are different. Any TGNC person seeking mental health care needs to be screened for symptoms of posttraumatic stress disorder. Some form of trauma is almost always present. It is better to discuss the long-lasting effects of trauma with TGNC patients and normalize their experience as being gender diverse in a largely cis-identified world.

Isolation

Of all the themes, isolation may be the one most commonly experienced within the TGNC population. Some TGNC people are lucky enough to find groups of others like themselves who can provide mirroring and emotional support. Many, however, are in places where few TGNC people live, and they may never come across anyone else who is gender diverse. This physical isolation creates emotional isolation. Therefore, it may be difficult for TGNC people to open up at the beginning of treatment. If patients are taught to hide their feelings and keep secrets about who they are, mental health clinicians will need to provide a lot of encouragement to undo those self-imposed rules. Not everyone enters mental health treatment ready to lie on a couch and free associate. Some people, especially those who are gender diverse, need encouragement to speak about sensitive topics for the first time and learn how they can express themselves free of ridicule or judgment in the office of an understanding mental health professional.

Resilience

Last, but not least, is a common positive theme associated with the TGNC community: resilience. Gender diverse people have many barriers and stigmas stacked against them. TGNC people learn to survive in a world that stigmatizes, discriminates, and even attacks them. Learning to survive as gender diverse in this world requires strength and resilience, which many TGNC people have. Being brave enough to be themselves and identify as their true gender is difficult and stressful, but your gender diverse patients will frequently be resourceful and capable in many ways.

SUMMARY

Working with TGNC people in a mental health setting requires the clinician to have some basic understanding of TGNC culture, treatment options, and specific needs. It is imperative for clinicians to treat the mental health symptoms that bring patients in for help, and all treatments should be conducted through the lens of gender diversity. Clinicians should maintain neutrality while applying their knowledge of medicinal and surgical interventions to provide treatment.

TGNC people deal with random attacks as well as intimate partner violence. They have high rates of suicide attempts and are at risk of substance abuse disorders as well as significant trauma. These high rates of mental health symptoms are most likely related to the way in which society views gender diversity and are not an inherent result of being TGNC.

With some preparation, the astute clinician can work with TGNC people. It is most important to have an open mind to the wide range of gender identities and learn to accept your patients for who they are and how they express themselves. All mental health professionals, both cisgender and trans identified, should be aware of their countertransference. Although it can sometimes be challenging to work within the world of TGNC people, it is intellectually stimulating and offers a superb opportunity to provide care to some of the individuals who have been most marginalized in society.

Key Points

- With training and supervision, most clinicians can provide individual and group treatment to TGNC people.
- Clinicians should be comfortable with gender diversity and fluidity and should have no expectations about what direction or how far patients may go in their transition.
- As mental health clinicians, we should be aware of how members of our specialties, particularly psychiatrists, have treated TGNC people in the past and do what we can to repair the relationship.
- Group therapy offers a valuable chance for TGNC people to meet and learn from others who share some of their life experiences.
- Suicide is common in the TGNC population, and patients should be regularly screened for safety.
- TGNC people are at risk of being attacked simply by leaving their home, which may make it difficult for them to get treatment.
- Consider intimate partner violence as well as a history of trauma in your clinical workup.

- Isolation remains a common theme among many of those who are gender diverse, and efforts to reduce patient isolation will help their overall mental health.

QUESTIONS

1. Leo is a 24-year-old man of trans experience. He has been seeing you in therapy for the past 3 months. He has yet to start taking testosterone and is unsure if he wants to because of the potential negative effects. He has been identifying as Leo only to you while in therapy; the rest of the world knows him at Laura. He continues to be worried about what would happen in his relationships with his family and wider social circle if he were to come out as a trans man. He knows his family would likely disown him, and his coworkers would likely be unsupportive. How should you approach this in therapy?

    A. Tell Leo that he is not ready to come out of the closet, and, given what you know of his family, he should probably stay in.
    B. Advise Leo that now is the time, and he should tell everyone in his life that he is a trans man. It's the only way for him to move forward.
    C. Meet Leo where he is at. Explore the pros and cons to coming out and tell Leo he should come out only when he is ready to do so.
    D. Bring Leo's family in for treatment. He can tell them his gender identity with you in the room for support.

2. Leo is now 28 years old and ready to start testosterone. He decides that it is time for him to make this choice, and he understands the risks and benefits of testosterone and is excited about the masculinizing effects it will have on his body. Three months after starting testosterone, Leo comes to you reporting increased sexual experiences and what he describes as an "increased libido." He is happy with his sexual activities but is concerned about how much he is thinking about sex. He has no problems with insomnia, pressured speech, racing thoughts, spending problems, or grandiosity. What should you say?

    A. Increased libido is a common effect of testosterone. Counsel him about what to expect while taking testosterone.
    B. He could be experiencing acute mania. Have him taken to the emergency room.

C. You've uncovered a sexual fetish. Ask more questions.
D. Advise him to decrease testosterone. The dose is probably too high.

3. Rebecca is a 31-year-old woman of trans experience. She is being treated for panic attacks and mild depressive symptoms. Her therapy with you is going well, but she remains afraid of leaving the house on occasion and misses therapy sessions. She sees on television other trans women being murdered and is worried this will happen to her. What should you tell her?

   A. Tell her that if she doesn't make at least three sessions out of each month you will discharge her from your services.
   B. Explain to her that she needs to see you every week in order to receive treatment.
   C. Increase her dose of benzodiazepines.
   D. Validate her concerns and explore ways she can get to treatment in a safe way.

4. Timmie is a 24-year-old man of trans experience. He is coming to see you to get a letter for top surgery. During the evaluation, you discover that Timmie is having multiple depressive symptoms and reports suicidal ideation. He has attempted suicide in the past by overdose and cutting his wrists and has an aunt who completed suicide. When asked more about his suicidal thoughts, Timmie says that he is unhappy with his body and once he has top surgery, those suicidal thoughts will go away. What should you do?

   A. Deny the letter for top surgery. Call 911 and have Timmie hospitalized.
   B. Do a suicide assessment and evaluate for treatment of depression. Timmie may still qualify for surgery, but he needs to understand that it might not cure his depressive symptoms.
   C. Provide the letter for top surgery. Timmie will probably get better afterward.
   D. Tell Timmie that you won't be able to evaluate him for top surgery until his symptoms of depression are under control. He will need to start medication first.

5. Chris is a 44-year-old gender-nonconforming person who comes to you for the first time for evaluation and treatment. Chris wants to restart testosterone, which he has taken in the past. During the course of the

evaluation, you note that Chris has auditory hallucinations that are fairly severe in nature. He also has strong paranoia that a chip has been implanted deep in his brain and that this chip is causing the hallucinations. Chris is homeless and has no access to food. He tells you testosterone is the most important thing to him right now. What steps should you take?

A. Evaluate and treat the psychotic symptoms. Explain to Chris that testosterone is possible, but you need more information first.
B. Deny any testosterone. It can make the hallucinations worse.
C. Provide him with testosterone. He doesn't seem to want treatment for the hallucinations.
D. Refer him to inpatient psychiatry.

ANSWERS

1. **The correct response is option C.**

   Leo should come out of the closet only when he is ready to do so. Pushing him out of the closet will not be helpful, and bringing in his family for a session will likely only make matters worse.

2. **The correct response is option A.**

   The increased libido sounds like a classic effect of taking testosterone. Leo has no other manic symptoms and is likely having a typical experience of someone on testosterone.

3. **The correct response is option D.**

   Rebecca has every right to be afraid, and cutting her off from services because of this realistic fear doesn't seem like the best or even an ethical option. Work with social services to find a way for her to get in and see you in a safe way.

4. **The correct response is option B.**

   Timmie is having depressive symptoms that need to be treated, but they seem to have been around for some time. He still needs to be assessed for suicidal ideation with the creation of a safety plan. If his depression and suicidal ideation appear chronic in nature and he is stable, he may still qualify for surgery.

5. **The correct response is option A.**

    Chris has a chronic and persistent mental illness that needs to be treated. He wants testosterone and probably should have it, but you need to make sure he is safe regarding his symptoms, is in stable housing, and is getting nutrition. Providing testosterone may help build rapport so you can get him connected with other services.

REFERENCES

Bockting WO, Miner MH, Swinburne Romine RE, et al: Stigma, mental health, and resilience in an online sample of the US transgender population. Am J Public Health 103(5):943–951, 2013 23488522

Brown GR, Jones KT: Mental health and medical health disparities in 5135 transgender veterans receiving healthcare in the Veterans Health Administration: a case–control study. LGBT Health 3(2):122–131, 2016 26674598

Budge SL, Adelson JL, Howard KA: Anxiety and depression in transgender individuals: the roles of transition status, loss, social support, and coping. J Consult Clin Psychol 81(3):545–557, 2013 23398495

Dhillon R, Bastiampillai T, Krishnan S, et al: Transgender late onset psychosis: the role of sex hormones. Aust N Z J Psychiatry 45(7):595–595, 2011

Drescher J: Gender policing in the clinical setting: discussion of Sandra Silverman's "The Colonized Mind: Gender, Trauma and Mentalization." Psychoanal Dialogues 25(1):67–76, 2015

Hoshiai M, Matsumoto Y, Sato T, et al: Psychiatric comorbidity among patients with gender identity disorder. Psychiatry Clin Neurosci 64(5):514–519, 2010 20727112

James SE, Herman JL, Rankin S, Keisling M, et al: The Report of the 2015 U.S. Transgender Survey. Washington, DC, National Center for Transgender Equality, 2016

Levitt HM, Ippolito MR: Being transgender: the experience of transgender identity development. J Homosex 61(12):1727–1758, 2014 25089681

McWilliams N: Psychoanalytic Diagnosis. New York, Guilford, 2011

Mustanski B, Andrews R, Puckett JA: The effects of cumulative victimization on mental health among lesbian, gay, bisexual, and transgender adolescents and young adults. Am J Public Health 106(3):527–533, 2016 26794175

Perez-Brumer A, Hatzenbuehler ML, Oldenburg CE, Bockting W: Individual- and structural-level risk factors for suicide attempts among transgender adults. Behav Med 41(3):164–171, 2015 26287284

Sevelius JM, Patouhas E, Keatley JG, Johnson MO: Barriers and facilitators to engagement and retention in care among transgender women living with human immunodeficiency virus. Ann Behav Med 47(1):5–16, 2014 24317955

Silverman S: The colonized mind: gender, trauma, and mentalization. Psychoanal Dialogues 25(1):51–66, 2015

Spicer S: Healthcare needs of the transgender homeless population. J Gay Lesbian Ment Health 14(4):320–339, 2010

Zelle A, Arms T: Psychosocial effects of health disparities of lesbian, gay, bisexual, and transgender older adults. J Psychosoc Nurs Ment Health Serv 53(7):25–30, 2015 26151148

9

TRANSITIONS AND DETRANSITIONS

If I didn't define myself for myself, I would be crunched into other people's fantasies for me and eaten alive.

Audre Lorde

IN THIS CHAPTER, I provide two case presentations: one of a person who is transitioning and the other of a person who is detransitioning. Many well-meaning clinicians who start to work with transgender and gender-nonconforming (TGNC) people will make the mistake of thinking that transitioning is a one-direction process with a distinct beginning and end. This is not the case.

In the first half of the chapter, I focus on the process of transition. When individuals decide to transition, it can mean any number of things. It can mean they are socially transitioning from one gender to another. Their transition may also involve hormones or surgical procedures. A person may complete one or all of the available options without referring to the process as transitioning. Individuals who transition from one gender to another may not refer to themselves as transgender.

The process by which someone transitions and the actions it includes will be, like almost everything else, an individual journey that is unique to each person. The timetable by which people make decisions regarding their gender can be short or spread over many decades. The decision to start hormones may happen because a person wishes to change particular aspects of their body, but others may avoid hormone treatment out of concern about the potential medical side effects. Surgical interventions are also relatively new and can come with complications. Why people choose one option over another will depend on how they define themselves and what they want out of life. These desires can change over time as well and may shift to include or exclude aspects of gender-affirming treatments.

Working with gender-nonconforming people will only highlight the arbitrary nature of these choices. How people see themselves and the changes they want to happen with their body, if any, will be unique to each person, and the treatment we provide as mental health professionals should remain person centered. It is easy to get caught up in the idea that transitioning is a stepwise process that involves moving from one change to another until a transition from one gender to another is complete. However, the directions and choices people make in their transitions can be in any direction. TGNC people represent a spectrum of gender presentations that may move and shift over time, and the job of a mental health professional is to remain open and respect the choices made by patients and help ensure that transitioning is done in a supportive and safe way.

In the second half of the chapter, I examine a somewhat controversial topic within the TGNC community and among their health care providers: detransitioning. Detransitioning typically involves transitioning back to a previously identified gender, although this is not always the case. It may include cessation of hormones, reversals of surgical procedures, name changes, and changes in overall gender identity. Not everyone who detransitions regrets transitioning in the first place, and, like transitioning, the process of deciding to detransition is a very individual and personal choice. Detransitioning in itself does not necessarily imply that mistakes were made, although that is a possibility. It means that what was previously right for someone in their life may not be the best choice for them anymore.

The idea of detransitioning is so anxiety provoking for so many people because it brings to light the potential for ambivalence and even misdiagnosis. Some studies have reported that up to 2% of TGNC people will decide to detransition (Dhejne et al. 2014). For the most part, these individuals tend to be TGNC young adults who started the transition process just a few years earlier. As mental health providers advocating for access to care and gender-affirming procedures, it can be scary to think that the care we provide might be seen by both patients and society as harmful down the road. As the pendulum swings from restrictive access to care and toward more patient autonomy, the number of TGNC people who decide to detransition can be expected to increase, but it is reasonable to believe they will likely remain the rare minority of gender diverse cases that a mental health professional will see. Also, along a similar vein, it is not unreasonable to hypothesize that just as the ex-gay movement became heavily publicized in the late 1990s and an increasing number people attempted to change their sexual orientation, they produced an ex-ex-gay movement of people who reverted back to their original identity of being gay.

It must be restated that the majority of TGNC people who decide to transition are very happy with their choices and report an improved quality of life after transition (Ruppin and Pfäfflin 2015). However, the possibility that someone may detransition is an outcome that clinicians should be ready for when working with a gender diverse population. Gender is a spectrum, and it can be fluid. Mental health professions should be mindful to advocate for less restrictive access to care but also safe care. It has been very difficult for gender diverse people to get access to gender-affirming care, and many have spent their lives fighting for respect and the rights of TGNC people.

TRANSITIONS

The idea of becoming more masculine, feminine, or gender nonconforming is what most people think of as being associated with transitioning. However, as stated earlier, the concept of transitioning is more of an umbrella term that can mean any number of actions individuals take to move themselves on a gender diverse scale.

From a psychological perspective, people improve once they have started transitioning. Before people identify as TGNC, while they are still in the "gender closet," they can have any number of psychological difficulties. Those who are not yet fully aware of their gender diversity can display classic symptoms of personality pathology, including mood lability, impulsivity, suicidal ideation, and self-harm. This frequently leads to misdiagnosis of a personality disorder. The majority of people with psychiatric symptoms prior to starting gender-affirming services improve following initiation of treatment (Ruppin and Pfäfflin 2015). It is unclear if the generally high satisfaction rate is related to previous Standards of Care implemented by the World Professional Association for Transgender Health (WPATH).

Those who are in the early stages of transitioning can present with different symptoms and coping strategies than those of people who have been transitioning over a period of time (Budge et al. 2013). People who are at the start of transitioning or understanding their gender diversity typically show more immature ego defense mechanisms, which may explain the frequent misdiagnosis and pathologizing that can occur with clinicians inexperienced in working with TGNC people. Once patients are in more gender-supportive environments, these symptoms subside for the most part. The initiation of hormones has even been associated with a second adolescence (Roller et al. 2015). A second adolescence is described by some patients in many ways like puberty, as a time when they experience physical and mental changes as they are growing into their changing body.

Regarding hormones in particular, research has shown a significant positive association between the initiation of hormone treatment and improvement of psychological functioning (de Vries et al. 2011; Heylens et al. 2014). Even patients with previously diagnosed mood and anxiety disorders showed improvements from hormone treatment alone (White Hughto and Reisner 2016).

Puberty suppression, which arrests the changes caused by puberty, is a new type of treatment offered to adolescents. This treatment provides more time for adolescents to explore their gender diversity, prevents symptoms of gender dysphoria related to body changes, and gives adolescents and their parents time to make a plan for any gender-affirming treatment options that will be sought out down the road. It also provides time to see if further changes in gender identity will take place (de Vries and Cohen-Kettenis 2012). Just as the initiation of hormones reduces psychopathology, the initiation of puberty suppression treatment improves psychological functioning as well (Costa et al. 2015; de Vries et al. 2011; Edwards-Leeper and Spack 2012).

Case Example

Tamika is a 48-year-old woman of trans experience. She has had a long transition process and remains, as she defines it, "somewhere in the middle." Tamika was assigned male at birth but felt she was female around puberty. Because she lived in a somewhat rural region, she hid her gender identity for several years until she could move to a more accepting place.

Tamika wasn't able to move, but she was able to explore more supportive environments by working as a truck driver. While on the road, she could express her female identity to everyone she came in contact with. She grew her hair long and wore female attire, although she described herself as "somewhat butch." She didn't exactly align with a classic feminine presentation but was also uncomfortable with her male body parts. For many years, Tamika led two lives. She identified as female when she was on the road but identified as male when she was back in her rural hometown. At home, she put her hair under a ball cap and wore more masculine clothing. She was also mindful about how she walked and talked when around her biological family.

While on the road, Tamika found a clinic where she could stop every few weeks to get estrogen injections. She felt that estrogen helped her body and mind align more with her gender identity. She took estrogen for about 5–10 years until her family finally confronted her about her "nontraditional" lifestyle. They continued to call her Trevor and wanted to know why she was not married yet. Tamika finally told them about her gender identity around the age of 30. Her family was not accepting of this at all and said they would not have anything to do with her if she was living as a woman.

Tamika spent some time away from her family, but she managed to reconnect with them even though they were still not accepting of her gender identity. She continued to see a therapist at the clinic where she received estrogen and reached a place in her life where she wanted to get top surgery. Tamika was in a bit of a conundrum because she knew if she had breast augmentation she would be happier with her body, but her family would likely not want to speak to her again. Tamika had been dating another woman of trans experience in a town she frequently visited, and they had been speaking at length about Tamika and her postponing any surgical procedures out of fear of being alienated from her family. Although her girlfriend was understanding of her difficult position, she was frustrated with Tamika for not making a permanent decision regarding top surgery. Tamika's therapist found herself becoming frustrated with Tamika as well. Some weeks she was ready to get a surgical consultation, and other weeks she said the decision would be too difficult and she was better off not pursuing any changes. Her ambivalence went on for years.

Tamika's presentation and case are not atypical. She has had to make difficult decisions in her life, and she was in the unfortunate position of having to choose between being comfortable with her body and gender expression and having an ongoing relationship with her family.

When you are working with a patient who is in a place of ambivalence, like Tamika, there are several topics that you should cover in treatment. The first would be defining what gender means for the patient. What does it mean to be male or female? What would her life be like if Tamika's family was more supportive? What is the meaning of top surgery for her? Does Tamika want top surgery because it will help align her body with who she feels like inside? How does her desire to have top surgery relate to her relationship with her girlfriend?

Whether or not a woman of trans experience, or any TGNC person, has top surgery is a personal choice. As with Tamika, a person does not come out of the closet, start hormones, and then proceed to surgery. The steps Tamika has gone through have taken years and are not unidirectional. She has been living both as a woman and a man depending on her location. Her response to having to go out of and back into the gender closet would be valuable to cover in treatment. Examining her defense mechanisms and how she handles the stress of being invalidated by her family and hometown will provide important information and may give insight into how to support her in treatment.

It would be worth exploring if Tamika's family situation is set in stone. Her family has said many times they would basically disown her if she were to live life as a woman in their presence. Tamika has had to hide her gender identity from her family for many years, and it's worth exploring what kind of information and understanding they have about TGNC people. Tamika may be open to letting you conduct an information session with them or refer them for family interventions. Although Tamika's family situation may seem unlikely to change, attempting to work on this aspect of Tamika's stress may be fruitful. Although Tamika has established a family of choice with her girlfriend, it is worth attempting to provide support and education to her biological family if she is open to it.

For Tamika, you will ultimately want to explore what she wants out of life. If she could have it her way, what would she envision? Would she like to have both her girlfriend and family living in the same town? What would it be like to express her gender identity with her family and be the person she wants to be? Over time, Tamika likely created a false self that she has used to interact with her family for years. This false self works almost like another personality and is used by a TGNC individual like Tamika to create safety by presenting themselves to others as those others want them to be (Winnicott 1965). TGNC people can consciously create a false self to be used for protection or to maintain relationships with people who are not accepting of gender diversity. Or, as can be seen in Chapter 11, "Plurality," a false self can be unconscious. In Tamika's case, she was largely aware of her defenses and used her false self as a way to maintain a relationship with her family.

In the end, Tamika is a woman of trans experience with difficult decisions to make. She may decide to continue to live her life the way it is as long as there are no changes with her girlfriend or with her biological family. Whether or not she decides to have top surgery does not mean she is or is not taking a next step or "moving forward." There is no real direction forward. Your goal as a mental health professional is to provide Tamika with the support and empathy she needs in order to make decisions for herself and live the healthiest and most satisfying life she can.

DETRANSITIONS

Case Example

Miguel is a 55-year-old gender neutral person who was assigned male at birth and who uses masculine pronouns. He grew up in the Midwest and spent much of his life knowing he was born in a body he was uncomfortable with. Around the age of 22, after the death of his mother, he was able to move to a city that offered hormone treatment and became engaged in gender-affirming care. Miguel was very happy with the results and lived his life as Melissa from the age of 22 until 52. Miguel also suffered from depression, which got particularly worse after the death of his mother, and he saw a therapist and psychiatrist regularly for treatment. His symptoms were more dysthymic and were largely treatment resistant.

Around the age of 50, Miguel started to have worsening symptoms of depression, stopped working, and had to leave his apartment for a homeless shelter. Over time, he was placed in permanent mental health housing. In the mental health housing, he was surrounded by people who were not knowledgeable about TGNC people and he was quickly targeted by the other residents and harassed almost daily.

Miguel decided to detransition. He stopped taking hormones and asked to be called Miguel instead of Melissa. He cut his hair short and wore male-

> identified clothing. He had some breast tissue that had developed from the years of taking estrogen, but he didn't want to make any further changes to his body.
>
> When Miguel was asked why he detransitioned, he said that he really didn't want to talk about it. When pushed for more information, he said that he was finished with that part of his life and thinks living as a man is best for him at this time. He was unsure if he would one day again identify as female, but for now he preferred to be seen as a cis male.
>
> Prior to Miguel's detransition, several efforts were made to treat symptoms that might potentially lead to detransitioning. Medication adjustments, supportive therapy, and advocating for him to be moved to different housing were not helpful. Miguel said that he was able to tolerate his placement and that he was afraid being moved might put him in a worse position. Over the next several years, Miguel stared drawing, made more friends in the housing, and continued monthly visits with his mental health team. He still calls himself transgender, but he is clear that he wants to live the remaining part of his life as male identified.

Miguel's case can be alarming to providers because it gives the impression that something wasn't being done correctly. Much of his life before age 50 can be seen as somewhat typical for some people of trans experience. He was able to get access to the treatment he wanted and was happy with the results. If he were less depressed, would he identify as Melissa again? Should more aggressive treatment have been provided to help his depression? However, multiple medication changes and trials were tried with Miguel, with no success. He was adherent to treatment and didn't mind his team attempting to provide care for him. Perhaps he was having unprocessed complicated grief from the death of his mother? This is unlikely, however, because he had identified as female for approximately 30 years. Despite all these hypotheses, Miguel's overall level of functioning increased after he decided to detransition.

Miguel was somewhat insistent that he didn't want to move, and it's unclear what trajectory his life would have taken had he been placed in a public housing system for people identifying as lesbian, gay, bisexual, transgender, or queer/questioning. When asked about this, Miguel said he was not sure, but he probably would have detransitioned regardless because that is what he thinks is right for him at this time.

WHEN IS A PERSON TRANSGENDER?

Is Miguel still transgender? He still identifies as transgender. Even though the gender he identifies with and the sex he was assigned at birth align, he still associates himself with the TGNC community, given his life trajectory. Miguel stated that he planned to live life as a male. If someone transitions from male to female and back to male, does that make that person transgender? It depends on how the person identifies. Keep in mind that the identity of the person's gender and gender experience lies with the individual. It is not the provider's place to label someone as transgender or cisgender. There are no rules about when and why someone identifies or stops identifying as transgender. Respect patients' decisions and continue to provide quality care regardless of how they identify.

WAS MIGUEL EVER TRANSGENDER?

Some might hypothesize that Miguel identified as female after the death of his mother as a coping mechanism for dealing with her death. The occurrence of his mother's death and the start of hormone treatment did coincide, but Miguel identified as female from early in childhood. If anything, the death of his mother may have given him the ability to move to a place where he could get gender-affirming care. Whether or not Miguel says he was transgender in the past is also up to him. A clinician can certainly say that he once identified as transgender.

PREDICTING WHO MIGHT NOT RESPOND WELL

Some research has looked at identifying people who might not respond well to gender-affirming treatments such as hormones or surgery. However, this group of individuals is so small that it has been difficult to do quantitative research in understanding why they detransitioned (Landén et al. 1998). Pooling this research shows a typical detransition rate lower than 5%. It may not come as a surprise that what we do know about those who detransition involves levels of social support and acceptance. In general, TGNC people who lack family support or have no other TGNC people in their social circle are the ones who may detransition (Landén et al. 1998).

There have also been correlations with poor outcomes of gender-affirming procedures in association with body type and older age (Eldh et al. 1997). The concern in stating such findings is that this might prevent older individuals with a lack of social support from getting gender-affirming therapies. This should not be the case. What you should take from this is that there might be some red flags that will lead you to more exploration with patients who are seeking out medical and surgical transitions. When doing an evaluation for letters of support, mental health professionals need to identify areas where a TGNC person might get better care and outcomes. Having a firm social support structure, particularly with other TGNC-identified people, will only increase the chances of positive outcomes from gender-affirming interventions.

A CASE FOR TRAUMA AND COPING

Trauma does not make someone transgender. A transgender identity is not a pathological result of previous trauma. TGNC people, for the most part, find their transition to be a positive reflection of who they are. In the past, the TGNC population was stigmatized and pathologized for their gender variance. All things considered, there are rare cases of people who decide to detransition and may say that their transition was a mistake in the first place. They might also say that the transition was a coping mechanism to help them in some other part of their life. It's possible that a cis woman who has experienced sexual assault might want to transition to male in order to prevent future assaults. A young adult who loses a parent may decide to transition to identify with that parent. Young gender diverse people might find solace and comfort in a group of transgender-identified teenagers. These are extreme cases, but they are within the realm of possibility. In situations such as these, good clinical evaluations are needed, with collaboration and consultation with a team of trans-affirming providers.

It is difficult for clinicians who pride themselves on being gender affirming to question patients about transition during probably one of the most vulnerable moments of their life. The entire point of providing TGNC-affirming care is to not stigmatize, to not pathologize, and to provide access to care. In-depth evaluations will give clues to potential red flags. Is the patient persistent, consistent, and insistent about their gender identity? A good biopsychosocial history will reveal most of that information.

For the majority of your evaluations with TGNC people, the need for gender-affirming treatments will be clear. However, some patients may suffer from conditions such as active psychosis, dissociative disorders, or obsessive-compulsive disorders that might call for further observation and evaluation. It is often the case that individuals experiencing these symptoms will still be able to make decisions about their gender identity and transitions, but good clinical care would tease apart any potential maladaptive coping mechanisms that might be at the heart of their decision to transition or detransition. Also, be mindful that patients may be at higher risk of suicide during these times. Some may be juggling between detransitioning and ending their life. Frequent check-ins may be needed while a person is detransitioning.

When conducting additional evaluation, be prepared to be criticized both by patients and by colleagues for what could be seen as putting up barriers to care and even transphobic behavior. At the end of the day our goal as clinicians is to do no harm. If you explain to patients your thoughts and why you want to lengthen the evaluation phase, they are likely to understand if they hear that you are coming from a place of compassion and concern for their safety. Good clinical evaluations and sessions will address the ambivalence that exists with all people on some level. Patients should know that just because they are ambivalent about treatment, it doesn't mean they will lose access to gender-affirming services.

SUMMARY

Transitioning is an umbrella term that can refer to any number of gender diverse presentations, including hormone treatment and gender-affirming procedures. The process is not unidirectional and can go fast or slow. Some people consider themselves to be transitioning their whole life.

Detransitioning is a controversial topic that highlights ambivalence and makes both TGNC people and their providers uneasy. Just because some people choose to detransition, it does not mean they were never transgender or gender diverse. It also should not impair others who wish to transition from having access to care. The purpose of talking about detransitioning is to prepare mental health professionals who work with TGNC people to be open to all possible avenues of transition and care.

When patients come to you asking for help to detransition, conduct a thorough evaluation, understand what is happening in their life that has led them to that decision, and manage your own feelings and thoughts around the detransition. If someone needs to be in therapy before further action is taken or should even be started on medication to treat psychiatric symptoms, that should be a shared decision of the patient and the provider.

People may identify as transgender and decide to get no treatment. Others might define themselves as gender nonconforming and have hormones and multiple surgical interventions. There is no standard case. Patients need to be met where they are, and we as providers need to listen to what they are telling us.

Key Points

- Gender transitioning is not a one-way process, and no specific time limit can be attached.
- Gender-affirming treatments are not a list of steps for patients to complete in transitioning.
- TGNC expression falls on a spectrum. Transitioning is an umbrella term that encompasses a number of gender-affirming options.

- Detransitioning is rare but can happen.
- Just because a patient detransitions doesn't mean they no longer or never identified as transgender.
- The presence of ambivalence does not mean that gender-affirming therapies are not right for a person.
- Approach each case individually.

QUESTIONS

1. Kathleen is a 35-year-old woman of trans experience who has been seeing you for treatment of dysthymia. She has been on hormone treatment for the past 7 years and her insurance is now paying for gender-affirming surgeries. She asks when would be the right time for her to get top surgery. What should you say?

    A. She should get top surgery right away because she has been on hormones for so long.
    B. When she gets top surgery is a personal decision that is up to her. Explore the pros and cons.
    C. She must have been taking hormones for at least a year before she can have top surgery, and she has surpassed that requirement, having taken hormones for 7 years.
    D. Top surgery should be done when patients are in their 20s.

2. Xavier is a 23-year-old man of trans experience. He has been talking with you in therapy about the possibility of having a phalloplasty. He is worried about the operation and is scared he will have complications. It seems he has a good understanding of the risks and benefits. In the end, he asks you to write a letter of support for the procedure. Should you write the letter?

    A. Probably. Ambivalence doesn't disqualify someone for surgery. Xavier may need to explore his ambivalence more to make an informed decision.
    B. No. He needs to be absolutely certain before having the procedure.
    C. Yes. He is old enough to decide and understands the risks and benefits. No other evaluation should take place.
    D. No. He is not old enough for phalloplasty.

3. Tom is a 45-year-old man of trans experience who has been seeing you in treatment for panic attacks. He has been taking testosterone for 15 years and has decided to stop. He says he just doesn't feel like he needs it anymore but plans to continue to identify as male. Which statement regarding Tom is true?

   A. Anyone who stops gender-affirming treatments is no longer transgender.
   B. Tom needs to be evaluated for depression immediately.
   C. Whether or not Tom identifies as transgender is up to him.
   D. As long as Tom still identifies as male, he is still transgender.

4. Codi is a 19-year-old woman of trans experience. She was kicked out of her parents' home a year ago because of her gender identity. She had never identified as female until the age of 16, when she made a group of friends who were gender diverse. She started hormones without medical supervision on her own at age 18 years and seems to understand the risks and benefits of estrogen. She now would like to be prescribed estrogen. Should she be given hormone treatment?

   A. No. She probably is relating to her friends and is not really transgender.
   B. No. It's unclear if she meets criteria for gender dysphoria.
   C. Yes. She is of age and can start hormone treatment as long as she understands the risks and benefits.
   D. Yes, although further evaluation may be needed.

5. Maureen is a 49-year-old woman of trans experience. She had top surgery about 5 years ago but has not had vaginoplasty. She has been taking estrogen for 20 years. For the past 3 years, she has been in individual therapy with you and has been asking about living life as a man again. She is thinking about detransitioning because it feels like it is right for her at this time. She is not suffering from any psychiatric symptoms and appears to be at baseline. What should be your response?

   A. Maureen might be suffering from an undiagnosed mental illness that is causing her to want to detransition.
   B. Gender is a spectrum on which people can shift back and forth. Explore all the possibilities with Maureen and provide support around discovering what is best for her.
   C. She can detransition but must identify as a male to do so.
   D. Have her hormone levels checked for insufficient quantities.

ANSWERS

1. **The correct response is option B.**

   There is no definite timeline or best time to have gender-affirming treatments, if at all. When and if to have surgical procedures is an individual's decision as long as they understand the risks and benefits of care.

2. **The correct response is option A.**

   A phalloplasty is a complicated procedure, and Xavier is right to be concerned about complications. He seems to meet criteria for a letter, but given his ambivalence, a few more sessions dedicated to exploring the pros and cons may help him.

3. **The correct response is option C.**

   Just because a person is taking hormones or having surgery does not mean they are or are not transgender. The identity of being transgender resides within the individual.

4. **The correct response is option D.**

   Codi meets criteria for hormone treatment; she understands the risks and benefits of treatment and is an adult. However, although there is no "typical" TGNC presentation, Codi's story does raise some cause for concern. Given her age and her quickness to identify as a woman of trans experience, it may be wise to do a few more sessions to explore the long-term effects of hormones and make sure Codi understands which changes are reversible and which are not. If she insists on having hormones, she meets criteria and should have access to them.

5. **The correct response is option B.**

   Although this is not a typical case, Maureen has every right to decide if and when she wants to continue hormones. The ultimate goal of any mental health care professional is to provide safe and supportive care to patients. Maureen would benefit from further exploration as to why she is detransitioning, but the choice is ultimately up to her.

REFERENCES

Budge SL, Adelson JL, Howard KA: Anxiety and depression in transgender individuals: the roles of transition status, loss, social support, and coping. J Consult Clin Psychol 81(3):545–557, 2013 23398495

Costa R, Dunsford M, Skagerberg E, et al: Psychological support, puberty suppression, and psychosocial functioning in adolescents with gender dysphoria. J Sex Med 12(11):2206–2214, 2015 26556015

de Vries AL, Cohen-Kettenis PT: Clinical management of gender dysphoria in children and adolescents: the Dutch approach. J Homosex 59(3):301–320, 2012 22455322

de Vries AL, Steensma TD, Doreleijers TA, Cohen-Kettenis PT: Puberty suppression in adolescents with gender identity disorder: a prospective follow-up study. J Sex Med 8(8):2276–2283, 2011 20646177

Dhejne C, Öberg K, Arver S, Landén M: An analysis of all applications for sex reassignment surgery in Sweden, 1960–2010: prevalence, incidence, and regrets. Arch Sex Behav 43(8):1535–1545, 2014 24872188

Edwards-Leeper L, Spack NP: Psychological evaluation and medical treatment of transgender youth in an interdisciplinary "Gender Management Service" (GeMS) in a major pediatric center. J Homosex 59(3):321–336, 2012 22455323

Eldh J, Berg A, Gustafsson M: Long-term follow up after sex reassignment surgery. Scand J Plast Reconstr Surg Hand Surg 31(1):39–45, 1997 9075286

Heylens G, Verroken C, De Cock S, et al: Effects of different steps in gender reassignment therapy on psychopathology: a prospective study of persons with a gender identity disorder. J Sex Med 11(1):119–126, 2014 24344788

Landén M, Wålinder J, Hambert G, Lundström B: Factors predictive of regret in sex reassignment. Acta Psychiatr Scand 97(4):284–289, 1998 9570489

Roller CG, Sedlak C, Draucker CB: Navigating the system: how transgender individuals engage in health care services. J Nurs Scholarsh 47(5):417–424, 2015 26243380

Ruppin U, Pfäfflin F: Long-term follow-up of adults with gender identity disorder. Arch Sex Behav 44(5):1321–1329, 2015 25690443

White Hughto JM, Reisner SL: A systematic review of the effects of hormone therapy on psychological functioning and quality of life in transgender individuals. Transgend Health 1(1):21–31, 2016 27595141

Winnicott DW: Ego distortion in terms of true and false self, in The Maturational Processes and the Facilitating Environment. New York, International Universities Press, 1965, pp 140–152

10

FAMILIES

> The bond that links your true family is not one of blood, but of respect and joy in each other's life.
>
> *Richard Bach*

THE WORD *FAMILY* can mean a host of different things, especially within the lesbian, gay, bisexual, transgender, and queer/questioning (LGBTQ) community. Although many people define family by blood relation, others may refer to a close collective social structure as their family. In this chapter, the word family could refer to a biological family, but it can just as likely refer to the social network that transgender and gender-nonconforming (TGNC) people create from the supportive group of friends they have in their life.

Working with families and couples is a regular part of the practice for many mental health professionals. Whether it be formal treatment targeting the family structure or supportive psychoeducational sessions regarding a family member in particular, mental health professionals need to be prepared to speak with family members about gender identity.

The practice of working with families can be particularly challenging. The main reason it is challenging is that with each additional person involved in a patient's care, there are more opinions, feelings, thoughts, and questions. Discussing a diagnosis such as major depression or schizophrenia can be difficult, with modern time constraints limiting both the length and frequency of sessions. Balancing time spent alone with the patient and time spent with the family can be complicated. Parents who might be paying for a child to receive services may demand time on their own with the provider. Maintaining an alliance with both the patient and all family members involved can be impossible at times, and mental health professionals might feel the familiar sensation that they are providing care to each and every person involved rather than just the patient. Maintaining boundaries while remaining aligned with all parties included is a skill that takes time and experience to acquire.

There is a host of information available through books, online resources, and face-to-face support groups and information sessions when families have questions about a family member's mental illness or treatment. The National Alliance of the Mentally Ill (NAMI) offers a plethora of support for both those suffering from a mental illness and their family members.

TGNC people bring a different perspective to family work. First, being gender diverse is not a mental illness. Although gender dysphoria is included in DSM-5 (American Psychiatric Association 2013), it is not labeled as a disorder. The problem this poses for families is confusion about nomenclature and where to find resources when the primary provider is unavailable. Although there are many resources providing information about TGNC individuals, there are also misinformation and opinions that are not based on research or anecdotal clinical evidence. Some family members may want to identify their loved one's gender diversity as "crazy." If family members want to find information to support their beliefs about TGNC people, they will. Referring family members to appropriate sources, such as the World Professional Association for Transgender Health (WPATH), even through a handout provided to the patient, can help rectify some common misconceptions. However, there may still be family members unwilling to accept that gender is a spectrum and that TGNC people should be respected for who they are.

FAMILIES OF CHOICE

A family of choice is exactly what it sounds like. It is a chosen family identified through attachment, support, and emotional connection rather than genetics. Unfortunately, many people in the LGBTQ world are estranged from their genetic families. Whether it be for religious reasons or because of individual bias, LGBTQ people are frequently abandoned at all ages by their biological families. It astounds many mental health professionals that family members can reject a loved one simply for having a diverse gender identity or sexual orientation. Many who work with the TGNC community will sadly notice a general lack of family involvement.

When TGNC people are rejected by their genetic family, and even sometimes when they aren't, they will form attachments to individuals in the community who offer the emotional and even financial support that their families do not. These attachments can be to other TGNC people, to people who are part of the larger queer community, or to those who seem to understand the TGNC community through previous relationships, experience, or education.

Families of choice should be identified to the mental health provider by the patients themselves. Once identified, they should be treated in the same way as any genetic family member. With the patient's permission, you can take calls from, answer questions by, and have joint sessions with the patient's family member of choice. These supports are extremely important to the mental health of TGNC people and can provide more healing and nurturing to a patient than any medication or therapy. They can provide valuable information and often have an understanding of when extra services are needed. Family members of choice should be a significant part of your treatment planning, and maintaining an alliance with them will increase the chances of your interventions having an effect. They can help prevent hospitalizations with their presence and encourage your patients to follow their treatment regimens and follow-up care in mental health, medicine, and surgery.

PARENTS

No parent is perfect, and parents shouldn't be held to that standard. It is also unreasonable to expect parents to be experts regarding TGNC people simply because they have a child who identifies as gender diverse. All parents can be both supportive and unsupportive. Their interaction with their TGNC children can range from supportive but confused to hostile. Many parents have good intentions, but these intentions can harm and alienate their children.

Case Example

Ramona is a 33-year-old woman of trans experience. She started to transition to female around the age of 29. After college, she spent her 20s studying auto mechanics and had worked several years in an auto shop. During this time, she was married to a cis woman in a heterosexual marriage, saying that it was important for her to get married and work because "that is what people do." In her late 20s, her marriage started to fall apart, which she said was mainly due to sexual incompatibility and her coming to the realization that she identified as female.

Ramona's parents were both in small business. They ran a store together in a moderate-size town and managed to make a good living for themselves raising two sons. Ramona, prior to transitioning, had a good relationship with her parents, citing them as a source of emotional support. When Ramona told her parents about her upcoming divorce and started to dress in more traditionally feminine attire, they started to get concerned. Ramona's paternal uncle had been diagnosed with paranoid schizophrenia many years previously and had been confined to an inpatient mental institution since then. He believed himself to be the new Moses and thought that God was telling him to eradicate nonbelievers from the face of the Earth. He never actually attacked anyone, but he made frequent threats to people around town and had been found with several guns and other weapons prior to his hospitalization. Ramona's uncle didn't respond to any treatments, and he was plagued with hallucinations.

Ramona's parents thought that she would be headed for the same fate. When Ramona found a trans-affirming primary care clinician and a psychiatrist to provide trans-affirming therapy, her parents wanted to speak with both providers. Wanting to stay on good terms with her parents, Ramona agreed. Her parents explained to both the primary care clinician and the psychiatrist that Ramona was probably suffering from schizophrenia like her uncle. They said that it wasn't normal for her to act like a woman and that she had never expressed these feelings before. They thought prescribing hormones to her was unethical given her condition and advised the psychiatrist to treat her for schizophrenia to prevent her symptoms from getting worse. Throughout the conversations, Ramona's parents continued to use her birth name and male pronouns.

Ramona met with her primary care clinician and her psychiatrist to discuss her parents' concerns. Ramona had never displayed symptoms of schizophrenia. She had no hallucinations, delusions, disorganization, or negative symptoms. However, she could empathize with her parents and their concern for her. She had seen what they went through with her uncle and had feared that coming out as trans to them might reactivate what they had previously experienced.

Despite her parents' protests, Ramona went ahead and started hormone therapy. Her parents were furious and wanted to know how her doctors could be so incompetent to both misdiagnose Ramona and provide inappropriate treatment. Ramona's primary care clinician and psychiatrist again spoke with Ramona's parents, explaining to them the reasoning behind their decisions. However, Ramona's parents refused to believe she was transgender.

Ramona's relationship with her parents started to fracture, but she had gained many friends in the TGNC community, and, once she heard their stories, hers also started to make sense. They had had similar interactions with their parents, and the shared stories helped decrease the amount of shame Ramona was feeling and gave her some hope that the relationship could be repaired.

After a year of hormone treatment, Ramona decided it was time for her to have a vaginoplasty to create a neovagina. She was very excited about the procedure, having experienced dysphoria about her genitals for some time. When her parents found out about the planned surgery, they were furious. They hadn't spoken to Ramona or her providers in several months and were upset the surgery was even being considered. They asked for an emergency meeting with Ramona's treatment team. Ramona, who was still trying to repair the relationship with her parents, agreed to the meeting.

Ramona's parents brought legal representation to the meeting, saying that Ramona was impaired and unable to make a decision regarding surgery. They claimed that Ramona had schizophrenia and should not have a vaginoplasty because her thinking she was a woman was delusional. Ramona's cli-

> nicians had prepared for this possibility and had had Ramona evaluated by two other clinicians, who both came to the same diagnosis and treatment plan. Ramona's mother, however, claimed she knew a psychiatrist who would diagnose Ramona with schizophrenia. The meeting ended with Ramona and her parents not speaking. Her parents were referred to the courts to decide about competency because Ramona's clinicians had already found her to have capacity around decision making.

Ramona's parents represent a somewhat extreme but common example of how many parents react when their child says they are TGNC. This is the same conversation mental health professionals had with parents of children identifying as gay or lesbian 20 years ago. Many parents will report that they never saw any signs or that their children never displayed gender-atypical behavior. However, although childhood presentation of gender diversity is common with TGNC people, it is not a requirement for the diagnosis of gender dysphoria. Presentations will vary depending on the environment and culture in which a child grows up. It may take years for individuals to piece together their feelings of gender diversity and come to identify with the TGNC community. Parents may expect a cookie cutter presentation like what they see in the movies or on television, but not all coming-out stories will be the same. Some children may present as gender dysphoric as children and in adulthood, whereas others may not. The largest group TGNC people you will likely come across are those who did not have a clinical presentation of gender dysphoria as a child but will retrospectively have memories of being gender diverse.

When parents are open to being involved, they can be just as supportive as the families of choice mentioned earlier. They have every right to express concern for their children and even make decisions for their children if they are underage. However, Ramona is in her 30s and involves her parents mostly to maintain a relationship with them. When parents do get involved and seem helpful, take the time to work with them and provide them with education resources regarding TGNC individuals. There are also organizations that can provide support groups so parents can connect and share experiences. It is crucial, however, to remember that the parents are not your patient. Studies have shown that TGNC people who come from unsupportive families have higher rates of suicide (Klein and Golub 2016). Sometimes, a healthy separation from a genetic family may be necessary in order to maintain the mental health of the TGNC person you are working with.

PARTNERS

Partners of TGNC people who knew their loved ones before they came out or transitioned can have experiences similar to those of parents. When a loved one identifies as TGNC, partners tend to question themselves more than their transitioning partner. They may wonder about their own sexual orientation and gender identity. They may feel as if they were lied to or misled. However, the feelings a person has about their gender identity can be kept from their conscious mind for years. It is important for partners to know that gender identity is an individual and very personal journey. There will be gender role changes that are new to both parties involved, and open communication and couple therapy may help guide the process.

Case Example

Iris is a 40-year-old woman of trans experience. She was previously married for 10 years to a cis female named Lauren. Iris had a problem with alcohol abuse for many years and eventually discovered that the alcohol was covering up how she felt about her gender identity. She tried hard to suppress it, but when she became sober, it was a reality she felt she had to face.

Iris previously worked as a baker and lived in a rural area with one close cis male friend named Larry. Iris and Lauren spent their spare time with Larry after work, and the three of them were very close. When Iris became sober and started to express her feelings of identifying as female, Lauren was supportive and said that she had always understood something to be different about Iris and that she was happy Iris was discovering her true self. Larry had different feelings. He thought that Iris was not really transgender and that this was her way of dealing with marital problems with Lauren.

Over time, Lauren and Iris decided to end their marriage. Although they were very close and remained friends, they were not romantically involved and hadn't been for some time. Iris continued to work as a baker, but the trio of Lauren, Iris, and Larry stopped hanging out. Larry continued to spend time with Iris, mostly poking fun at her transition. He refused to call Iris by the correct name and used male pronouns. Iris had transitioned for some time and presented in a very feminine way, but when she and Larry went out, he still referred to her as male. This confused people at the restaurants and stores they went to because everyone saw Iris as female.

Matters became more complicated when Lauren and Larry started to have a romantic relationship. They began seeing each other and excluded Iris. Having become distant with two of her biggest supports, Iris started to make new friends, some of them TGNC identified. Lauren remained somewhat supportive but was confused because of the feelings she had developed for Larry. Lauren had to navigate being supportive of Iris while she was romantically connected with Larry, who was dismissive of Iris.

This love triangle illuminates several ways that partners can both be supportive and make situations more complicated. Lauren obviously loves Iris and wants to be supportive of her. She also may have confused her feelings for Iris and transferred them to Larry, the other male in her life. It's possible that Lauren and Larry had harbored feelings for each other for some time, but the timing of their romance starting as Iris transitions makes the picture fuzzy. Larry's dismissiveness of Iris's gender identity comes across as abusive. Iris wants to stay connected to Larry but finds it difficult to do so because of the way she is being treated. It's possible that Larry's actions might stem from guilt over developing a romantic relationship with his best friend's wife. Lauren and Larry would probably both benefit from someone to discuss their feelings with. That way, they can maintain their relationship and still be supportive of Iris. Iris would also likely benefit from continuing to expand her social circle to include a family of choice who understands her gender identity and can help her as she discovers who she is.

Some partners involved with TGNC individuals can be extremely supportive. Relationships of all kinds have their challenges. TGNC people might minimize the impact their transition is having on their partner through an open and honest nonjudgmental dialogue, and exploration of relationships is needed to understand the dynamics that our patients face day to day.

CHILDREN

The effects of a transitioning parent on their children need continued exploration. Transitions of any kind, whether they be work or relationship based, can have impacts on the functionality and behavior of children. It's unclear what the effects are of having a parent transition from one gender identity to another; however, what is well known is that having a supportive parent, regardless of gender, is of critical importance to the welfare of any child.

Case Example

Tyrus is a 38-year-old man of trans experience. He transitioned around the age of 30 after his husband died from cancer. He had kept his gender identity secret from his husband because he wanted to maintain their relationship and because of their shared son, Jeremy. Jeremy was around 3 years old when his father died and 4 years old when his mother started transitioning.

Tyrus was worried about what would happen with Jeremy as he transitioned. He started to see a therapist weekly for supportive psychotherapy and was prescribed testosterone by his primary care clinician. He decided to not include Jeremy in a family session but went to therapy to help him understand how to best handle the parent-child relationship.

Jeremy called Tyrus "Mommy" for a few years after the transition began, but around the age of 8 years, he started to understand that Tyrus wanted to be called "Daddy." Because of Tyrus's physical presentation, the other parents and children in Jeremy's school identified Tyrus as male. They thought Jeremy was making a mistake by calling Tyrus "Mommy." Tyrus had explained to the other parents that his partner had died but saw no reason in outing himself to the community. He was worried that outing himself as transgender would have ripple effects on Jeremy and his friendships.

Tyrus and Jeremy had several discussions over the years, and Jeremy came to understand what transgender means and why Tyrus identifies as

> male. For Jeremy, Tyrus represents both "Mommy" and "Daddy," and their relationship is quite close. He is now 14 and participates in the local school LGBTQ organization as a straight cis male providing support and friendship to trans-identified students.

Children are somewhat less rigid than adults. In many ways, they can handle the transition of a parent better than a parent can handle the transition of a child. Depending on the ages of the children, they may not understand the change in appearance or reasons why someone would transition. Children use their friends' parents as models and compare them with their own parents. Knowing that other children in his class may typically have a Mommy and Daddy would make Jeremy think that he too should also have both. Not all families are this way, however, and it is best for children to understand that the term *family* can have several meanings and that not all families are made of a cis male married to a cis female with 2.5 children. Some families are made up of one parent or even three or more. Some might have only cis males or cis females. Some may have TGNC parents as well. This is not news for most mental health professionals, but these ideas of family diversity should be discussed with children, especially when they ask.

Tyrus is a good example of a parent who is dealing with several stressors at once. He lost his partner to cancer, has started his own transition, is raising a child, and is navigating being TGNC in a largely TGNC-phobic world. People like Tyrus have extra stressors that most people don't think about. Other parents, teachers, and students will react differently to a parent who is TGNC. A TGNC parent outing themselves is subject to stressors from multiple angles.

SUMMARY

When a mental health professional thinks about families, especially families that include a member who is TGNC, it is best not to make any assumptions about who is part of a patient's family and who they depend on for emotional support. Because many TGNC people have been rejected by their families and communities, they have to go out and create a family of choice full of emotionally supportive friendships and romantic relationships.

As people come out as TGNC and transition, their family members are going to have reactions, both positive and negative. Parents will respond to children, partners will respond to partners, and children will respond to parents. These are some of the major familial connections that will be affected, but anyone considered part of someone's family can function as both a stress and a support depending on the interaction.

Families, particularly families of choice, should be included when forming a treatment plan for TGNC people. They can be a source of great support for many people, but they can cause detrimental stress to others. Mental health professionals should not ignore this major aspect of patients' lives. Ignoring the dynamics of families interacting with TGNC people will likely lead to treatments that are less than effective.

Key Points

- All families are diverse, and no one structure models an ideal family makeup.
- Children need one supportive parent, regardless of gender, in order to function well.
- Family dynamics can be complicated when working with TGNC people.
- A family of choice consists of nongenetic relationships with people who are emotionally supportive and provide a social structure.
- Parents of TGNC people can be both a support and a hindrance to care.
- Parents may report they never saw signs that their child was gender nonconforming.
- Partners of people who are transitioning may question their own gender and sexual orientation.
- Children of TGNC parents are likely to understand gender diversity differently as they age.
- TGNC parents face transphobia from schools, parents, teachers, and students.

QUESTIONS

1. You've been asked to provide an evaluation for surgery for Stacy, a 28-year-old woman of trans experience. She came out around the age of 24 after taking some time to understand her gender identity. She lives a somewhat sheltered life and came to understand her feelings only after meeting other people of trans experience. After meeting with her, you find that she is highly functioning, works as a real estate agent, has multiple friendships, and has never had a formal psychiatric history. Stacy

said she received the support of many of her friends, and although she respects therapy, she never felt she needed that level of care. You find her to have no major psychiatric symptoms. She wants breast augmentation and clearly understands the risks and benefits. After you provide her with a letter of support, her father calls. He is angry and says his son is delusional and he can't believe that someone would approve him for surgery. He thinks his son is psychotic. What should you say?

A. Stacy is high functioning and meets WPATH Standards of Care for top surgery.
B. Ask the father to clarify. The two of you should discuss his concerns and share information with each other.
C. Call Stacy and tell her you need to retract your letter.
D. Tell the father that you don't have permission to speak and can't confirm that you've met with anyone; however, you will hear his concerns.

2. You've been working with Bobby, a 45-year-old man of trans experience. He has been seeing you in therapy for symptoms of major depression. He recently transitioned somewhat late in life after taking some time to understand his gender identity. He is still married to a cis man named Dustin. Dustin comes in for an information session with Bobby and asks to speak to you a few minutes alone. Bobby agrees. Once alone, Dustin tells you that he loves Bobby very much but he finds himself less and less attracted to him as he becomes more male in appearance. He wants to make the marriage work and wonders if his sexual orientation depends on Bobby's gender identity. What should you say?

   A. Tell Dustin that if he still loves Bobby he must be a gay man.
   B. Tell Dustin that he is a straight man and will probably fall out of love with Bobby eventually. They should probably end the marriage now.
   C. Explain to Dustin that sexual orientation is a spectrum and it's unclear how the relationship will progress. Encourage him to communicate more with Bobby.
   D. Tell Dustin he's probably always been bisexual and things could still work out.

3. Aiko is a 24-year-old woman of trans experience admitted to an inpatient unit where you are working. She had a suicide attempt secondary to worsening depression. She grew up in a very abusive household and had to leave her parents' house after they kicked her out for being trans-

gender. You get a call from the front desk that several people are waiting outside to come in and see Aiko during visiting hours. It seems to be both of her parents as well as some of her friends. Aiko can have only two visitors. Who do you let in to see her?

A. Her parents are her family and should be allowed to see her first.
B. Her friends are more important to let in because they are probably more supportive.
C. Ask Aiko who she would like to see.
D. Nobody should see Aiko until she has recovered more.

4. Khaldun is a 30-year-old man of trans experience. He has been seeing you in therapy for the past year. His grew up in a religiously conservative country, and his parents are unaccepting of his gender identity. They threw him out of their house when he was a teenager. They were physically abusive when he was a child. Khaldun greatly respects his parents and would like to reconnect with them. The last time they spoke, they told him never to contact them again. How would you approach this in therapy?

   A. Khaldun should do whatever is necessary to make the relationship with his parents work.
   B. Process with Khaldun his motivations as to why he wants to connect with his parents.
   C. Tell Khaldun his parents were very abusive and he probably shouldn't be in contact with them.
   D. Tell Khaldun he seems to be masochistic.

5. Augustina is a 48-year-old woman of trans experience. She has been seeing you in therapy for the past year after coming to realize later in life that she identifies as a woman. She has three adult children who live in other states. They are all very independent, and she typically sees them only on holidays. Augustina is divorced from her children's mother, who also lives in a different state. Augustina thinks she is ready to tell her children about her gender identity. When she sees them during the upcoming holiday season, she wants to see them in the clothing in which and by the name with which she feels comfortable. She is asking your opinion about the matter. What should you say?

   A. Choosing when to come out to family is a very personal decision. It sounds as if Augustina has put a lot of thought into this, and you support whatever decision she thinks is best.

B. Tell her she should definitely come out to her children. Better now than to put it off.
C. It's probably best that she not tell them. Maybe they aren't old enough to understand.
D. Ask her if she has told her ex-wife yet.

ANSWERS

1. **The correct response is option D.**

If your patient is an adult and you don't have permission, you shouldn't be speaking to anyone about their case unless it is an emergency. Even though this person claims to be Stacy's father, you don't know that for sure. You should respect your patient's privacy but be willing to hear concerns from family members without giving out any information.

2. **The correct response is option C.**

Sexual orientation is a spectrum just like gender identity. You don't really know Dustin or his experiences in life. How he defines his sexual orientation is up to him. It's nice that he loves Bobby so much, however, and only time will tell how the two will work out romantically.

3. **The correct response is option C.**

Aiko will probably know best who she needs to see. Ask her who she prefers for visitors. Given her current state, she would likely benefit from seeing people who are more supportive.

4. **The correct response is option B.**

On the basis of what you know about Khaldun and his history, contacting his parents would lead to further conflict. It's probably best to process with him his motivation. Although it is understandable that he would want his relationship with his parents to be repaired, they seem to have made it clear they don't want anything to do with him.

5. **The correct response is option A.**

There is no right time or place to come out. Augustina appears to be making an informed and thoughtful decision about coming out to her children. She hasn't brought up interest in coming out to her ex-wife and is more focused on her children currently.

REFERENCES

American Psychiatric Association: Diagnostic and Statistical Manual of Mental Disorders, 5th Edition. Arlington, VA, American Psychiatric Association, 2013

Klein A, Golub S: Family rejection as a predictor of suicide attempts and substance misuse among transgender and gender nonconforming adults. LGBT Health 3(3):193–199, 2016 27046450

11

PLURALITY

They would always say that I am not right for this clinic, but really, these clinics were not right for me.

Emilia

THE PHENOMENON OF plurality is unknown to most mental health clinicians. Most professionals know this condition as *dissociative identity disorder* (American Psychiatric Association 2013), although plurality and dissociative identity disorder are not exactly the same. Being plural, or having two or more people existing in one body or space, is just one part of the diagnosis of dissociative identity disorder. Many people who are plural do not experience distress from the existence of others within themselves.

The diagnosis of dissociative identity disorder still remains controversial, but for those clinicians who have seen it and worked with it, the existence of dissociative states is without question. Most recent estimates place the prevalence of dissociative identity disorder at 1.5% (Johnson et al. 2006). The presence of plurality is likely higher. There are communities of plural people, particularly online, who have developed a culture and words for what they (emphasis on *they*) experience. Some of the vocabulary involved will be included later in this chapter.

The idea of plurality becomes important when working with some transgender and gender-nonconforming (TGNC) people. Many TGNC people have had traumatic backgrounds, some severely so, and it would make sense for some of them to have dissociative states. These dissociative personalities can have different gender identities, making the evaluation and treatment of gender dysphoria more complex. However, although dissociative identity disorder and plurality are frequently associated with trauma, there are those who are plural and report no history of trauma. The case presentation in this chapter describes someone with severe trauma, but this is not a definitive or universal reason for the existence of plurality.

Many clinicians have probably already worked with plural people and are unaware of it. Changes in personality structures can be subtle and difficult to appreciate, and symptoms such as these are not typically brought up in a general mental health evaluation. Dissociations, like so many other topics in this book, typically occur on a spectrum. For practitioners who are skeptical of dissociative states, consider that to a certain extent, dissociations are universally experienced: on one end of the spectrum, and most commonly experienced, are minor dissociative states that occur when individuals are bored or want to disconnect from their immediate environment. This is colloquially known as *daydreaming.*

On the other end of the spectrum, people might dissociate so much that they become a different person altogether. Those who have experienced sexual or physical abuse may turn to this defense as a way of protecting themselves from experiencing the full force of repeated traumatic events. Going in and out of states of awareness or consciousness is fertile ground for new personalities to appear.

Case Example

Emilia is a 50-year-old who uses *she* and *her* as pronouns. She has a long psychiatric history, with multiple past hospitalizations secondary to suicidal ideation and some suicide attempts. She was born to a single mother who was mentally ill, and Emilia had to be placed in foster care from the time she was an infant. Unfortunately, the foster care she was placed in was not a safe environment. Her foster parents were physically abusive, and at the age of 6 years, Emilia had to be placed in a group home. Life in the group home was also very traumatic for Emilia. The director of the group home was physically abusive, and Emilia was sexually abused by other adults in the home. As a result, she had many behavioral problems, which only led to more physical abuse. Despite all of these struggles, Emilia graduated from high school and was accepted into college. Finally, at the age of 17, she moved away from the group home and into a dormitory.

In her early 20s, Emilia had difficulty staying in school. She experienced worsening mood lability, impulsivity, quickness to anger, and frequent suicidal ideation, symptoms consistent with chronic posttraumatic stress disorder (PTSD). At age 26, she was hospitalized for the first time after a suicide attempt she made by overdosing on over-the-counter medication. Emilia went in and out of hospitals and outpatient clinics. At different times she was diagnosed with PTSD, schizophrenia, borderline personality disorder, and bipolar disorder but never dissociative identity disorder.

Given the severity of her symptoms, Emilia was passed from clinic to clinic. Many of the clinicians referred her out for more specialized services, saying that her symptoms were not appropriate for outpatient services. Emilia made some progress with behavioral treatments but was known to have "good days and bad days." After a variety of treatments, both medication management and psychotherapy, were tried, she was ultimately referred to psychoanalysis for very intensive care.

Emilia went to psychoanalysis 4 days a week. Her analyst, seeing Emilia so frequently, discovered her dissociative symptoms. It became apparent that Emilia had at least five other personalities, or *alters*, who were part of her overall presentation. Emilia was assigned female at birth, but she identified as gender neutral. Many of the personalities she embodied were male identified. They were of different age ranges, and, in retrospect, it was apparent that they presented themselves during different stages of Emilia's life.

The first personality she developed was a toddler, the second a young girl. The third was a teenage boy. Two adults, both of whom were male identified, followed. Emilia's shifts in and out of these personalities were mostly subtle. Slight changes in her voice or the way she carried herself were evident during sessions. The most severe dissociative symptoms occurred when traumatic events took place. Her personality would shift entirely, and she had no recollection of the events that occurred while she was presenting as the alter.

After several years of analysis, Emilia's symptoms started to stabilize. She became less labile and reactive. She understood her dissociative states and was able to handle better the transition between them. Her alters were still present, but they were more part of a larger picture of Emilia rather than replacements for Emilia. They existed together and would depend on each other during stressful times.

Regarding gender identity, Emilia said that she felt like a boy most of the time but also at times felt like a girl. She was assigned female at birth and did not desire to take hormones or have gender-affirming procedures of any kind. She had some thoughts about masculinizing her body but mainly was concerned about her ability to pass as male. She said that if the procedures were better she would do them, but she didn't have confidence in medicine's current ability to help her physically transition.

Emilia is a good example of someone who lives a dissociative life. Although some of what she has experienced is pathological, do not be quick to assume that her symptoms need to be or should be treated. For many people with a background of trauma, and for some who don't have a background of trauma, the alters who are with them in their dissociative lives can provide a sense of comfort and stability. For Emilia, many of her alters were able to handle stressful situations that were too much for her to deal with.

OPEN AND CLOSED SYSTEMS

The plural person can be referred to as a *system* that is a collection of parts making up a whole. These systems can be open or closed. Emilia is a closed system. She said she discovered people living inside her but thought they had always been there. In contrast, in an open system, people may come and go throughout someone's life. Alters may be present at some points and absent at others (E of NS 2017).

FRONTING AND BLENDING

Fronting can be understood as a representation of who controls the system, that is, the person to whom you are speaking. Emilia was typically the person fronting her system. If an alter is present at a particular time, that alter might be the one fronting. It is possible to "co-front" as well, with two or more alters present at the same time. It's as if you are speaking to both alters simultaneously. There can also be a diffusion of alters at the same time, which is referred to as *blending*. In blending, some of the characteristics of alters are mixed with others (E of NS 2017).

HEADSPACE

Headspace is an interesting concept. It refers to the space inside the head of the plural person. It is where the alters reside. Some plural people can have quite extravagant headspaces, which can be described as parks, cities, forests, or even entire universes. Emilia doesn't have a headspace; she thinks the alters are inside her, but there is no defined space in which they reside (E of NS 2017).

IS THIS PSYCHOSIS?

Is the plural person psychotic? Maybe, but probably not. Many plural people have no symptoms of psychosis, although their clinicians may believe the experience of alters to be a psychotic symptom. There are no negative symptoms, hallucinations, or disorganization. Although some clinicians might say that the presence of alters can be considered a delusion, I would argue that these potential delusions are usually helpful and supportive of the individual. They bring comfort, not distress.

IS THIS A PERSONALITY DISORDER?

Is a diagnosis of personality disorder appropriate for a plural person? Maybe, but also probably not. Although plural people can have personality disorders, many do not. Personality disorders are distinguished by lifelong symptoms and characteristics, but plural people may not be plural until later in life. The types of personality disorder many clinicians would associate with plurality are the Cluster B group—borderline, histrionic, narcissistic, and antisocial. I would argue that there is a lack of symptoms other than dissociation in plural people in general. Symptoms of mood lability, impulsivity, and suicidal ideation are frequent in both people with personality disorders and those who have experienced chronic trauma (Herman 1992). Emilia has a significant history of trauma in her life, but she lacks the symptoms that would otherwise characterize her as having a personality disorder. As stated previously, it is quite common for plural people to have experienced trauma, but this is not always the case.

GENDER DYSPHORIA

Where does all this fit with gender dysphoria? The simple answer would be to say that it's complicated. One way to look at a case like Emilia's would be to see her and her alters as one large system that makes decisions together. When it comes to informed consent for gender-affirming treatments, it is best to view plural systems in a gender-nonconforming way. A system can have a variety of genders present, and the group might choose to masculinize or feminize the body in certain aspects through hormones or gender-affirming procedures.

When working with a plural person, it is best to be transparent about your confusion as a mental health professional about what to do. Although most clinicians are comfortable with capacity evaluations for gender-affirming treatments, working with a plural person can make the conversation and assessment complicated. Sharing with your patient your dilemma will likely encourage them to provide you with information that makes your evaluation easier.

Emilia may be in a plural system, but she is the person leading the system the majority of the time. During assessment, she was the one who was deciding if the system would pursue hormone treatment or gender-affirming surgery. In other cases, however, this process might not be so easy. In the case of co-fronting, two people might be present the majority of the time and could disagree about gender-affirming treatments. This situation is rare, but if it does happen, I would encourage you to view it as a manifestation of the person's ambivalence and treat that ambivalence as you would with any other patient. Explore the pros and cons of treatments, what it means to be male or female, and the permanence and long-term implications of any decisions.

Emilia identifies as female but also has considered masculinizing her body to align with the alters inside her plural system. Her reason for declining gender-affirming treatments was that she said she wasn't happy with the current treatments available. This could be viewed as an accurate reflection of reality but also an intellectualizing of ambivalence. Emilia might one day decide to pursue treatment options available to her.

SUMMARY

Plurality is a more patient-centered approach to what has historically been referred to as dissociative identities. This is not the same as the DSM-5 diagnosis of dissociative identity disorder (American Psychiatric Association 2013). Plurality makes up just one part of the larger diagnosis and does not necessarily cause distress. Although many people who are plural have a history of trauma, there are just as many who do not. A plural system is a collection of all the alters present. With some people these alters might come and go, whereas with others they are static and waiting to be discovered.

When working with plurality, it is necessary for clinicians to be open and transparent with patients about their decision making regarding gender-affirming treatments. Plural people need treatment and assessments just as any patient would. They also may need access to gender-affirming treatments. Approach plural people with a sense of humility and curiosity. Discuss with them what gender means for each of the alters present and whether there will be a shared decision making when pursuing treatment options available.

Clinicians should communicate closely with each other if they are part of a team treating a plural person. All mental health professionals involved should be aware of plurality when it is present so that an appropriate evaluation can take place. These evaluations may need to happen over time so the clinicians can look for the three major hallmarks of someone who can provide consent for treatment: insistency, consistency, and persistency.

Key Points

- Plurality refers to what many mental health professionals know as dissociative identities.
- Plurality is not the same as dissociative identity disorder but makes up one part of it.
- Many plural people are quite happy with the alters present inside them.
- Plurality is not necessarily caused by trauma, although trauma can be part of the overall picture.
- Plurality becomes complicated when clinicians are working with gender dysphoria.
- It is important for mental health professionals to be open and transparent with plural people about their

understanding of plurality and how it affects their assessment process.

QUESTIONS

1. Peppy is a 27-year-old man of trans experience. He was referred to you for an evaluation because his primary care clinician is worried he might be having a psychotic break. After knowing his doctor for 4 years, Peppy disclosed to him about the other people he has living inside him. They have been present much of his life and are supportive when he needs them. What should you do when you meet Peppy?

   A. Prescribe an antipsychotic to treat his delusions.
   B. Tell the primary care doctor Peppy is just fine and doesn't need mental health care treatment.
   C. Recommend Peppy for inpatient treatment.
   D. Do an evaluation.

2. What is a common name for another personality or person who is part of a plural state?

   A. A dissociative disorder.
   B. An alter.
   C. A delusion.
   D. A headspace.

3. Tanner is a 22-year-old man of trans experience. After he was found in his room alone talking to himself, Tanner was taken by his family to a psychiatric emergency room where you are the consultant. When you first see him, he appears to be internally preoccupied, and his family tell you that he has been slowly isolating himself over the past 6 months. What should you do?

   A. Admit Tanner to the hospital.
   B. Do an evaluation.
   C. Start antipsychotic medication.
   D. Refer him to outpatient gender-affirming therapy.

4. Jenni is a 44-year-old woman of trans experience. She has known you for about 6 months and has revealed to you her plurality. You have evidence of at least two other distinct personalities. Jenni identifies as female, but

each of her alters is gender neutral. Jenni is ready to get top surgery and asks you for an evaluation. She understands the surgery and follow-up care required. She has no other major psychiatric symptoms except some mild mood disorder symptoms. Which response is correct?

A. Jenni meets the criteria for gender dysphoria and appears to be stable.
B. Jenni may need to explore a little more the long-term implications of gender-affirming surgery for her alters.
C. Jenni may need further observation in order to be safe.
D. Discuss with Jenni the complicated nature of your decision and ask her for more information.
E. All are correct.

5. In a plural person, when two or more people are typically present most or all of the time, this can be referred to as which of the following?

   A. Co-fronting.
   B. Pan-gender.
   C. Alteration.
   D. Fronting.

ANSWERS

1. **The correct response is option D.**

   Peppy sounds like he is a plural person, but as a mental health professional, the only way you can provide good care is to do an evaluation. Be careful not to make judgments until you have done a thorough evaluation.

2. **The correct response is option B.**

   An alter is another name for a distinct personality in a plural person.

3. **The correct response is option B.**

   Just like the first question, this might seem obvious at first glance, but the only way to provide good care is to do a proper evaluation before a decision is made.

4. **The correct response is option E (all are correct).**

   If you work with gender diverse people, at some point you may come across this scenario. All responses are technically correct, and whatever you decide will be a clinical judgment call. Building trust and having discussions about gender and long-term outcomes is probably the best way to approach this case.

5. **The correct response is option A.**

   Co-fronting is the existence of two or more alters present simultaneously.

REFERENCES

American Psychiatric Association: Diagnostic and Statistical Manual of Mental Disorders, 5th Edition. Arlington, VA, American Psychiatric Association, 2013

E of NS: What is plurality? Plurality Resource, 2017. Available at: https://pluralityresource.org/plurality-information/. Accessed June 11, 2017.

Herman J: Trauma and Recovery, 1st Edition. New York, Basic Books, 1992

Johnson JG, Cohen P, Kasen S, Brook JS: Dissociative disorders among adults in the community, impaired functioning, and axis I and II comorbidity. J Psychiatr Res 40(2):131–140, 2006 16337235

12

SEXUALITY

A promiscuous person is a person who is getting more sex than you are.

Victor Lownes

FOR THE MENTAL HEALTH professional, talking about sex and sexuality tends to be rather commonplace. However, for those in treatment, the topic of sex tends to be the one that makes them feel the most vulnerable. Usually, people feel a great deal of shame and are embarrassed to expose their sexual thoughts and actions to their therapist. It can take years of therapy before patients talk about their sexual intimacy, and even then it might be more of a superficial discussion. The topics in this chapter apply not just to transgender and gender-nonconforming (TGNC) people but to anyone with whom you are having a discussion on sex and sexuality.

When working with TGNC people, it is important to make room in your sessions for discussion and exploration of sex and sexuality. Additionally, keep in mind that the topics discussed in this chapter will likely apply not just to TGNC people but to most people. For the TGNC population, this topic will be particularly sensitive. Concerns about the body, a potential history of trauma, being objectified, and their fear of what their therapist might be thinking are just a few of the reasons talking about sex is difficult. Many patients may not want to talk about their sex life, and we should by no means ask them to talk about sex if they are not ready to do so. However, mental health clinicians need to communicate to their patients that sex and sexuality are a perfectly appropriate topic in mental health treatment. For many people, their therapist or psychiatrist is the only person in their life with whom they can discuss these concerns without fear of judgment. For that very reason, sex needs to always be on the table as a potential area of exploration.

TALKING ABOUT SEX

First and foremost, before the topic of sex and sexuality can enter a therapy session, a safe space needs to be developed. Psychoanalysis has been good at creating safety. Spending several hours with their analyst a week, patients become comfortable expressing thoughts as they free associate. Lying on the couch may provide additional encouragement for patients to talk about sensitive topics because the expressions on the other person's face during the discussion have been removed. When patients sit face to face with the therapist, every facial movement of the therapist can be interpreted and projected on. Mental health professionals should be mindful of their internal thoughts and beliefs about sex that come up as well as the content of the therapy session.

In order to have discussions with TGNC patients—or any patient—regarding sex, mental health professionals need to first be aware of their own sex, gender, and sexuality. For mental health professionals to talk about sex, they need to first be aware of what assumptions and perspectives they are bringing into the room. Making assumptions about gender, sexuality, and sexual acts tends to be a rookie mistake in the mental health world. Even if your gender and sexuality match those of your patient, your intimate lives can be very different. It's good practice to take the stance that we know absolutely nothing about our patients' sex life and sexuality. This would apply to all patients and is a good starting place in treatment. Even the most well-analyzed patients still might have a hard time recognizing their own impulses and desires.

The lesbian, gay, bisexual, transgender, and queer/questioning (LGBTQ) community is one that has traditionally been pathologized and stigmatized by mental health professionals. Many TGNC people are looking for therapists who are trans affirming. Displaying that you have some basic knowledge of the TGNC community and are open to a diverse expression of gender and sexuality is crucial to building the foundation of trust necessary in therapy. Although some TGNC people might identify as heterosexual and monogamous, topics such as open relationships, poly relationships, pansexuality, and kink are all possible within the TGNC community, just as with any other community. It is important for therapists to be aware of the feelings and ideas they have about nontraditional and queer lifestyles. With a constant bombardment of messages from the world we live in being mostly cis and heterosexual, therapists should be aware of their own potentially unconscious thoughts related to diverse lifestyles. As stated in Chapter 8, "Gender-Affirming Mental Health," these thoughts can manifest as internalized transphobia. Only when we are aware of our own gender diverse dialogue will we be able to help our patients in the most supportive and empathic way.

USE OF WORDS IN ESTABLISHING TRUST

When seeing patients weekly in analysis, individual therapy, or even in psychiatric medication visits, regularity and time are needed to establish trust. In addition, the words we use can have a significant impact in the creation of a safe environment. Medical terminology such as *penis* or *vagina* can be used but should be avoided if patients provide you with their own vocabulary. Using the patient's words is the first way to validate the patient and to communicate that you are both listening to them and respecting their language. If a patient says a word that you are unfamiliar with, don't ignore it or feel ashamed you might not understand. Simply tell the patient that you hear all kinds of words to describe body parts and sex acts throughout the day and ask if they would mind clarifying what they mean so that you can make sure you understand them clearly. After you have clarified the vocabulary, continue to validate the patient by using their vocabulary in future statements.

Traditional words for body parts might also be rejected within the TGNC community. Each individual has their own way of thinking and experiencing their body. For example, someone who has had a vaginoplasty might not refer to the body part as a vagina. They may not even think of their body part as a vagina. Asking questions from a place of curiosity, respect, and compassion will provide better treatment and make you a better therapist.

SEXUALITY

Sexuality in the TGNC community is as diverse as gender. Sexual orientation and gender identity are separate, but they interact with each other. The idea that heterosexuality means being attracted to the opposite and homosexual means being attracted to the same should be questioned. It is up to the person in front of us to decide how they will be defined (Rowniak and Chesla 2013).

Case Example

Ichiro is a 30-year-old man of trans experience. He was assigned female at birth and raised as a girl until adolescence. Around puberty, Ichiro started to have gender dysphoric symptoms as he began to develop breast tissue and had a period for the first time. He had identified more as masculine from early life but was unaware of gender diversity and assumed he was just a tomboy. In his early adolescence, Ichiro started to identify as more of a butch lesbian and had two lesbian relationships. His butch identity made him more comfortable and lined up with his behavior and feelings about himself. However, although he continued to have dysphoric symptoms, it wasn't until he was almost 20 years old that he decided a male identity would make him most comfortable. In college, he started hormone treatment, changed his name to Ichiro, and identified with male pronouns. He continued to be attracted to cis females, and in his relationship in college he identified as a heterosexual male.

Ichiro was very happy with the effects of testosterone. His voice changed, he started to grow hair on his body, and his libido increased. Over time, Ichiro noticed his sexual attraction shifting slightly from cis females to both trans and cis males. He started to explore sex and his sexuality with men and ended up having a long-term relationship with another trans man that has lasted for 7 years. Ichiro still has some sexual feelings for cis women. At times he identifies as bisexual, and other times he identifies as a gay man.

Ichiro is a good example of how gender and sexuality are both diverse and not static. People can change over time. Ichiro used his gender identity and who he was attracted to as a guide for identifying his sexual orientation. A clinician who is not aware of the gender and sexual orientation spectrum might not think to ask about changing feelings. As Ichiro shifts from lesbian relationships to gay relationships, his relationship dynamics may change as well. His risk factors for sexually transmitted diseases also might change, signifying the importance of a primary care clinician or other medical professional being aware that assumptions regarding a patient's sexual behavior should never be made.

Sexual orientation is not defined simply by whether someone identifies as male or female and whether that person is attracted to men or women. A trans man being attracted only to trans men tends to identify as gay, but this isn't always the case. The label placed on a person's sexual behavior typically has no bearing on that behavior. If a person is labeled as a gay man, does that mean he has sex only with other cis gay men? And if so, what sexual activities does he participate in with other gay men? A man of trans experience might identify as a gay man but have insertive penile-vaginal intercourse with another trans man. Both trans men may have had a metoidioplasty or a phalloplasty to create a phallus, and neither of them may have had a vaginectomy to remove vaginal tissue. The label doesn't always align with the body parts. Only with clear conversations with patients about what they are doing and with whom they are doing it will we have a better understanding of their individual sexuality (Alegria 2011). It is also possible for sexual orientation to shift as someone's gender shifts. Because someone is attracted to cis men or trans men at one point doesn't mean that attraction can't shift to cis women and/or trans women at another point in time. Sexual orientation is fluid just as gender identity is (Levitt and Ippolito 2014).

THE BODY

The nature of gender dysphoria lies in the discomfort a person has with their body or sex assigned at birth in relation to their gender identity. Men of trans experience may or may not have dysphoria around breast tissue, their vagina, or the shape of their body. Women of trans experience may or may not have dysphoria around their penis, testicles, or body hair. TGNC people who are more comfortable with their bodies will be more comfortable with sex. Understanding which parts of the body align with their gender identity exists within the mind of the patient. Only through exploration and understanding can we discover how patients see themselves and how they would like to be seen by others.

For a group with diverse gender identities and sexual orientations, the types of sexual behaviors and activities can be numerous. A cis-heteronormative society will value penile-vaginal intercourse as "real sex" in the same way that a gay-normative culture will value penile-anal intercourse as "real sex." The truth is that many cis straight and gay people don't have penile-vaginal or penile-anal sex. If they aren't having this type of sex, does that mean any physical activity they are having with another person would not be labeled as sex? Of course not. How people define sex is a very personal thing. Some people call kissing and cuddling sex. Some people say that if nobody had an orgasm, you didn't have sex. There are as many opinions about what is and isn't sex as there are people. The sex lives of TGNC people should be seen as equally diverse and individualistic.

With the addition of hormones or surgical procedures, TGNC people will experience sex and sexuality in a new and different way. Some people describe sex with their new body as a new kind of virginity, and exploring their sexuality with this new body can be an exciting and scary experience (Rowniak and Chesla 2013).

For men of trans experience, the presence of breast tissue is generally dysphoric. As described in Chapter 16, "Transmasculine Top Surgery," many trans men wear binders to flatten their chest and help shape their body. Top surgery for trans men is a common procedure, and trans men are typically well aware of the pros and cons of the different types of procedures. Their views of themselves change for the positive after top surgery, and general satisfaction with top surgery is exceptionally high.

Phalloplasty is generally less popular. It is an invasive procedure with the possibility of many complications. Many trans men are content after having top surgery and do not wish to pursue bottom surgery of any kind. Some may want a vaginectomy, but the procedure is also not universal by any means. Many trans men are satisfied with their vagina, and many clinicians may be surprised to learn of trans men who like to receive penetrative vaginal sex. The concept of what is masculine has been challenged by sexual and gender diversity. Can cis gay men who enjoy penetrative anal sex be masculine? Of course. Along the same lines, many men of trans experience who identify as masculine may enjoy penetrative vaginal intercourse. Age-old ideas of who is the top or bottom, masculine or feminine, dominant or submissive, should be reevaluated, especially when working with the LGBTQ community.

Women of trans experience follow a similar pattern. The presence of breast tissue and the shape of the body signal both consciously and unconsciously to others that they are speaking with someone who identifies as female. Many women of trans experience desire transfeminine top surgery, but at the time of this writing, insurance companies are still not paying for transfeminine top surgery unless estrogen has shown no breast growth over the previous year of treatment. Many trans women are rightfully frustrated when treatment for such a major dysphoric symptom is refused because it is not "medically necessary."

Trans women, like trans men, have a mixed relationship with bottom surgery. Many trans women have strong dysphoric feelings around their penis and testicles. There are a handful of documented cases of trans women not having access to care and attempting to perform a penectomy on themselves. There are also some women of trans experience who do not have dysphoric symptoms around their penis and enjoy giving penetrative penile-anal or penile-vaginal intercourse. Trans women who have a vaginoplasty might also not be comfortable with or desire receptive vaginal intercourse. Just because someone has a certain body part, it doesn't mean they want to use it for sexual activities. Similarly, a TGNC person with a body part that is thought of as male or female may or may not have dysphoric feelings around that body part.

Regarding gender-conforming and nonbinary people, the body, mind, and sexuality can be very diverse, and typical boxes for male and female are broken down. As with any patient, there will be no way to know what a person feels and thinks about a particular body part without having a conversation about it. Nonbinary people may want transmasculine or transfeminine top and/or bottom surgery. Their views of sex and sexuality will likely not conform to traditional roles. Thoughtful exploration will continue to be a key for both the therapist and the patient in the discovery of sex and sexuality.

FURTHER SEXUALITIES

The idea that only three sexualities (heterosexual, homosexual, and bisexual) exist is outdated, and their meanings are largely lost when it comes to the TGNC community. With the diversity of sexual orientations, genders, and sexualities present in the world, there is a growing list of names to describe them. The vocabulary around gender and sexuality can be daunting, and keeping up with the latest phrases and words is practically impossible. However, there are some major terms to be aware of, including *pansexual* or *omnisexual.* These terms refer to people who are attracted to all genders and displays of gender identity. A pansexual person might be attracted to cis or trans men, cis or trans women, gender-nonconforming people, and gender binary people. Those attracted to TGNC people can also be described as *transamorous*. There are no rules when it comes to attraction, and applying a label to patients with regard to their sexual orientation will likely not capture the diversity of sexuality present.

POLYAMOROUS RELATIONSHIPS

Relationships don't always exist in a dyad. There are also nontraditional relationships in which three or more people are participating. These relationships can be emotional and sexual. The LGBTQ community overall is probably more comfortable with nontraditional relationships because they have been excluded from participating in traditional government-respected relationships for so long. The same historical ideas of what a romantic relationship or marriage should be don't apply as much. Straight and cis people also participate in nontraditional relationships, and popular culture is starting to accept this.

Polyamorous people are typically emotionally or sexually invested in more than one person at a time. Sometimes, all the people involved are interested in each other, and at other times there may be individual connections within a larger group. The more people involved, the more complicated the relationships can get. Three people in a relationship, also known as a *throuple*, may find that in some ways their lives are made easier by it. Not only is there an additional person to share emotional and sexual intimacy with, but for those who live together, their financial stability is stronger with shared expenses split three ways.

Many mental health professionals feel uncomfortable working with people who are in nontraditional relationships. This is frequently because it makes them question their own life and relationships. Countertransference can be quite strong, and when working as clinicians, we must always be aware of our feelings around a patient's choice and understand how our views of the world might influence our interaction with our patients and their choices. Although some might believe that a traditional monogamous heterosexual lifestyle is the best possible relationship, this is certainly not true for everyone. However, it's unclear if a poly relationship will bring someone more happiness, more satisfaction, or more stability. Explore relationship possibilities with your patient and be aware of your own inexperience with or feelings about nontraditional relationships.

ASEXUALITY

Just as we need to be open with and supportive of TGNC people and their relationship choices, there is also a need to support and understand those who have no interest in a relationship. Sigmund Freud said, "Love and work are the cornerstones of humanness." Although this might be somewhat true, each person will have their own definition of what love and work is. There are some people who have no romantic feelings and few to no sexual thoughts. Romantic feelings for some people are different from sexual feelings. *Aromantic* people desire close friendships and may have partners who are more like a best friend. Do not pathologize people who don't desire romance and be careful not to try to diagnose people as having a mental illness just because their experience of relationships is different from yours.

Many TGNC people have experienced trauma. Some have experienced repeated sexual trauma. For reasons of safety, they may not want to engage in a romantic or sexual relationship with another person. This is different from the aromanticism described above. When discussing relationships and sex with patients, make a clear distinction between what they desire and what they may or may not feel safe participating in. An aromantic person may have no desire to be in a romantic relationship, and this is ego-syntonic for them. A person with a history of trauma may fear a romantic relationship because of a previous abusive relationship, although they may still desire to be in a relationship. This would typically be ego-dystonic for that person.

COMMUNICATION

Much like the communication between a therapist and a patient, the communication between those in a romantic relationship or sexual relationship may need assistance. Navigating sex and sexuality is difficult for almost everyone, and talking about sex is even more so. For TGNC people, they are talking not only about their own body and how it might be changing over time but also the bodies of their partners.

For better or worse, traditional concepts of sex and sexuality will come into question. When visualizing a sexual act between two people, most people have in their mind an example of a traditional heterosexual cissexual relationship. These sexual relationships have been depicted in movies, television, and pornography. How about a depiction of someone who is TGNC with a cis male or female? What about two or three people who are TGNC? The rules around sexual positions and actions are no longer present.

Heterosexual cis people have decades of mirroring as a guideline when experiencing sex for themselves. Even before television and the movies, they could witness displays of affection from heterosexual couples interacting in public. This is not true for the LGBTQ community overall and for the TGNC community in particular. There is no guidebook for every romantic and sexual interaction. Who pays for a meal? Who buys the presents? Who gets down on one knee? Who initiates sex? Who gives and who receives? These are questions that the TGNC community will need to navigate with their partners. Frequent and specific communication is best. TGNC people should be encouraged to talk with their partners in an open and honest way, all the while respecting each other's word choices, desires, and feelings.

KINK

Kink is a form of sexual expression outside the typical concept of what sex is and should be. Many connect the word to bondage, domination, and sadomasochism (BDSM), but it is a larger term that represents any sexual activities that are outside of what is thought of as traditional or "vanilla" sex. BDSM might include bondage, spanking, tickling, and even some torture. It is probably the most well-known form of kink and may or may not include sexual arousal. People have different ways of expressing their sexuality to each other, and forms of kink might provide a safe way of doing so. Experimenting with forms of sexual expression should be encouraged as long as it is safe.

Case Example

Anthony is a 25-year-old man of trans experience. He has been dating two different men over the past year, and he identifies with the BDSM community and kink. For him, he says, kink includes some bondage and light consensual slapping and name calling. He likes his partners to be more dominant. Anthony has come up with a safe word with his partners, and they know if he says the safe word that consent has been withdrawn and any activities need to stop. Anthony likes kink play only when it is related to his sexuality. In his daily life, he does not like to be called names or dominated.

Whatever individuals' sexual proclivity, if they are going to engage in BDSM or kink, clear boundaries need to be set with communication about what is and is not OK. People frequently use a "safe word" that when said means that actions have gone too far or a break is needed. It is appropriate for a mental health clinician to be sex positive but at the same time express concern for a person's well-being. Navigating that line can sometimes be difficult for any clinician. When speaking with your patients about sex or kink, always come from a place of wanting what is best for them all around.

SUMMARY

Human sexuality is as diverse as gender identity. They are separate but interact with each other. Someone's gender identity does not necessarily define that person's sexual orientation. A person's gender expression and who they are attracted to as well as how they define their sexual orientation are all individual choices and feelings. As clinicians, our job is to listen and understand without applying our own judgments or rules. Relationships, sex, and sexuality in the TGNC population are very diverse. This allows both patient and clinician the freedom of knowing there are no traditions or guidebooks to go by. Each TGNC person will need to listen to their own thoughts and desires in order to discover their personal sexuality.

Key Points

- Gender identity does not define sexual orientation, and sexual orientation does not define gender identity.
- Clinicians who work with the TGNC population should become comfortable talking about sex and sexuality.
- Don't force patients to talk about sex but let them know it's an appropriate topic to discuss.
- When talking about sex and body parts, use the words your patient uses.
- Ask clarifying questions when necessary and try not to make assumptions.
- Be aware of your own countertransference around topics such as polyamory, kink, and asexuality.

QUESTIONS

1. If a woman of trans experience is attracted to cis females only, what does that mean regarding her sexual orientation?

   A. She is straight because she was assigned male at birth.
   B. She is a lesbian because she is a woman who likes women.
   C. It depends on what she does sexually with other women.
   D. She is how she defines herself to be.

2. Miranda is a 50-year-old woman of trans experience. She has been seeing you in therapy for the past year to help with symptoms of depression. Lately, with treatment her depressive symptoms have been improving and she has been having romantic and sexual partners again. In her ses-

sion today she says she and her partner were having a great time last night and she really enjoyed the muffing. You don't know what muffing is. What do you say?

A. Let the comment slide so as not to offend Miranda with your questions.
B. Assume muffing means some sort of sex act.
C. Tell Miranda to pardon your ignorance but you've never heard the term muffing and you are hoping she will explain it.
D. Tell her she should use common words in therapy so you can understand her.

3. Nathan is a man of trans experience who has been seeing you for treatment of social phobia and panic attacks. He has been in an intimate relationship with another man of trans experience and they are both into kink and BDSM. Nathan's partner, Kyle, likes to tie him up and spank him with a paddle. No bruises are ever left and the couple both seem to enjoy the interaction. What should you say as a therapist?

   A. It seems as if they are both enjoying themselves and it appears to be a healthy expression of sexuality.
   B. Nathan is clearly dealing with PTSD issues from childhood trauma. Explore his history more.
   C. BDSM is safe only if a safe word is being used. Ask Nathan his safe word.
   D. Ask him why they don't have other forms of sex.

4. Anita is a 44-year-old woman of trans experience. She is currently working as a lawyer and has been seeing you to help treat her insomnia. There are no other psychiatric symptoms. She does not have a romantic relationship but has a diverse group of friends with whom she is very happy. When asked about her romantic life, Anita says she has no interest in dating or sex and likes her life the way it is. How should you respond to this?

   A. Anita has been clear she is currently happy with her life, and there are no red flags in her presentation. Treat her insomnia as she has requested.
   B. Anita is dealing with commitment issues, probably because she works too much.
   C. Anita probably has sexual trauma in the past, and that explains her lack of sexual desire.

D. Anita may be dealing with major depression that is causing her to have no interest in sex.

5. Anton is an 18-year-old man of trans experience who uses the pronoun *they*. They are currently in college and navigating sexual relationships in addition to the stress of school. They come to you because they are concerned about their sexual orientation. Anton finds themselves attracted to both cis and trans men and women. They have had sexual relationships and seem to have no clear preference. They are worried that they don't know who might be best to have a romantic relationship with. How should you respond?

   A. Anton may be suffering from mania. Evaluate them further.
   B. Anton is likely pansexual. Explore with them what they want out of a relationship.
   C. Anton should decide if they like men or women more in order to navigate the dating world better.
   D. Anton is likely confused, and these are passing feelings.

ANSWERS

1. **The correct response is option D.**

   How someone defines their sexual orientation is ultimately up to them. Putting people into boxes as you see them typically does not help.

2. **The correct response is option C.**

   If a patient uses a term you are unaware of, ask what it means. It is impossible to know the wide variety of self-expression and new words.

3. **The correct response is option A.**

   Healthy sexuality can exist in a wide variety of forms. Nathan and his partner are happy and there is clearly no harm being done. It doesn't sound like a safe word is needed. Nathan should be validated and encouraged.

4. **The correct response is option A.**

   Anita came to you for treatment of insomnia. Treat her insomnia. She may be aromantic, but that is not completely clear.

5. **The correct response is option B.**

   Anton seems to fit the definition of pansexual, although they might not define themselves that way. If they are having concerns about what they want out of a relationship, then explore that topic with them. The gender identity of Anton's partner seems like it won't be the deciding factor in who they would like to see romantically.

REFERENCES

Alegria CA: Transgender identity and health care: implications for psychosocial and physical evaluation. J Am Acad Nurse Pract 23(4):175–182, 2011 21489011

Levitt HM, Ippolito MR: Being transgender: the experience of transgender identity development. J Homosex 61(12):1727–1758, 2014 25089681

Rowniak S, Chesla C: Coming out for a third time: transmen, sexual orientation, and identity. Arch Sex Behav 42(3):449–461, 2013 23179238

Part III

Primary Care and Hormone Treatment

13

PRIMARY CARE

> In a society that has yet to fully accept transgender individuals, one of the most valuable things a provider can offer is compassion and acceptance.
>
> *Maycock and Kennedy (2014, p. 79)*

MANY MENTAL HEALTH professionals outside of the medical field shy away from thinking about medical diagnoses. If patients present with what appears to be a physical illness, they are quickly referred back to their primary care doctor for further evaluation and treatment. This may be suitable for the majority of patients clinicians come across in their practice because of the number of primary care clinicians available. However, lack of awareness on the part of the mental health professional of typical physical conditions in the transgender and gender-nonconforming (TGNC) community can be detrimental to the overall well-being of gender diverse people. Part of working with TGNC people is understanding and advocating for their physical and mental well-being.

Ruling out a physical diagnosis is paramount in any psychiatric diagnosis, and I would hazard to say that many mental health professionals take this step for granted. Symptoms of major depression, for instance, can actually be problems related to the thyroid or even a precursor to pancreatic cancer. For patients with serious and persistent mental illness, a yearly physical is recommended, and regular lab work is necessary when monitoring psychiatric medications.

For the TGNC community, there are many levels of complexity regarding maintaining physical health that the majority of the cis world never has to think about. Going to a primary clinician requires that gender diverse people out themselves. Primary care doctors must know their patients' gender status as well as their body in order to provide proper care. To a certain extent, this is true for every patient, but the typical patient does not worry about the reaction of a primary care doctor to them being a cis male or cis female. Many TGNC people avoid primary care altogether out of fear of discrimination (Sevelius et al. 2014).

The majority of the TGNC community can get adequate health care from a general primary care clinician if the clinician is open to working with gender diverse people. Conditions such as high blood pressure, diabetes, and high cholesterol (ailments that affect many people) can be treated by a generalist. If clinics made it easier for TGNC people to access care, some of these major medical ailments could be treated, and overall morbidity and mortality with TGNC people would improve. However, there seem to be two main categories of blind spots in the general medical physical when it comes to TGNC people: standard screenings that relate to particular body parts and knowledge of sexual health and risk factors.

ACCESS TO CARE

As stated in previous chapters, the most detrimental problem facing TGNC people is access to care. Walking into a primary care office for a general physical can be anxiety provoking and stressful. The majority of primary care clinicians are not educated about TGNC care and are unaware of how to proceed with standard treatment when it comes to gender diverse people. From the start of treatment, TGNC people must fill out paperwork requiring them to disclose their gender identity, which may raise questions and change the way they are treated by clinic staff.

In addition to dealing with a lack of TGNC-competent primary care clinicians, many TGNC people do not have access to health insurance. When they do have health insurance, certain screening tests or treatments may be denied because of the gender status on their insurance card. Whoever bills the insurance for the primary care visit must match the gender on the insurance card to the bill being submitted. These nuances further cause frustration on the part of the TGNC patient and the clinic staff.

Access to care is exemplified by the case of Robert Eads. Robert was a man of trans experience born in 1945 who transitioned in his 40s. Around 1996 it was discovered he had ovarian cancer. Ovarian cancer is difficult enough to treat and endure, but Robert had further problems in that he sought treatment from more than 12 doctors, and they all refused to treat him. Apparently, the reasons for their refusal had to do with fears that their reputations would suffer from working with a person of trans experience. By the time Robert found treatment, the cancer had spread, and he died. This case highlights how prejudice and ignorance can cause a TGNC person fatal harm. Robert's story is best summed up in the documentary film *Southern Comfort* (Davis 2001).

THE TGNC PHYSICAL

For a TGNC person, going to a primary care visit and disrobing can exacerbate dysphoric symptoms felt about particular body parts. In addition, many TGNC people have a history of trauma, some of it sexual in nature. TGNC patients are frequently subjected to unnecessary intrusive questions and examinations because providers are curious about TGNC people (Ellis et al. 2015; Kosenko 2011).

What makes the general physical anxiety-producing for both the provider and the patient is that the very nature of the physical requires discussion of sensitive topics about the body. As a provider, giving more information than necessary about what you are doing and why you are doing it is probably a good rule of thumb. A clinician must be aware of the patient's physical anatomy in order to make a clinical judgment about how to proceed with standard screenings and treatment planning. Primary care clinicians will have to be particularly mindful of the words they use to describe certain body parts and explain to their TGNC-identified patients why they need to be examined. It is important for clinicians to be aware of their body language and convey nonjudgment with their body language (Quinn et al. 2015).

To make matters more complicated, TGNC people might need different treatment depending on whether they are receiving hormone therapy and whether they have had certain gender-affirming procedures. The primary care visit requires an individual approach, and the provider should not make assumptions about a person's identity or physical anatomy. An individual approach might serve the general population in getting good medical care, but for a TGNC person it is a requirement.

GENERAL SCREENINGS

It takes a primary care residency for most mental health professionals to be aware of all of the facets that go into providing primary care. That being said, mental health providers can and should be aware of particular instances specific to TGNC people. Knowing this information and discussing it with either the TGNC person or their medical provider could prevent medical harm and even save someone's life.

Case Example

Kristie is a 54-year-old woman of trans experience. For the majority of her life, she lived in a place that didn't offer trans-competent health care, hormone treatment, or even trans-affirming mental health care. She spent a large portion of her life in the closet and unable to identify as female out of fear of what her family and community might do.

At the age of 50, Kristie was able to move away from her town and find a mental health clinic that provides gender-affirming care. She was not, however, able to find a primary care clinician experienced in working with gender diverse patients. She started to see both a psychiatrist and a social worker for treatment of symptoms of major depression. After about 6 months of treatment, her symptoms of major depression improved.

More than anything, Kristie wanted to have a vaginoplasty. She hadn't been receiving hormone treatment because she could not find a clinician who would prescribe estrogen or spironolactone. She had been working much of her life in real estate and had managed to save up enough money to pay for a vaginoplasty with her surgeon of choice. The surgeon required Kristie to get a standard physical and blood work, and her psychiatrist and social worker provided letters of support for the vaginoplasty.

A primary clinician was found to provide Kristie with a standard physical and basic lab work. Kristie's surgeon had noticed some lab work missing and ordered it himself. After performing a physical and reviewing the blood work, Kristie's surgeon discovered that she had prostate cancer and had to cancel the procedure. Radiation would be required to shrink the tumor before a vaginoplasty could be attempted. Kristie's primary care doctor had not thought to screen Kristie for prostate cancer because she hadn't made the connection that Kristie still had a prostate that needed screening.

This case is a good example of how multiple systems can fail a TGNC person. It took Kristie years to find gender-affirming mental health treatment, and she never did find trans-competent primary care. Had her primary care clinician been aware of her physical anatomy and not made assumptions regarding her gender identity, a standard prostate cancer screening would have been provided. Kristie's mental health team should have also been mindful of her lack of trans-competent primary care and helped to facilitate proper treatment. A psychiatrist should have access to lab work done by a primary care doctor, and in this case, knowledge of the needs of TGNC primary care should have alerted the psychiatrist to the absence of prostate cancer screening. TGNC people are generally less likely to get screened for common cancers because of lack of access to and inability to find trans-competent care (Vogel 2014). Also, it is not common knowledge, but the prostate is not typically removed during a vaginoplasty procedure (Wichinski 2015), so prostate cancer screening is necessary even after the surgery has been performed.

Providing good mental health care is difficult without competent physical health care. Whether or not patients are receiving hormone treatment and what gender-affirming surgeries they have had will affect which screening tests they need. Largely, this will be left up to the primary care provider, but it is still important for mental health professionals to keep these screenings in mind and talk about them with their patients in order to make sure they are receiving quality health care. Certain types of cancer disproportionally affect the LGBTQ population, and primary care providers should be sure to screen for these (see Table 13–1) (Quinn et al. 2015). A general useful rule is that if the body part is present, it should be checked.

TABLE 13–1. Cancer screenings needed for TGNC patients

Assigned male at birth	Assigned female at birth
Anal cancer	Anal cancer
Breast cancer	Breast cancer
Testicular cancer (without orchiectomy)	Cervical cancer (without vaginectomy)
Prostate cancer	Endometrial cancer (without hysterectomy)
Lung cancer	Lung cancer
Colon cancer	Colon cancer

Source. Quinn et al. 2015.

SEXUAL HEALTH AND HIV

The topic of sex and sexual health is already difficult for many primary care providers. Even mental health professionals, who should be comfortable having conversations about sex and sexuality, shy away from this topic. It is not typical or advisable to discuss anatomy during a first mental health session with a TGNC person, but if it is brought up by the patient or if several weeks go by and a good rapport has been built, then sex and sexuality should be talked about.

Mental health professionals should know that TGNC people are particularly vulnerable with regard to their sexual health. HIV and sexually transmitted diseases can go undetected because primary care clinicians don't have the time or mindfulness to discuss sexual practices and anatomy with their gender diverse patients.

The range of sexual activity within the TGNC community is as diverse as the people themselves. Some TGNC people do not engage in sexual intercourse. Those who do may engage in certain activities that put their sexual health at risk. Trans women, for example may be attracted only to other trans women. Depending on whether or not they have had bottom surgery, they may be having insertive or receptive penile intercourse. This could put them at risk of sexually transmitted diseases (STDs) in the mouth, penis, or anus. However, a primary care doctor may not know to talk to a woman of trans experience about who she is having sex with and what sexual acts are happening. In addition, there is limited information available to providers about STD and HIV transmission rates with a neovagina (van Griensven et al. 2013). Traditional prevention efforts may not apply to the TGNC population (Kosenko et al. 2013).

TGNC people are also at risk of sexual abuse and sexual assault, and it's understandable they may be uncomfortable discussing these topics in a brief primary care visit. Some TGNC people have been exposed to the world of sex work and have clients who pass on to them STDs and HIV. Those TGNC people who do engage in sex work are trying, usually as a last resort, to make enough money to survive, to pay for housing, medical treatment, hormones, and gender-affirming surgeries. If their clients demand that a condom not be used, the decision made is one of putting oneself at risk versus not having enough rent money for the month. Sexual health practices must be discussed in a nonjudgmental way, with the risk factors surveyed and treatments offered in the most objective way possible.

Case Example

Tabor is a 29-year-old man of trans experience. He previously had identified as a butch lesbian and came to understand over time that he was born male and should live his life as one. Although he connected with the butch lesbian culture, for him, his identity had always been male, and he was trying to find a way to make how he feels fit with his sex assigned at birth. He became connected with an endocrinologist who provided an evaluation for hormone treatment. The endocrinologist then communicated to Tabor's primary care clinician the recommended dose of testosterone. Tabor wanted to start with a low dose of testosterone because he is a very anxious person and was worried a higher dose might activate his anxiety.

After 2 months of hormone treatment, Tabor was surprised that his menstrual periods had stopped. He was happy with the result but didn't expect it so soon. He noticed that he would occasionally have some spotting of blood, but not anything like his usual periods. He started seeing a therapist to help him with anxiety and over time decided to have top surgery. He had been binding for several years and thought now was the time to have the procedure.

Things then became more complicated. Tabor's surgeon asked him to get a physical prior to the surgery, so Tabor went to see his primary care clinician. His lab work appeared normal. The surgeon also ran a panel of lab work and discovered that Tabor was pregnant. The surgery was canceled, and Tabor was referred to an obstetrician for evaluation. To make matters worse, the obstetrician discovered that Tabor also had cervical cancer.

Tabor's primary care doctor was astounded. Several assumptions had been made, which had led to Tabor missing some important examinations and lab work. The primary care clinician sat down with Tabor to discuss his sexual health in more detail. Tabor did identify with the butch lesbian culture, but he had been having receptive penile-vaginal intercourse for years. He reported that he probably was more bisexual, but he was afraid of outing himself to his lesbian friends out of fear of being ostracized. After identifying as male, he continued to have unprotected receptive penile-vaginal intercourse but didn't believe pregnancy was possible because he was taking testosterone.

Tabor is another good example of how the system can fail a TGNC person if the primary care clinician is not competent to work with gender diverse people. Tabor's experience of hiding his bisexuality from his friends is not uncommon. Groups of gay- and lesbian-identified people can become very closely attached, and if someone in the group has sexual experiences outside of the definition of the group, they can be ridiculed and even cut off from the group. For many young people, having a family of choice that might also reject them for their sexual practices is more than they can bear. There are multiple types of closets and reasons why people would hide their sexuality from different groups of people.

If sex and sexuality had been discussed more in depth during the primary care visit, the clinician would have discovered that Tabor was having unprotected receptive penile intercourse and was at risk for pregnancy and STDs. Standard doses of testosterone make pregnancy rare but not impossible. Years of unprotected sex may have put Tabor at higher risk for cervical cancer. Had the primary care physician known this, he would have recommended a pap smear or standard gynecological visits.

However, Tabor likely would have had a hard time following these recommendations. It is very difficult for a man of trans experience to walk into a gynecologist's office for an annual visit. The staff and other patients will wonder why a man is in an office typically meant for females. There are few gynecologists who work with men of trans experience, which limits a trans man's ability to receive appropriate care. Gynecologists need to be prepared to ask questions about anatomy that uses the language of the patient. It is traumatizing for some trans men to have to go through a traditionally female exam. To provide more access, the idea that it is a traditionally female exam needs to be changed to an exam for people with uterus, cervix, and vagina. The gender identity of the person is irrelevant to the risk. It's the body part that must be screened and examined.

WHAT CAN A MENTAL HEALTH PROFESSIONAL DO?

Mental health professionals who work with TGNC people should take it on themselves to know their patients' sexual histories and sexual practices. Not all TGNC people will want to discuss these topics with their mental health provider, but some form of conversation needs to happen even if the patients provide no information about themselves. Mental health professionals should educate their patients about risks of STDs, HIV, and cancer. It must be made clear that when it comes to these risks, gender identity does not matter as much as the body part that dictates screenings.

Knowing a patient's sexual history, the mental health clinician can brainstorm ways in which the patient can access care in a way that feels physically and mentally safe for them. If the patient is open to the idea, the mental health clinician can discuss risk factors with the patient's primary care clinician. If the therapist talking with the primary care doctor about risk factors is what will prevent medical problems, then it should be done. Conversations about sex and sexuality can be uncomfortable and even more so with TGNC people who might have dysphoric symptoms around certain body parts. It is necessary, however, to advocate for our patients' health in this way. Mental health professionals should practice ways to make these conversations more comfortable and encourage patients to open up about their sexual lives. Our goal is to provide nonjudgmental and empathic listening. What better way to communicate that empathy than during such a delicate conversation?

SUMMARY

People who are TGNC have multiple barriers in getting adequate health care. Having primary care clinicians who are competent in working with TGNC people seems to be the area where the most improvement can take place. Having a trans-friendly office environment and staff who respect pronouns and gender identities will make the visit to the general practitioner's office easier. Primary clinicians should do what they can to make TGNC people feel more comfortable in the medical office environment and be aware of the potential for past trauma and current dysphoria around specific anatomical structures.

Primary care clinicians should be encouraged to use the word choice that patients provide in describing body parts. This will help decrease the stress and anxiety that occur when TGNC people talk about their bodies. Clinicians should always prepare patients for anxiety-provoking physicals and make time to discuss sexual risk factors and anatomical structures in need of general screenings. The more transparent the primary care clinician can be, the better care the TGNC person will ultimately receive.

Mental health professionals should recognize that talking about physical health screenings and sexual practices is necessary with all patients but particularly for TGNC people, who might not get adequate screenings elsewhere. We can use our conversational expertise to discuss sensitive topics and advocate for our patients with their primary care clinicians or other specialists. These small steps can have an enormous impact on the lives and health of our patients.

Key Points

- Lack of access to TGNC-competent health care is the biggest risk facing the health of TGNC people.
- Lack of trans-friendly health clinics provides another barrier to TGNC people getting appropriate care.
- TGNC people have been turned away from care simply because they are gender diverse.
- Even well-intentioned primary care clinicians may have blind spots about the particulars of TGNC medical care.
- Clinicians should not make assumptions about what anatomical structures are present in their patients.
- Clinicians should not make assumptions about the sexual practices of their patients.
- Only by creating a safe environment and asking questions can clinicians understand the appropriate treatment needed for their TGNC patients.
- Mental health professionals have a duty to advocate for their TGNC patients getting appropriate health care.
- Mental health professionals can offer their advocacy skills and communicate sensitive topics to other clinicians working with their TGNC patients.

QUESTIONS

1. Scott is a 55-year-old man of trans experience. He has been seeing you as a therapist for several years for treatment of anxiety secondary to long-term history of trauma. He is taking testosterone, and lately, he has been having worsening symptoms of depression. He has been losing weight despite not changing his diet and reports that he has a dull pain in his stomach. He has also noticed he has shortness of breath, which

has been going on for the past year. He goes to his primary care doctor for a regular checkup and reports that he normally gets his heart and lungs listened to. When you ask him about a genital exam, he says he never had bottom surgery and because of past experience is too traumatized to go to a gynecologist. How should you proceed?

A. Tell Scott to go see his primary care clinician as soon as possible.
B. Tell him to go see a gynecologist as soon as possible.
C. Tell him to see a psychiatrist to get treatment for major depression.
D. Offer to discuss his symptoms with his primary care provider. This could be a serious medical problem.

2. Corey is an 18-year-old man of trans experience. He has been seeing you in therapy for the past 6 months for treatment of anxiety and depression. He isn't ready to start testosterone yet and is not sure if it's the right decision for his body. He said he probably doesn't need testosterone anyway, because his periods just stopped on their own 2 months ago. He was so happy that this happened without him having to do anything. How should you proceed?

   A. Congratulate Corey and validate his happiness.
   B. Ask Corey about his sexual practices and tell him to get a pregnancy test.
   C. Refer him to a gynecologist.
   D. Tell him that you're not an expert and he should see a primary care doctor.

3. Verna is a 50-year-old woman of trans experience. She came out at an early age and has been taking estrogen for many years. She had top surgery with breast augmentation 20 years ago and had a vaginoplasty within the past 10 years. She has been seeing you for therapy to help with her current relationship and navigating her sexuality. She comes to you one day concerned that she felt a bump in her breast while she was showering. She didn't think much of it and says she doesn't think it's a big deal because she was assigned male at birth and men don't get breast cancer. What should you tell her?

   A. Cis men and trans women can get breast cancer. She should have a mammogram and consult with a surgeon.
   B. Verna is right: if she was assigned male at birth, breast cancer is unlikely.

C. The implant from top surgery is probably out of place. Nothing to worry about.
D. Verna should talk to her primary care clinician.

4. Rodrick is a 23-year-old man of trans experience. He came out during his teenage years and started testosterone 5 years ago. He ultimately had top surgery and a phalloplasty. He describes himself as pansexual and a top sexually (that is, he likes to have penetrative, not receptive, sex). He is excited to be exploring his sexuality. He said he hasn't been to his primary care doctor in a year and is avoiding going. When you ask why, he says it's very embarrassing. One of his partners was fingering him in the anus last week and felt a small bump. He told his doctor he only tops and is afraid his doctor will get angry with him for experimenting. What should you say?

   A. Advise Rodrick to see his primary care doctor as soon as possible because he could have anal cancer.
   B. Thank him for telling you. Ask him about his sexual practices, and tell him that it could be any range of things. Offer to call his doctor for him.
   C. Tell him to wait and see if the bump gets larger or goes away.
   D. Tell him he should be worried about his doctor being angry. He shouldn't lie about his sexual behavior.

5. Ashley is a 25-year-old gender-nonconforming person who uses the pronoun they and has been seeing you for PTSD symptoms. They were assigned female at birth and take testosterone. Their appearance is traditionally masculine, although they see themselves as living as neither gender. They tell you they are upset because their older sister was recently diagnosed with cervical cancer and they have never had a gynecological exam. They have their vagina, cervix, and uterus. Ashley wants to get an exam but is extremely worried about what people will think of them in the office and what the gynecologist will say to them. What should you do?

   A. Tell Ashley they will need to build up the courage to go on their own. You can help them with anxiety-reducing techniques.
   B. Tell them they are too young to have a problem and shouldn't worry about it.
   C. Tell Ashley's primary care doctor to do the examination.
   D. Tell them you'll work something out, either with a friend escorting them or with a case manager. Either way, you'll help facilitate the visit.

ANSWERS

1. **The correct response is option D.**

   Scott's condition sounds serious, and he could be having symptoms of cancer. Scott would have gone to a doctor on his own if he were able to, and at this point you need to facilitate Scott's receiving an examination and treatment. If Scott agrees, call his primary care doctor while he is with you and connect him to care before he leaves your room.

2. **The correct response is option B.**

   Corey probably doesn't understand that the cessation of his periods could indicate pregnancy. Assumptions shouldn't be made about someone's background knowledge or sexual practices. Further exploration is needed, and Corey needs to have a pregnancy test.

3. **The correct response is option A.**

   Cis men and trans women can absolutely get breast cancer. You should provide Verna with information about breast cancer and advise her to tell her primary care doctor and get a mammogram as soon as possible. A surgeon may be needed to provide treatment.

4. **The correct response is option B.**

   Rodrick needs to be informed about the risk factors associated with anal sex, especially unprotected sex. Just because he identifies as a top doesn't mean he doesn't also have receptive anal intercourse. This could be a hemorrhoid, an STD, cancer, or something else. He is scared of his primary care clinician for a reason that is unclear, but you need to facilitate an examination taking place.

5. **The correct response is option D.**

   With Ashley's family history of cervical cancer, they are right in wanting a gynecological exam. Because of Ashley's history of trauma and given the severity of their symptoms, you will need to go above and beyond what you would normally do with patients in order to get them care. Connecting Ashley with a social worker or case manager may be necessary. Brainstorming potential friends that could go with them is also a possibility.

REFERENCES

Davis K: Southern Comfort. HBO documentary, 2001

Ellis S, Bailey L, McNeil J: Trans people's experiences of mental health and gender identity services: a UK study. J Gay Lesbian Ment Health 19(1):4–20, 2015

Kosenko K: Contextual influences on sexual risk-taking in the transgender community. J Sex Res 48(2–3), 285–296, 2011 20336575

Kosenko K, Rintamaki L, Raney S, Maness K: Transgender patient perceptions of stigma in health care contexts. Med Care 51(9):819–822, 2013 23929399

Maycock LB, Kennedy HP: Breast care in the transgender individual. J Midwifery Womens Health 59(1):74–81, 2014 24224502

Quinn GP, Schabath MB, Sanchez JA, et al: The importance of disclosure: lesbian, gay, bisexual, transgender/transsexual, queer/questioning, and intersex individuals and the cancer continuum. Cancer 121(8):1160–1163, 2015 25521303

Sevelius JM, Patouhas E, Keatley JG, Johnson MO: Barriers and facilitators to engagement and retention in care among transgender women living with human immunodeficiency virus. Ann Behav Med 47(1):5–16, 2014 24317955

van Griensven F, Na Ayutthaya PP, Wilson E: HIV surveillance and prevention in transgender women. Lancet Infect Dis 13(3):185–186, 2013 23260127

Vogel L: Screening programs overlook transgender people. CMAJ 186(11):823–823, 2014 24982296

Wichinski KA: Providing culturally proficient care for transgender patients. Nursing 45(2):58–63, 2015 25585225

14

TRANSMASCULINE HORMONES

To me the definition of true masculinity—and femininity, too—is being able to lay in your own skin comfortably.

Vincent D'Onofrio

TRANSMASCULINE MEDICINAL TREATMENT, or hormone therapy, consists primarily of testosterone, or simply "T" in the transgender and gender-nonconforming (TGNC) community. For those clinicians who have been fortunate enough to work with men of trans experience and have seen the effects of hormone therapy over time, many will tell you the effects can be dramatic. It's interesting how one particular hormone in the body can have such an effect on the shape, sounds, behavior, and overall appearance of a person. It's also important to note that the other effects of testosterone have been greatly exaggerated, and a general lack of knowledge and experience working with testosterone has prevented many trans men from getting medicinal treatment for gender dysphoria.

Medicinal treatment with testosterone is just one way people who are TGNC can make changes to their bodies. People who are gender binary, gender nonbinary, or gender nonconforming and even women of trans experience may want to add testosterone to their treatment for a variety of reasons. Men of trans experience may want to take testosterone for a period of time; others may take testosterone for life, and others may decide to never take it. Some insurance companies and government agencies will say that a person needs to take testosterone for a certain period of time before they can get gender-affirming surgeries or have their gender marker changed on their identification. Medicinal treatment and surgical treatment are optional services available to TGNC people. Treatment should never be forced on someone simply because they fall outside of a gender binary spectrum and want affirming care.

Many psychiatrists will prescribe mood stabilizers and antipsychotic medication with multiple side effects and need for lab monitoring, but when it comes to testosterone, a chemical already found in the human body, they become anxious and shy away from providing care. However, as a mental health clinician, you certainly don't need to be a chemist or endocrinologist to understand and talk about testosterone with your patients.

LACK OF ACCESS

The primary problem with testosterone for men of trans experience is not the potential side effects but the lack of access to the medication in the first place. The psychological damage of someone not having access to hormone treatments and the methods that people go through in order to get hormones are far more detrimental to a person than having safe access to care from a knowledgeable provider.

For many trans men who live in areas with no access to care, the only way to get hormones is off the street. There are steroids available on the black market that will provide TGNC people with the desired effects they are looking for but at a cost. Some reports say as many as 25% of trans men are getting hormones from nonmedical sources (Rotondi et al. 2013). When people purchase testosterone instead of having it prescribed, it's impossible to know exactly what they are getting. There is also the aspect of having no access to clean needles to inject the hormone. Sharing needles and doses of testosterone puts trans men at risk of exposure to HIV, hepatitis, and a number of bloodborne illnesses.

Many primary care providers will say they don't feel comfortable prescribing testosterone to trans men because it is dangerous. These same providers will prescribe testosterone to a cis male who is suffering from erectile dysfunction with very few questions asked. This is largely because primary care providers don't feel comfortable assessing a patient for gender dysphoria. They say it is a mental health diagnosis and should be left to mental health professionals. However, although it is true that gender dysphoria is listed in DSM-5 (American Psychiatric Association 2013), ICD-10-CM includes gender identity disorder as a medical diagnosis.

The presence of gender dysphoria doesn't equate to hormone treatment; a TGNC person must also understand the risks and benefits of treatment. To put it another way, it's not the job of the clinician to label someone as having gender dysphoria and prescribe them medication such as testosterone. It's the job of the clinician to provide gender-affirming care by understanding a person's gender variance, providing education about the risks and benefits of hormone treatment, and offering testosterone as one option of care should the patient feel it is right for them and their body.

WHAT IS TESTOSTERONE?

Testosterone is an androgen or anabolic steroid, a hormone found in the human body of both males and females. Although testosterone is present in higher concentration in cis males, the ovaries of cis females also make testosterone. In cis men it is made by the testes and is responsible for a wide range of physical effects and some sexual behaviors. It peaks in the blood at different times in development and slowly decreases as people age.

It isn't necessary for a mental health clinician to understand the chemical formula or biochemical synthesis of testosterone. What is necessary is to understand the risks and benefits of testosterone use. As mental health professionals, we must understand the basics because we will likely need to advocate that our patients get access to hormones and educate patients, families, and other clinicians of the potential positive and negative effects of using testosterone. To understand testosterone and to be comfortable both prescribing it and seeing patients who take it, you can break down the effects into physical and psychological benefits and drawbacks.

EFFECTS ON THE BODY

The effects of testosterone on the cis male body are fairly well understood. Research focusing on the physical effects on the trans male body is growing but remains sparse. Testosterone, like other hormones, takes time to have effect on the body. TGNC people who start taking testosterone should be educated that changes will start to occur in the short term, but long-term effects may take months to years.

Many practitioners are anxious about prescribing testosterone because they don't understand how it will change a person over time. The hormone affects individuals differently as would any medication, but there are some overarching themes. These themes include changes to a person's hair, muscles, fat, skin, voice, and cis female sex organs (Figures 14–1 and 14–2).

Hair

The presence of body hair in particular areas is a subtle signal that the mind reads as traditionally masculine. Trans men who start testosterone will notice changes to their hair over time. Depending on the person, hair can start to grow more readily on the face; under the arms; on the chest, stomach, and legs; and around the genitals. The distribution and development of this hair

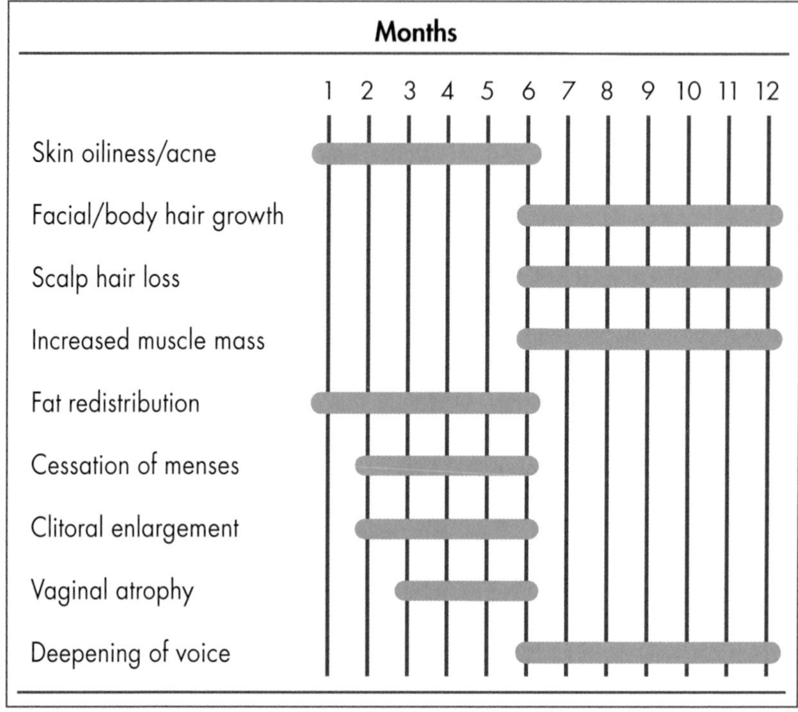

FIGURE 14–1. Onset of effects of testosterone in hormone therapy.
Source. Hembree et al. 2009.

has been said to be similar to what happens with a cis male during puberty (Ettner et al. 2016). Beard growth can take months to years.

The shape of a cis male hair pattern when compared with a cis female hair pattern has subtle differences (Figure 14–3). These differences communicate unconscious messages of maleness or femaleness. Hair around the scalp will start to recede, especially around the temples. Alopecia, or hair loss, has been associated with testosterone in cis men and is frequently a worry among individuals who are taking testosterone. Hair loss or baldness can occur in up to 50% of those who take testosterone (Ettner et al. 2016). Some trans men will forgo testosterone to avoid this potential side effect.

Muscles

Testosterone is known to cause an increase in muscle mass and a decrease in levels of body fat overall (Van Caenegem et al. 2015). Many cis men take forms of steroids or synthetic testosterone to develop muscles, and this mental connection to cis men using illicit steroids has probably made it

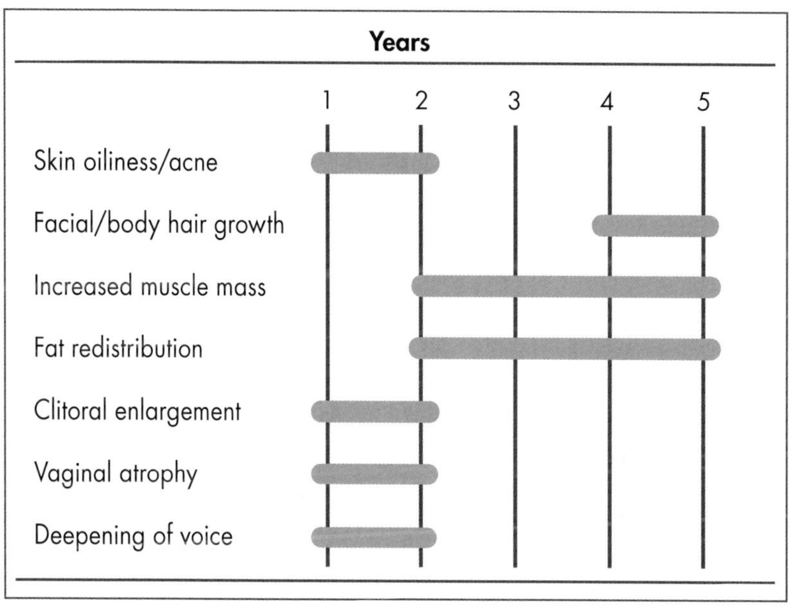

FIGURE 14–2. Maximum effects of testosterone in hormone therapy.
Source. Hembree et al. 2009.

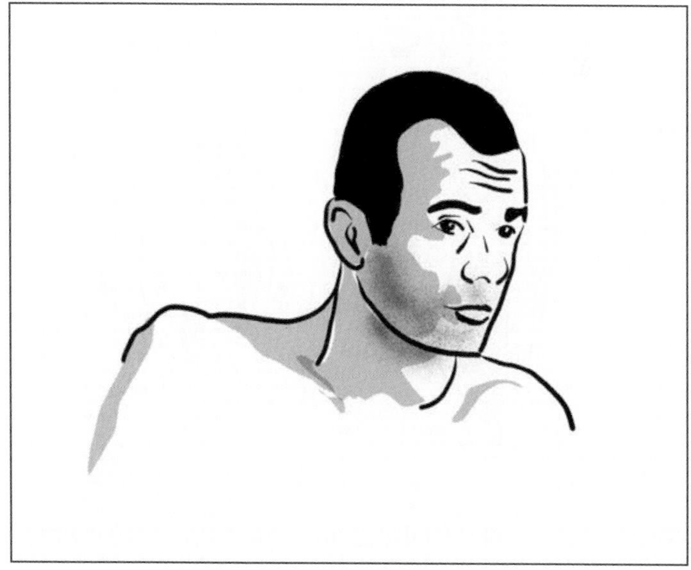

FIGURE 14–3. Stereotypical masculine appearance.

more difficult for trans men to get access to testosterone. Correlating the physical effects of steroid use with the effects of a trans man taking testosterone likely exaggerates the risks and discourages practitioners from providing hormone treatment. The steroids cis men take are not in standard prescribed doses and are not followed medically. Trans men may tell you that testosterone can have an effect on their physical abilities to run faster, lift more, and have more stamina, but you will not see these changes with cis males taking the same dose of testosterone unless they have an androgen deficiency.

Fat

The bodies of cis males and cis females also differ in the way that fat is distributed (Figure 14–4). Cis men tend to carry extra fat in their stomachs. Cis females store extra fat in their hips and breasts. Trans men taking testosterone will generally notice a change in fat distribution over time. Their hips may shrink, and more fat will be stored in the abdominal region. However, not everyone will notice this result. Testosterone is also noted to be associated with an overall increase in a person's body mass index (Deutsch et al. 2015).

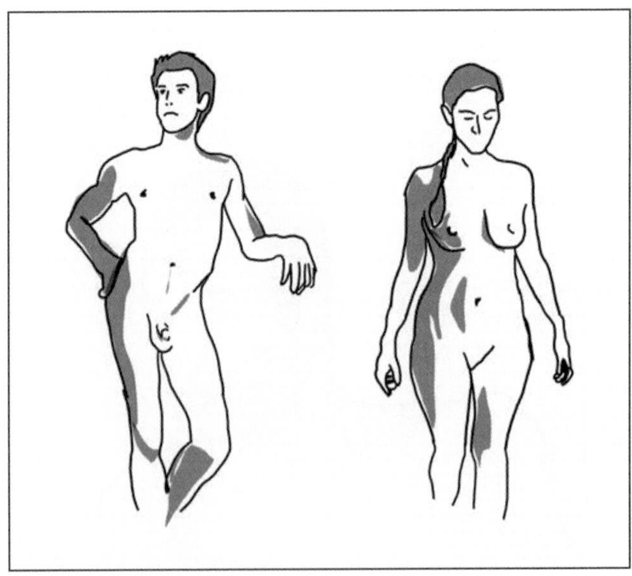

FIGURE 14–4. General fat distribution for males and females.

Skin

Just as a cis male going through puberty will have a surge of testosterone and an increase in acne, trans men can expect oily skin to be a common side effect of testosterone use. Depending on the age of the trans man, it can be disconcerting because acne is so visible to the world around you and frequent acne in someone who is postadolescence will likely raise questions from people who are unaware of that person's gender identity. Trans men should expect, although not tolerate, questions about acne. Typical treatment of acne in someone on testosterone is the same as it would be for anyone else.

Voice

Trans men typically are happy with their voice deepening, and some will report a scratchiness in their throat soon after starting testosterone. Slight changes in a person's voice can make a big difference in the way the world perceives them. The timbre of someone's voice is an immediate cue to that person's gender identity. As the length of the vocal cords changes, the sound produced by them may lead to a person on the other end of a phone call automatic replying with "Mister" instead of "Miss." Voice changes, once they have occurred, are permanent.

Cis Female Sex Organs

Trans men taking testosterone can expect changes to cis female sex organs over time. First, the clitoris will enlarge. This is important for the metoidioplasty procedure, as explained in Chapter 18, "Transmasculine Bottom Surgery." A small percentage of trans men report enough clitoral enlargement that penetrative sexual intercourse is possible (Ettner et al. 2016).

The vagina will start to atrophy, or shrink, over time. For most people, menses, or periods, will stop, usually in 2–6 months (Hembree et al. 2009). However, not everyone who takes testosterone will notice a decrease or cessation in menses. This change, like any other, is not guaranteed. Surgical procedures such as a hysterectomy may need to be done if menstruation is having a continued negative dysphoric effect on a man of trans experience.

There are no notable changes to the breasts that occur with testosterone use.

Case Example

Bailey is a 20-year-old man of trans experience. He identified as male from a young age. His parents were supportive of his identity, and Bailey was always known to his friends and teachers as male. When puberty started, Bailey used a binder to help flatten his chest, but he wanted to masculinize like the other boys in his class, who were growing beards and changing shape while Bailey was developing more like a cis female. He was very upset by this and began to experience depressive symptoms, including depressed mood, hopelessness, decreased energy, and social isolation. His parents found a gender-affirming therapist on the Internet who provided psychoeducation about potential treatment options. One option mentioned was puberty suppression, or decreasing Bailey's estrogen and progesterone levels to prevent further development and dysphoric symptoms. However, there was no clinic in the state or even in the larger region that could offer these services. Bailey was having a period monthly, which was a reminder of his body and how uncomfortable he was with its makeup, and his symptoms of depression worsened.

When Bailey turned 18, he moved to college and a larger city that offered trans-affirming care. His primary care doctor prescribed testosterone as Bailey had wanted for a long time. The doctor discussed with him the potential risks and benefits of treatment and did basic lab work and a physical to make sure Bailey was healthy. A nurse provided him with his first testosterone injection, and Bailey continued with a gender-affirming therapist to help him with symptoms of gender dysphoria and depression.

After a few weeks, Bailey started to notice an itching around his vocal cords. His skin started to become oily, and he began to develop mild acne. He noticed fat changes in his body and the movement of fat more from his hip region to his stomach. Bailey was already somewhat thin, so fat changes were minimal overall.

After 7 or 8 months of treatment, Bailey was noticing regular facial hair growth and more hair on his chest. His voice had continued to drop, and he was very happy that people automatically assumed he was a cis male when speaking to him on the phone. His hairline changed, receding slightly. He noticed that people at his college and new friends automatically referred to him as male. These changes made Bailey very happy, and his symptoms of depression started to improve. He and his therapist began discussing potential surgical options for him, including top surgery.

EFFECTS ON THE MIND

Testosterone's effects on the mind are not as well researched as the physical effects. Most of what is known about testosterone and how it affects the mind is through conjecture or anecdotal evidence. However, just because these changes are not well researched doesn't mean that they can be discounted. One noted and well-documented change with the addition of testosterone is increased libido (Meriggiola and Gava 2015). This typically is a positive result but can be troublesome for people who might have a history of sexual trauma or who remain socially isolated with no comfortable way to express their sexual energy. Trans men might report their increased libido as something they are both happy with and troubled by simultaneously. This ambivalence can be quite common. Along that same vein, testosterone usually leads to a reversible loss in fertility. Sometimes, however, the loss of fertility is irreversible. Because a person taking testosterone has the potential to become infertile, there should be a discussion about long-term fertility (Meriggiola and Gava 2015).

From a psychiatric symptom point of view, many clinicians attribute the emergence of psychiatric symptoms to the start of testosterone use. Some unfortunate trans men develop schizophrenia or bipolar disorder, and inpatient clinicians are quick to point to testosterone as the cause. These clinicians stop the hormone while the patient is receiving treatment, and the patient is then discharged to care with recommendations that testosterone be discontinued. It's interesting to note the quickness to blame a hormone, which is already present in both cis male and cis female bodies, as the cause of serious mental illness. These same clinicians would likely never question the presence of testosterone as the cause for illness in a cis male patient and would never recommend chemical or physical castration as a treatment. Testosterone as a cause for psychosis or mania is a red herring. Trans men or gender-nonconforming people who are receiving testosterone need to be evaluated and clinically assessed just as any cis person would be. TGNC people can develop psychotic, manic, and depressive symptoms just as any other patient, and in my experience, the chance of these symptoms being due to their hormones is low.

Some trans men receive large doses of testosterone in order to obtain the physical effects they desire, such as the cessation of menses. This can lead to supraphysiological levels of testosterone in the body. Serious mental illness has not been associated with high levels of testosterone, but some patients may report increased levels of anxiety, alertness, or activation. Although testosterone doesn't cause these symptoms necessarily, it might exacerbate them if the dose is too high. It's worth considering a discussion with both the patient and prescriber if you note that the patient seems more jittery after initiation of testosterone. Standard reference ranges for testosterone levels in the blood of trans men have been difficult to obtain because of lack of research (Roberts et al. 2014).

A change in the ability to focus has also been reported. Testosterone may increase attention and concentration but on one particular task at a time. Some trans men might say that testosterone made them "dumber" in that they can no longer multitask like they used to. There is only anecdotal evidence for these reports, but they may have merit when considering learning differences in cis males and cis females.

Finally, there is the question of sexual orientation. Some studies have reported that how far along a person is in their transition might correlate to that person's sexual orientation (Rowniak and Chesla 2012). Trans men may initially report being attracted to only cis women, but after months to years of testosterone treatment, they may start to be attracted to trans men and cis men. Many people might say that testosterone can make you gay. This raises many questions, including larger questions about what it means to be gay. When gender identity and sexual orientation are thought of as being on a spectrum, the idea of homosexuality starts to lose its meaning. Also, there is a chance that an increased libido makes it possible for someone to tap into attractions they didn't notice or appreciate before.

MONITORING

Before patients start testosterone, they should be aware of potential risks, and they should be monitored during treatment (Table 14–1). Monitoring for safety while a patient is taking testosterone is no more difficult than monitoring for any number of chronic conditions. General lab work is done before a patient starts testosterone to evaluate blood levels, liver and renal function, lipid levels, and glucose (Steinle 2011). Several recommendations have been made about how often lab work should be done, but it is generally agreed that it should be done quarterly in the first year of treatment and then about two times per year thereafter. A physical is generally done too, but in one study that applied a harm reduction model in reference to lack of access to care, some experts felt that not requiring a physical exam prior to starting hormones might mitigate the risks of a patient turning to the black market for hormones (Vardi et al. 2008).

Erythrocytosis, an increase in red blood cell volume, can be a concern with patients taking testosterone because it can lead to damaging effects on the blood vessels over time. As with any medication, the liver and kidneys need to be regularly monitored. Lipid, or cholesterol, and glucose levels may increase, and they also need to be part of a regular checkup. There have been some reports that testosterone can cause cardiac problems in the long term, but recent research has disproven this theory, and testosterone appears to have no major cardiac effects over time (Gooren 2014).

FORMS OF TESTOSTERONE

Testosterone comes in two major forms: intramuscular and transdermal (Table 14–2). Intramuscular, or parenteral, is the most popular route. Intramuscular testosterone comes in a small vial, and storage in health care facilities can be difficult because it is considered a controlled substance. Most patients need to pick it up and take it to their medical clinic where it is injected. Over time, patients can choose to learn how to self-administer the hormone, requiring fewer clinic visits. An average dose is 200 mg every other week. Testosterone levels typically peak after injection and reduce until the next dose (Meriggiola and Gava 2015). The dose and frequency of the injection can change depending on provider and patient preference.

TABLE 14–1. Monitoring guide for testosterone

Monitor the following prior to starting hormones and every 3 months for the first year:

- Testosterone (both serum testosterone and free testosterone)

  For injectable testosterone, measure midway between injections for an ideal range of 350–700 ng/dL.

  For oral testosterone, measure at least 3–5 hours after the dose was taken.

- Estradiol (should be below 50 pg/mL)
- Complete blood count
- Liver function tests
- Lipid profile
- Hemoglobin A1C
- Blood pressure
- Weight

After 1 year, switch to twice yearly monitoring.

Consider a bone mineral density test as needed if clinically appropriate.

Mammograms and pap smears should be continued if tissue is present.

Source. Adapted from Hembree et al. 2009.

TABLE 14–2. Routes of administration of testosterone

Route	Dosage
Oral testosterone undecanoate[a]	160–240 mg/day
Testosterone enanthate or cypionate intramuscular	100–200 mg every 20 weeks or 50% weekly
Testosterone undecanoate intramuscular[a]	1,000 mg every 12 weeks
Transdermal gel 1%	2.5–10 g/day
Transdermal patch	2.5–7.5 mg/day

[a]Not available in the United States.
Source. Adapted from Hembree et al. 2009.

Transdermal dosing is also available. Although a patch can mimic cis male levels of testosterone, the application can result in a rash or irritated skin and can be difficult to maintain. It also leaves the wearer open to questions if the patch is noticed, and the patch has a tendency to get damaged when it becomes wet through bathing or even sweat.

INFORMED CONSENT

When a TGNC person is ready to start testosterone, the most important thing a clinician can do is to make sure the patient is well informed of the risks and benefits of treatment. The benefits of treatment include changes to a person's body to treat symptoms of gender dysphoria. Changes to a person's hair, muscle mass, fat distribution, voice, libido, and cis female sex organs are all potential benefits of treatment. Potential risks or drawbacks to treatment include hair loss, oily skin, erythrocytosis, and lipid and glucose changes. The ultimate goal of treatment is to both suppress endogenous hormones (estrogen and progesterone) and maintain testosterone within a range typical for cis males (Hembree et al. 2009).

After patients have been fully informed of these changes, the timeline during which the changes occur, and the permanence of the changes, they can make an informed decision about whether or not they think testosterone is right for them and their body. It's very important that patients have time to ask questions and that they clarify that they understand all the risks and benefits. With the business of modern medicine tending to result in shorter visits, mental health clinicians may need to advocate that these primary care visits are not rushed and that they warrant special care and attention. It is common for patients who seek testosterone treatment to have read articles or watched videos about possible outcomes, and TGNC patients are sometimes more informed about the risks and benefits of treatment than are their providers.

It should also be noted that the World Professional Association for Transgender Health (WPATH) Standards of Care do not suggest that someone be in psychotherapy or have a psychiatric evaluation prior to starting hormone therapy. Although mental health treatment can largely benefit anyone who receives it, including TGNC people, forcing someone to go to mental health treatment prior to receiving access to hormones is inappropriate and can lead to more harm.

SUMMARY

The transmasculine hormone testosterone is also referred to as medicinal or hormone treatment for TGNC people who wish to have masculinizing effects on their body. Testosterone has been shown to help significantly with symptoms of gender dysphoria. Given that testosterone has been widely prescribed, its physical effects, both positive and negative, have been documented. The psychological benefit of taking testosterone are still being studied, but its effect on the relief of gender dysphoric symptoms is clear. Its negative effects on mental health have been exaggerated, and the harm of not having access to testosterone is much greater than the difficulties of medical monitoring and administration.

Key Points

- Testosterone administration for trans men is also known as medicinal or hormone treatment.
- The effects of testosterone do not happen immediately but occur over months to years.
- The most harmful aspect of hormone treatment is lack of access leading to unsupervised use and the potential for sharing needles.
- Individuals taking testosterone can expect positive results, including an increase in hair growth, a lower voice, increased muscle mass, changes in fat distribution, cessation of menses, clitoral enlargement, and an increased libido.
- Potential drawbacks to testosterone include alopecia and oily skin.
- Intramuscular injections are the most common form of administration of testosterone.
- Patients start testosterone after reviewing the risks and benefits of treatment and making an informed choice about whether or not testosterone is right for their body.

QUESTIONS

1. Gerry, a man of trans experience, is 22 years old and is about to start testosterone. You have been seeing him and providing gender-affirming treatment for the past 2 years. His girlfriend, Rachael, a cis female, asks to come to a session with Gerry to talk about what to expect from testosterone. Rachael, who is very happy in their relationship, expresses

concern that she has heard starting testosterone will turn Gerry gay and he won't like cis women anymore. Gerry has already tried to reassure her, but he would like you to provide her with your professional mental health opinion. What's the most appropriate thing to say?

A. On the basis of your experience, you think there is a good chance, that Gerry will turn gay, and he and Rachael should prepare for his shift in sexual orientation.
B. There is no evidence of someone's sexual orientation changing from testosterone use.
C. Gerry might notice an increased libido and find himself attracted to a wider range of gender identities, and his sexual interests can broaden. How Gerry defines his sexual orientation will ultimately be up to him.
D. Gerry will probably end up bisexual, not gay. Rachael has nothing to worry about.

2. Jaime is a 24-year-old man of trans experience who comes to you after taking testosterone for 1 month. He has been panicking because his voice hasn't changed and he thinks testosterone hasn't worked for him. People still call him "Miss" over the phone, and he is disturbed by the feminine sound of his voice. How should you counsel Jaime?

A. If Jaime's voice hasn't changed yet, it likely won't. He should practice acceptance and learn to live his life with the voice he has.
B. Changes to the voice of a person taking testosterone can take months or years. Reassure Jaime that changes can still take place, and you'll continue to support him along the way.
C. The voice isn't typically affected by testosterone administration.
D. Tell him to ask his primary care doctor to increase the dose. It's probably not high enough.

3. Graham is a 30-year-old man of trans experience who recently came out to his family. He wanted to tell his family about his gender identity before starting hormone treatment. His mother was terrified and said that there was a history of heart disease in the family, and she thought Graham was basically killing himself by starting treatment. Graham wants your opinion about testosterone effects on the heart. What should you say?

A. There are potential effects, mostly an increase in red blood cells called erythrocytosis. Major heart disease due to testosterone has not been supported by research. Graham should make sure he gets regular blood work and checkups. It's all about weighing the risks and benefits of treatment.

B. Heart disease has been shown to be worsened by testosterone injections. Advise Graham that he is taking his life in his hands by starting the hormone.

C. There is absolutely no cardiovascular risk associated with testosterone treatment. Graham has nothing to worry about, but he should still get regular blood work done.

D. Testosterone can cause heart attacks, just like what happens with cis men and steroid use.

4. Toby is an 18-year-old man of trans experience who has been taking testosterone for 6 months. He has been seeing you for treatment of social phobia and wanted to talk with you about the fact that he continues to have his period despite starting testosterone. He's very distraught and doesn't know what to do. Any suggestions?

   A. If he is still having his period, that likely won't change. Maybe he should get a hysterectomy.
   B. It can take years for his period to stop. Tell him to give it more time.
   C. Analyze the meaning behind his periods and why he is so upset by them.
   D. There should have been some effect on his period by now. Encourage Toby to discuss a dose increase with his primary care doctor. Offer to advocate for him.

5. Billy is a 23-year-old man of trans experience who has been taking testosterone 200 mg every 2 weeks for 3 years. He is in graduate school and has been under a large amount of pressure. Lately, he has started to hear auditory hallucinations of someone telling him he looks like a girl. Billy has a family history of schizophrenia. He shows up in an emergency room and is admitted so that antipsychotic medication can be administered. You are the resident on the unit, and your attending physician wonders why you continued Billy's testosterone. He thinks it's the reason Billy is having hallucinations. What should you say?

   A. Apologize to the attending, telling him it was an oversight on your part and you'll stop the hormone immediately.
   B. Tell Billy that the team thinks testosterone is causing his hallucinations. Ask him if he would like to stop taking it.
   C. Inform your attending that Billy has been taking testosterone for 3 years, and it likely has nothing to do with his psychotic symptoms.

D. Compromise with your attending and the patient. Lower but do not stop the testosterone.

6. You have been working in a medical clinic as the mental health care provider. Primary care physicians seek out your advice, and you work mainly to help patients who have mental health concerns. Travis is a 31-year-old man who recently came out as trans and would like to start testosterone. The primary care doctor would like you to evaluate Travis to make sure he is "really transgender." He suggests you do at least 3 months of therapy with the patient before he will agree to prescribe testosterone. How should you advocate for Travis?

   A. Therapy is not a requirement for hormone treatment. Informed consent is. Educate the primary care doctor on this matter and tell him you'll be happy to see Travis for therapy if Travis is asking for mental health services.
   B. The doctor has made a suggestion, so you should probably follow it. See Travis for 3 months and explore his gender identity.
   C. Travis likely does need therapy. People don't typically transition at age 31.
   D. Travis doesn't need therapy if he just wants hormones. Refuse to see the patient.

ANSWERS

1. **The correct response is option C.**

   Sexual orientation and gender identity are very personal. Gerry is involved with Rachael, and there is no reason to believe he will stop having feelings for her. It is possible that his attraction to other gender identities may broaden, but how he chooses to define himself will ultimately be up to him.

2. **The correct response is option B.**

   It's still pretty early in treatment. Jaime shouldn't expect many changes after 1 month of injections. He's likely to experience a change in his voice, but he needs to give it more time. There is no reason to change the dose of testosterone until it has had time to work.

3. **The correct response is option A.**

   What we do know about the physical effects of testosterone is that it can cause erythrocytosis, or an increase in red blood cells. This can damage blood vessels over time but is easily avoided with regular checkups. Major heart disease has not been shown, and having no access to testosterone will likely be more dangerous to Graham than receiving hormone therapy would be.

4. **The correct response is option D.**

   Six months is a decent amount of time to notice changes to menses. The dose of testosterone may need to be increased, and Toby should definitely talk to his prescriber about it. Offer to advocate for him.

5. **The correct response is option C.**

   The correlation between testosterone and serious psychiatric conditions has been greatly exaggerated. Billy is probably dealing with the emergence of schizophrenia, and it's unfortunate that testosterone is being blamed for it. He has a 3-year history of taking the hormone without any problems. Stopping testosterone or even decreasing the dose would be insensitive and potentially harmful to a patient in such a fragile state.

6. **The correct response is option A.**

   Therapy is absolutely not a requirement for hormone treatment. Putting up unnecessary barriers likely has more to do with personal prejudice than sound clinical judgment. It's possible that there is a miscommunication, so you should ask the primary care doctor what he means by "really transgender." You also want to be available to provide therapy if Travis himself is requesting it for a mental health concern. Advocating for our patients in these moments is some of the most important work we as mental health providers can do for the TGNC population.

REFERENCES

American Psychiatric Association: Diagnostic and Statistical Manual of Mental Disorders, 5th Edition. Arlington, VA, American Psychiatric Association, 2013

Deutsch MB, Bhakri V, Kubicek K: Effects of cross-sex hormone treatment on transgender women and men. Obstet Gynecol 125(3):605–610, 2015 25730222

Ettner R, Monstrey S, Coleman E (eds): Principles of Transgender Medicine and Surgery, 2nd Edition. New York, Routledge, 2016

Gooren LJ: Management of female-to-male transgender persons: medical and surgical management, life expectancy. Curr Opin Endocrinol Diabetes Obes 21(3):233–238, 2014 24755998

Hembree WC, Cohen-Kettenis P, Delemarre-van de Waal HA, et al; Endocrine Society: Endocrine treatment of transsexual persons: an Endocrine Society clinical practice guideline. J Clin Endocrinol Metab 94(9):3132–3154, 2009 19509099

Meriggiola MC, Gava G: Endocrine care of transpeople part II. A review of cross-sex hormonal treatments, outcomes and adverse effects in transwomen. Clin Endocrinol (Oxf) 83(5):607–615, 2015 25692882

Roberts TK, Kraft CS, French D, et al: Interpreting laboratory results in transgender patients on hormone therapy. Am J Med 127(2):159–162, 2014 24332725

Rotondi NK, Bauer GR, Scanlon K, et al: Nonprescribed hormone use and self-performed surgeries: "do-it-yourself" transitions in transgender communities in Ontario, Canada. Am J Public Health 103(10):1830–1836, 2013 23948009

Rowniak S, Chesla C: Coming out for a third time: transmen, sexual orientation, and identity. Arch Sex Behav 42(3):449–461, 2012 23179238

Steinle K: Hormonal management of the female-to-male transgender patient. J Midwifery Womens Health 56(3):293–302, 2011 21535376

Van Caenegem E, Wierckx K, Taes Y, et al: Body composition, bone turnover, and bone mass in trans men during testosterone treatment: 1-year follow-up data from a prospective case-controlled study (ENIGI). Eur J Endocrinol 172(2):163–171, 2015 25550352

Vardi Y, Wylie KR, Moser C, et al: Is physical examination required before prescribing hormones to patients with gender dysphoria? J Sex Med 5(1):21–26, 2008 18173763

15

TRANSFEMININE HORMONES

I love the smell of estrogen in the morning.

Katie Couric

JUST AS TESTOSTERONE has in many ways become synonymous with transmasculine hormones, estrogen is generally what people mean by *transfeminine hormone* or hormone replacement therapy. Providing transfeminine hormones is slightly more complicated because three prescriptions are considered—estrogen, progesterone, and spironolactone. Estrogen and progesterone are hormones found in cis males and cis females just like testosterone. These two hormones are not only responsible for the physical appearance of what is classically defined as female, but they also regulate the menstrual cycle and the potential for pregnancy.

When a woman of trans experience starts hormone treatment, she generally is given both estrogen and spironolactone. The addition of progesterone is debatable in that it's unclear if it provides beneficial effects. A later section in this chapter is devoted to progesterone, what it does in the body, and some of the pros and cons to consider in treatment.

Spironolactone is a testosterone blocker. All of the masculinizing effects of testosterone are blocked when someone starts spironolactone. Muscle development, hair growth, and sex drive all decrease once spironolactone is started. How long a person should take spironolactone is up for debate. A section is devoted to this topic later in the chapter as well.

Regardless of whether a woman of trans experience takes only estrogen and spironolactone or the two hormones plus progesterone, the effects happen over months to years. There are no fast effects when it comes to feminizing the body. Some patients and clinicians report that it can take up to 3 years to see a full effect from the regimen. Patience and persistence are required, and supportive reassurance is a frequent intervention used by mental health professionals.

ESTROGEN

Lack of Access

Just as with testosterone, the most potentially dangerous part of estrogen is lack of access to it. Because so many women of trans experience have no access to knowledgeable trans-affirming providers, they have no choice but to get estrogen off the street. In some surveys, close to 70% of trans women have reported ordering feminizing hormones from the Internet and not under medical supervision (Mepham et al. 2014). When hormones are taken without supervision, it's unclear exactly what chemical or chemicals people are putting into their bodies. Another danger is that estrogen can also be given intramuscularly, which means that trans women without access to sterile needles might be sharing them. Lack of access to both estrogen and sterile needles can further a trans woman's risk factors of acquiring HIV, hepatitis, and other bloodborne illnesses.

What Is Estrogen?

Estrogen is a hormone in the body that is responsible for a number of physical changes. It's best to think of estrogen as a growth hormone, just like testosterone. Physical characteristics of what most people think of as feminine are usually the result of estrogen. Hair, skin, fat, muscles, breasts, and sex organs are all affected by estrogen. In cis men, extra testosterone is converted into estrogen. Many clinicians are anxious about prescribing hormones that are already present in all of our bodies, but the only difference is the amount of the hormone and ultimate concentration, and this is what causes the physical effects.

Effects on the Body

The effects of estrogen on the trans female body include changes to hair, muscles, breast development, fat storage, skin, voice, and cis male sex organs (Figures 15–1 and 15–2).

Hair

One of the main benefits of estrogen is its effect on body hair. Many women of trans experience are happy to see that their body hair becomes softer and thinner. This is likely due to combined treatment with spironolactone. Some

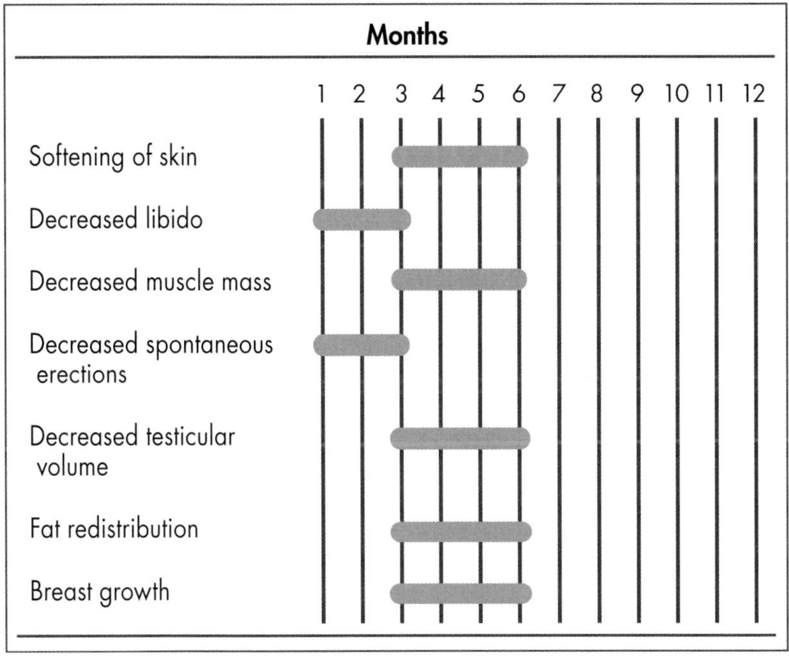

FIGURE 15–1. Onset of effects of estrogen in hormone therapy.
Source. Hembree et al. 2009.

trans women will say the parts of their body that used to be hairier have thinned out or stopped producing noticeable hair altogether. Chest and stomach hair becomes sparser, and hair on the legs becomes thinner, softer, and easier to shave (Ettner et al. 2016). Regarding the scalp, there are reports that women of trans experience who were previously balding showed some scalp hair regrowth after starting estrogen and spironolactone (Stevenson et al. 2016).

The beard or facial hair, however, is a bit more complicated. In most people, it doesn't seem to respond to either the addition of estrogen or the blocking of testosterone. For many trans women, this will be a source of dysphoria and frustration, as the presence of facial hair is a classic automatic signal to onlookers' brains that they are talking to a male. Depending on the person's genetic makeup, facial hair can grow fast, thick, and dark. This will require daily, and sometimes twice daily, maintenance to prevent any facial hair from showing. Electrolysis potentially can provide relief, but it can be expensive and is rarely paid for by insurance, and some people respond better to electrolysis than others. Patients may become distressed over the continued presence of facial hair, and their mental health clinicians should

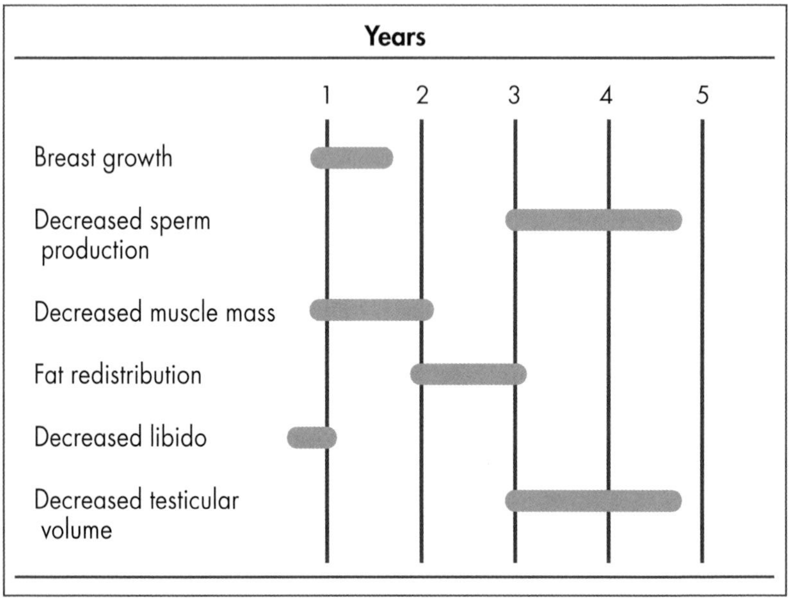

FIGURE 15–2. Maximum effects of estrogen in hormone therapy.
Source. Hembree et al. 2009.

inform them that this occurrence is a common one within women of trans experience and that it isn't related to hormones or dosing.

Muscles

In cis women, muscles typically aren't as defined as with cis men. The softness and roundness to the shape of the body represent a more classic feminine physique. Although current society might encourage muscle development and being toned, many women of trans experience are pleased when their arms and legs become rounder and less defined. They report it makes them feel more feminine and decreases dysphoric feelings. Muscles themselves become softer and less bulky. These are typically considered positive results of estrogen treatment and what many are aiming to achieve by taking estrogen.

Breast Development

Estrogen is well known to cause breast growth in cis women and women of trans experience. The amount of breast growth can highly depend on the person, their body type, and how long they have been taking estrogen. The amount of breast growth can be described as moderate. Some people may experience a large amount of breast growth; others might not. The younger a person is when starting estrogen and initiating the suppression of testosterone, the better the results. It usually takes up to 2 years to have the full effects of estrogen on the breasts, and after 2 years there will likely be no further growth (Maycock and Kennedy 2014).

Insurance companies are still quick to deny top surgery for trans women, saying the surgery is unnecessary. They claim that estrogen causes breast growth, and this should be sufficient. However, every woman of trans experience responds differently to estrogen, and the amount of distress that occurs from not having breasts can be psychiatrically significant. What an insurance company might claim is an elective procedure could be crucial for a woman of trans experience who has gender dysphoria.

Fat

Estrogen has been identified as what leads to a more pear-shaped body or hourglass figure in cis women. Estrogen increases fat storage in the body, and the collection of more fat deposits under the skin makes the body rounder and softer. Some people report specifically that the face, arms, and shoulders are affected. With estrogen present, fat is moved away from the stomach area and more to the hips and thighs. Each person responds differently over time, but the effects of estrogen can add extra dimension to what is thought of as feminine body features. The overall body mass index of women of trans experience seems to stay unchanged from estrogen over time (Deutsch et al. 2015).

Skin

Just as testosterone is responsible for making the skin oilier and can cause acne, estrogen can dry out the skin and give it a softer appearance. Women of trans experience taking estrogen report these changes over months to years but typically are happy with the result.

Voice

It's pretty clear that estrogen has no effect on the voice. Testosterone can drop the voice in pitch over time, which happens when the vocal cords lengthen. However, estrogen cannot shorten the vocal cords and thus will have no effect on the pitch of a person's voice. Many women of trans experience seek either voice training or surgical intervention to change the timbre of their voice.

Cis Male Sex Organs

The presence of estrogen can cause particular changes in cis male sex organs. The testicles have been noted to shrink in size, and the production of testosterone decreases and potentially stops. The prostate also gets smaller.

The only potential unwanted effect that this can cause is that the prostate surrounds part of the bladder, so shrinking of the prostate can lead to mild incontinence, which has been reported to improve over the course of 1 year of treatment (Ettner et al. 2016).

Case Example

Patricia is a 36-year-old woman of trans experience. She grew up in the deep South and spent most of her life working in construction. As a teenager, she worked in the family business and became skilled in several aspects of construction, including electrical systems, plumbing, and painting. She is quite good at these skills and continues to make a living that way.

Because Patricia has worked so many years in construction, she has developed a muscular physique. All the bending, lifting, and hard labor caused her to naturally develop a muscular body. Although she was quite a skilled laborer, she had a difficult time with substance abuse, particularly alcohol. For several years, she used alcohol to suppress the fact that she knew she was really a woman and had been born in a body that doesn't reflect that. She had problems with binge drinking, blackouts, and tremors from withdrawal.

Around the age of 32, Patricia became sober and told her friends and family her gender identity. Neither family nor friends were accepting of this, and they told her that they didn't believe it because she had never said anything before. Patricia, like many other TGNC people, had had to hide her true gender identity out of fear of isolation, abandonment, and even the threat of death. Had she revealed herself to be a woman of trans experience earlier in her life, she may have been attacked or killed by people in her small community. She described herself as a "professional" at convincing others she was a man.

Patricia started to seek treatment in the closest city she could find. It was a 4-hour drive, but she was willing to commute to the city to get trans-affirming care. She started taking estrogen and received supportive psychotherapy to provide her with validating treatment given the lack of understanding in the community in which she lived.

After starting the estrogen, Patricia began dressing in more feminine clothes, grew out her hair, and changed the tone of her voice with practice. She could express her femininity while at her doctor's office or with her therapist, but otherwise she had to go back to her more masculine persona when she was back with her family and friends. This lasted only so long, however, and Patricia started wearing more feminine clothes to work, with her long hair visible from under the hat she used to hide it. Her coworkers also noticed her voice changing and made fun of her, calling her a "sissy."

Over time, estrogen started to change Patricia's body. Although she remained somewhat muscular in build, her body became less defined. She grew wider in the hips and took on a slightly hourglass shape. Her skin became softer, and she noticed less hair all over her body. She had never really grown much facial hair, so she was happy that frequent shaving was not a problem. She still had symptoms of dysphoria, however, because her face remained mostly unchanged. She was hoping the effects of estrogen would soften her facial features, but after 3 years of treatment, there were no major changes to her jawline or the shape of her face overall.

Patricia had a difficult time staying with the estrogen treatment. Her regimen required her to get an intramuscular injection every 2 weeks. Given that she had to drive several hours each way, she attempted to schedule visits with her primary care doctor, therapist, and nurse all on the same day. She had to ask for time off work every 2 weeks, and her boss became rather frustrated at her absences. He also figured out where she was going given her changes over time, and the reason for her absences only made him angrier.

Patricia had previously been known as Paul, and her coworkers and friends continued to call her Paul. Patricia wore women's clothing to work, wore her hair down, and spoke in a more feminine voice. When she and her coworkers went to restaurants, the wait staff who came to know her called her Patricia and used the pronoun she, but her coworkers and boss continued to misgender her and use the incorrect name. It created confusion with the wait staff and others she met because they saw her as female and thought her coworkers were playing a joke.

Patricia was happy overall with the effects of hormone treatment. Estrogen helped change her body in ways that made her feel more feminine. Although it didn't change her appearance as much as she had hoped, she was still enjoying the changes it did make, which helped her body feel more in touch with the Patricia she had always known herself to be.

Effects on the Mind

Estrogen has very complicated effects on the brain and mind overall. Although the details of these effects are too numerous to review, there are large changes that take place in patients receiving estrogen, and familiarity with these changes is important when working with TGNC people.

Estrogen has effects on a trans woman's mood. Some say that it leads to more depressive symptoms. Others say it has more of an antidepressant effect. In a general sense, the presence of estrogen does seem to result in the person receiving it feeling more emotions. Some patients might report being more tearful at times or being aware of their feelings more. However, there are many women of trans experience who notice no mood changes, and they might even describe themselves as less emotional after starting hormone therapy. Although some of these changes might be stereotypical in nature, there is a common theme, and the complex effects of estrogen on the brain remain complicated and specific to an individual's genetic makeup. There is very little to no research on this topic, and much of what is known is either from direct patient feedback or online communities and blogs.

With the increase of estrogen in the system, there is a decrease in testosterone. A decrease in testosterone can lead to a decrease in sex drive. Some trans women have reported that their attraction toward individuals changes. Before they started taking estrogen, their physical attraction had been more visually based, whereas after taking estrogen, they noticed that they became attracted to different aspects of their love interest and that the emotional relationship with their partners became more pronounced. For some people, even a low-dose testosterone replacement may be needed to help with sexual interest. Although this is not true for every trans woman taking estrogen, it is an interesting phenomenon related to hormones in general (Ettner et al. 2016).

Monitoring

TGNC people who want to start hormone therapy should first have baseline lab work done, including blood counts, liver and renal function, lipid levels, and glucose. The main potential side effect of estrogen use is blood clots. Just as with a cis woman taking birth control medication, the presence of estrogen could potentially lead to blood clots. The actual occurrence of these clots is low, and risk factors such as smoking or family history should be taken into account (Ott et al. 2010). Women of trans experience who are older or have a history of clotting might require extra monitoring and lower levels of estrogen.

There is also concern that estrogen might increase the risk of tumors and breast cancer (Ettner et al. 2016). However, although there is evidence that women of trans experience who take estrogen have a higher chance than their cis male counterparts of developing breast cancer, they do not have the same risk as a cis female. Nevertheless, women of trans experience taking estrogen should receive routine breast exams just as any cis female would.

With the drop in testosterone, sperm production also decreases. Women of trans experience who have a desire to one day have children should be counseled about sperm storage or freezing their sperm before they start hormone treatment (Maycock and Kennedy 2014). Even if estrogen is stopped in the future, there is a chance that sperm production will not start again. The cost of freezing a person's sperm is quite high, however, and many women of trans experience will not be able to afford these services.

Generally, it takes about 6 months for trans women to reach physiological levels of estrogen in their bodies (Deutsch et al. 2015). This means that after about 6 months of treatment, their estrogen and testosterone levels should mimic those of a cis female.

Forms of Estrogen

Estrogen is an umbrella term for a hormone that comes in multiple forms. Estradiol is the form that is given in hormone therapy because it is the most potent and common form found in a cis woman's body. It can be given via oral, transdermal, or intramuscular routes. Some clinicians and patients say that the transdermal route seems to best mimic a cis female's hormonal system, but patches can create irritation, fall off, and can get damaged. The intramuscular route is frequently selected just as with testosterone, and over time the patient is taught to give self-injections approximately every 2 weeks. Larger

TABLE 15–1. Monitoring guidelines for estrogen

Monitor the following prior to starting hormones and every 3 months for the first year:

- Estradiol (do not exceed 200 pg/mL)
- Testosterone (should be below 55 ng/dL)
- Electrolytes (if patient is taking spironolactone)
- Complete blood count
- Liver function tests
- Lipid profile
- Hemoglobin A1C
- Blood pressure
- Weight

After 1 year, switch to twice yearly monitoring.

Consider a bone mineral density test as needed if clinically appropriate.

Do not forget a prostate exam as clinically indicated for cis males.

Source. Adapted from Hembree et al. 2009.

doses plus the addition of spironolactone may be required in order to decrease levels of endogenous testosterone (Spack 2009). Guidelines for monitoring estrogen are provided in Table 15–1.

Informed Consent

Estrogen is not just a prescription to treat someone who is transgender; many people at multiple points on the gender spectrum may want to take estrogen for its feminizing effects. All patients who want to take estrogen should be made aware of the risk factors. Thromboembolism, or blood clots, should be covered, as well as the slightly increased chance of breast cancer. Patients also should be made aware of the potential for permanent cessation of sperm production. A thorough informed consent conversation will also cover the potential psychological effects, including decreased libido and changes in mood.

SPIRONOLACTONE

Spironolactone is most commonly known as a diuretic or water pill. It is also a testosterone blocker and is given alongside estrogen in the first 6 months of treatment. After 6 months of treatment, the levels of testosterone usually drop significantly and spironolactone is no longer needed. This is highly dependent on prescriber and patient preference. Each person will respond differently, and some may choose to remain on the medication for a longer period of time.

Given that spironolactone was originally meant to be a diuretic, an obvious side effect is dehydration. Some trans women report craving water and salt when being treated with spironolactone. It is also known as a potassium-sparing diuretic, which means higher levels of potassium might be found in the bloodstream. Regular lab work would alert the prescriber to potential side effects, and patients taking this medication should be encouraged to get regular medical follow-ups. Spironolactone is given only in oral form.

PROGESTERONE

Progesterone is the other feminizing hormone. Some clinicians even describe it as an anti-estrogen. There is debate about whether or not progesterone should be given alongside estrogen in women of trans experience. Progesterone counteracts some of the effects of estrogen, for example, reducing the risk of breast cancer or blood clots. There is also some anecdotal evidence that it helps provide an overall sense of calm and relaxation. Some patients believe that it helps with breast development and feminizing the body, but many clinicians would say that it really affects only the uterus and is not important in trans women.

SUMMARY

There are three main forms of treatment offered as hormonal or medicinal treatment to women of trans experience or any TGNC person seeking feminizing effects on the body. Estrogen, progesterone, and spironolactone can be given depending on the effects desired. Although these chemicals have been studied in detail, research into their effects on women of trans experience is severely lacking. The long-term effects as well as particular side effects of the medications need to be observed. Dosing levels and their correlation to overall physical and mental health should be studied as well. Whatever the particular effects may be, it is clear that feminizing hormones provide a great deal of psychological relief to those who are having dysphoric symptoms and wish to feminize the body.

Key Points

- Feminizing hormone treatment is basically estrogen along with spironolactone.

- The main harm that can come from hormone treatment is lack of access, not the hormone itself.
- Estrogen can have major physical and psychological effects, including changes to breast tissue, fat distribution, skin, and hair.
- Changes from estrogen take months to years.
- Feminizing hormone treatment will not have any effect on a person's voice.
- There are potential side effects to these medications, and patients should be encouraged to get regular checkups and lab work.
- It is debatable whether or not progesterone should be given along with estrogen.

QUESTIONS

1. Lorie is a 34-year-old woman of trans experience. You've been seeing her for several months, and she started hormone treatment with estrogen about the same time she began therapy with you. Although she is happy with the effects of estrogen overall, she is having continued dysphoric symptoms around her beard growth. She has to shave twice a day to hide her facial hair and is wondering how long it will take for her facial hair to stop growing. What's your response?

    A. It takes months to years for estrogen to have its full effects. Ask Lorie to be patient.
    B. Facial hair typically doesn't respond well to estrogen or spironolactone. She will likely need to seek out electrolysis.
    C. It's unclear whether or not the facial hair will respond to treatment. She should ask her primary care clinician.
    D. Lorie can use makeup to conceal her facial hair. Discuss this option with her.

2. Cherise, a 25-year-old woman of trans experience, was recently seen for a medical evaluation to start feminizing hormone treatment. She has been having agoraphobia and panic attacks because every time she leaves her apartment, kids in the neighborhood scream at her and throw rocks because they have witnessed her transition over time. In addition

to the anxiety caused by leaving her house, she is worried about some of the risk factors of estrogen treatment. She desperately wants to be taking the hormone but heard she could get breast cancer. Her mother has breast cancer. She asks you what she should do.

A. She should start estrogen. It probably won't cause breast cancer and she'll likely be just fine.
B. A history of breast cancer in the family is a contraindication to estrogen use. Break the bad news that she cannot take estrogen.
C. There is no evidence one way or another that estrogen causes breast cancer. Tell her she'll have to decide on her own with the help of her primary care clinician.
D. Although there is a slight increase in the risk of breast cancer with estrogen use, it is still well below that of the cis female population. Given her history, Cherise should alert her primary care physician and have regular breast exams. The benefits of estrogen to her will likely outweigh the risks.

3. Silvia is a 27-year-old woman of trans experience. She is seeing you to help her with an application for supportive housing but wants to know if you can help her with some questions she didn't have time to ask her primary care clinician. She started estrogen 6 months ago and is curious about how it will affect her voice over time. What's your answer?

   A. Unfortunately, estrogen probably won't have an effect. Give her referrals for voice lessons and tell her you can speak to her about her voice more in supportive therapy if she would like.
   B. Her voice will change about 1 year after starting hormones.
   C. Tell her she has to have surgery to change her voice. That's the only true option.
   D. It's unclear what will happen to her voice. More time is needed.

4. Phyllis, 47-year old woman of trans experience, recently started taking estrogen, progesterone, and spironolactone for feminizing hormone treatment. She has multiple medical problems and a history of cardiac arrhythmia in her family history. Lately, she has been experiencing intense thirst and is putting salt on all her meals. What should you tell her?

   A. It's unclear. Phyllis should go to her primary care clinician.
   B. She's probably suffering from anxiety, and that is causing the intense thirst. Give her an anxiety scale and provide cognitive-behavioral therapy.

C. It's likely that the spironolactone is causing her symptoms, and with her cardiac history she should have lab work done. Refer her to an urgent care appointment.
D. Progesterone is well known to cause intense thirst and dehydration. Tell Phyllis to stop taking it.

5. Sofia is a 33-year-old woman of trans experience who has been seeing you for 3 years for treatment of posttraumatic stress disorder secondary to a long history of physical abuse because of her gender diversity. Her symptoms have been resolving with gender-affirming treatments, and she has been taking estrogen for more than 2 years now. She is disappointed in the growth of her breasts, reporting little to no change since starting estrogen. She normally packs her bra to make herself look more feminine. Her insurance has told her that breast augmentation is not a medically necessary procedure and is not an option for her. She's unsure what steps to take next. What's your advice?

   A. After 2 years, maximal breast growth from estrogen has probably been reached. Sofia needs to be referred for surgical consultation, and her insurance should be informed that breast augmentation is a medically necessary procedure for this patient.
   B. Two years is not enough to know what will happen with breast growth. She should wait and see for a few more years.
   C. Her dose of estrogen isn't high enough. She should contact her primary care clinician and ask for an increased dose.
   D. She should receive analysis about her concern about breast size. It probably represents an internalized transphobic thought she is having.

6. Akira is a 27-year-old woman of trans experience. She is about to start estrogen but heard that it can affect sperm production. She would like to have her own biological children one day and is unsure what to do. She also wants to start taking hormones as soon as possible because she has been waiting several years to get access to a trans-affirming provider. How should you counsel her?

   A. The estrogen may affect her sperm production, but if she ever wants to have children she just needs to stop the estrogen and she will start making sperm again.
   B. She will have to decide between having a biological child and taking estrogen.

C. Estrogen doesn't affect sperm production. She will need to make a decision only when it comes time to have vaginoplasty.
D. Her sperm production will be affected, and changes may be permanent. She should be advised that freezing her sperm is an option, and she should probably decide before she starts estrogen.

ANSWERS

1. **The correct response is option B.**

   Facial hair typically doesn't respond to estrogen or spironolactone. There is no point in waiting, and Lorie's distress is due to a particular issue. Electrolysis is an option for her at this point. Advising her about makeup is inappropriate unless she asks you about it specifically.

2. **The correct response is option D.**

   Breast cancer is possible but unlikely. Explain to Cherise that her chances of getting breast cancer are very low, but to be safe she should do regular breast exams and see a primary care clinician for regular checkups.

3. **The correct response is option A.**

   The voice doesn't typically respond to estrogen. The vocal cords lengthen with testosterone, causing a deeper voice, but they can't shorten with estrogen. Although surgery is an option, a less invasive approach would be voice lessons. You should also offer to provide supportive treatments in therapy around the distress caused by her voice.

4. **The correct response is option C.**

   Spironolactone is a diuretic and can cause water loss and increased potassium levels in the blood. Given her cardiac family history, Phyllis might need a checkup and blood work just to be safe. Although this isn't an emergency, she should probably see someone urgently.

5. **The correct response is option A.**

   After 2 years of estrogen treatment, maximum breast growth has probably been reached, and the lack of further growth is not due to the dosage. Although undergoing analysis and exploring body concerns are a long-term goal, Sofia is having a not uncommon lack of breast growth from estrogen. Analyzing this concern will come across as invalidating. She should have access to breast augmentation, and your primary goal at this point is to advocate for your patient.

6. **The correct response is option D.**

   Akira should expect estrogen to affect sperm production and also expect this effect to be permanent. It is appropriate to discuss the option to freeze her sperm. Although vaginoplasty would definitely make it impossible to have a biological child, don't assume she even wants a vaginoplasty. Remember that all medications and procedures are options available to patients. Exploring her long-term plans and goals is important at this time.

REFERENCES

Deutsch MB, Bhakri V, Kubicek K: Effects of cross-sex hormone treatment on transgender women and men. Obstet Gynecol 125(3):605–610, 2015 25730222

Ettner R, Monstrey S, Coleman E (eds): Principles of Transgender Medicine and Surgery, 2nd Edition. New York, Routledge, 2016

Hembree WC, Cohen-Kettenis P, Delemarre-van de Waal HL, et al: Endocrine treatment of transsexual persons: an Endocrine Society clinical practice guideline. J Clin Endocrinol Metab 94(9):3132–3154, 2009 19509099

Maycock LB, Kennedy HP: Breast care in the transgender individual. J Midwifery Womens Health 59(1):74–81, 2014 24224502

Mepham N, Bouman WP, Arcelus J, et al: People with gender dysphoria who self-prescribe cross-sex hormones: prevalence, sources, and side effects knowledge. J Sex Med 11(12):2995–3001, 2014 25213018

Ott J, Kaufmann U, Bentz EK, et al: Incidence of thrombophilia and venous thrombosis in transsexuals under cross-sex hormone therapy. Fertil Steril 93(4):1267–1272, 2010 19200981

Spack N: An endocrine perspective on the care of transgender adolescents. J Gay Lesbian Ment Health 13(4):309–319, 2009

Stevenson M, Wixon N, Safer J: Scalp hair regrowth in hormone-treated transgender woman. Transgender Health 1(1):202–204, 2016

Part IV

Surgical and Nonsurgical Gender-Affirming Procedures

16

TRANSMASCULINE TOP SURGERY

to the little boy i never got to be, while everyone was grieving over the loss of a daughter, i still mourn for you.

FOR MEN OF trans experience, transmasculine top surgery is a common surgical option. Aesthetically, a flat chest tends to be a desire for trans men and even many gender-nonconforming or gender fluid people, although there are those who don't desire a flat chest (Figure 16–1). The dysphoric symptoms that can come with having breasts when you don't identify as female can be significant. Breast tissue starts to develop during the early stages of puberty, and as the breasts increase in size, trans men begin efforts to bind their chest to give it the appearance of being flat.

For those who don't regularly think about the presence or absence of breasts on their body, it may be surprising how frequently the chest is used as a signal for gender. Just like hair, face, and voice, the chest adds another cue that people look for when they are automatically and unconsciously assigning gender to those around them. When a person appears to be androgynous or gender neutral, I've heard comments from strangers and colleagues alike using the presence of breasts to be the deciding factor in how they assign gender. As much as people may deny it, we assign gender all day long, and a flat chest is one major cue that sends signals within our brains that say "man."

Many trans men will bring up the dysphoria around their chest from the start of treatment. Try to imagine all the situations you might be in where your chest is exposed. You can be modest in covering up your lower half, but the top half of the body being either covered or not covered is yet another cue that we use to assign gender. Trans men are put in all sorts of awkward situations in which they have to expose their chest, from high school and dorm showers to locker rooms, swimming pools, and beaches. Some will say they dislike the summer or warm

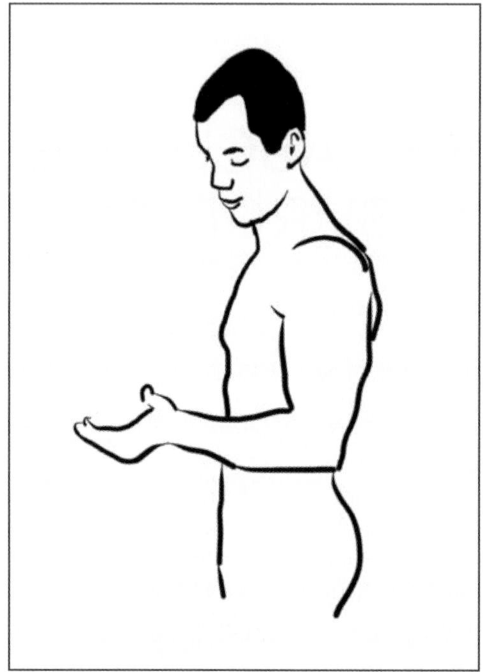

FIGURE 16–1. A flat chest generally communicates maleness.

geographic areas that require them to wear less clothing. Colder weather affords heavier clothing and more cover-up. Most adolescents in general are uncomfortable with their bodies, but a young trans man has to worry about his clothing and how it will signal his gender status to others. There is a struggle to find clothing that both sends the right signals regarding a person's gender identity and is also personally appealing and comfortable to the wearer.

BINDING

Binding is a colloquial term that describes the act of using a material to flatten or bind the chest area. The device that is used to do this is commonly called a *binder* (Figure 16–2). A binder can be made of any type of material but it is generally some form of spandex or synthetic stretchable fiber. It comes in many shapes depending on what the wearer is looking for. It can be in the form of a tank top, a T-shirt, or just a wrap that fits around the chest.

Trans men aren't the only group of people who have used binders. The "fashion" of bodies has changed throughout history, and cis women have been known to bind their breasts depending on the culture and time. In some places and times in history, it has been considered fashionable for cis women to appear flatter and not hourglass shaped. Even cis men in today's culture may wear binding garments in an effort to meet the unrealistic body expectations placed on them.

Binders are meant to be tight and worn during the day only. Wearing a binder at night or for long periods of time can be dangerous. The blood flow to the area being constricted will decrease, which can lead to fluid buildup, blood clots, dermatological conditions, and even fractured ribs (Asexual Visibility and Education Network 2017). Although binders are meant to be tight, they are not meant to be painful. The wearer should be able to breathe without discomfort, and only stretchable and breathable material should be used. Masking tape or other adhesive replacements for binders don't move with the body and can harm the wearer. Getting binders on and off can be a challenge. There are Web sites dedicated to binders and their use, and the act of binding is widely talked about in the trans male community (TransGuys.com 2017).

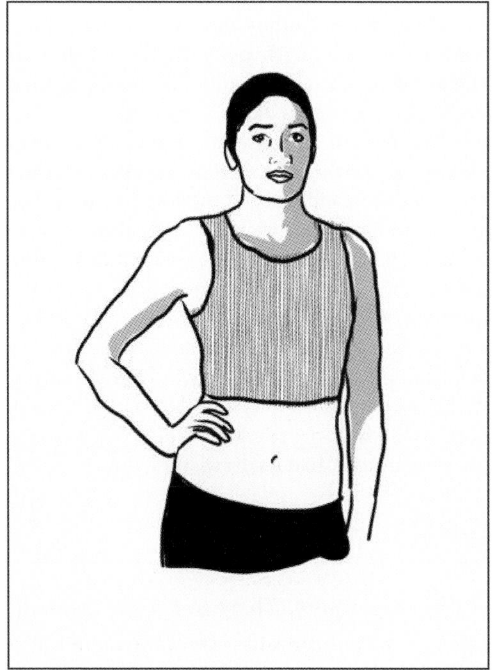

FIGURE 16–2. Example of a binder.

Case Example

Nathan is an 18-year-old man of trans experience. He identified as male from an early age and grew up in a supportive family who encouraged him to dress, play, and go by male pronouns as he saw fit. He was known by his family, friends, and teachers to be a boy throughout elementary school, and it wasn't until junior high that dysphoric symptoms started to arise. Around the age of 14, he started to have breast growth. A trans-competent provider was not available where he and his family lived, and there was no clinic to supply puberty suppression treatment. Also, Nathan's family was lower middle class, and they had little access to insurance and therefore wouldn't have been able to afford puberty suppression even if they did have access to it.

To Nathan's knowledge, there was no other trans teenager at his small suburban school. Nathan noticed that the other cis boys in his class were starting to develop facial hair, their voices were dropping, and they were becoming more muscular. As Nathan's breasts continued to get larger, he went to his mother for advice. His mother was understanding and called the lesbian, gay, bisexual, transgender, and queer/questioning (LGBTQ) center in the city closest to where they lived. She explained about her son, his concerns, and their lack of access to care. The knowledgeable LGBTQ center staff member was able to inform Nathan's mother about binding and gave her online references to read more about it.

Nathan and his mother ordered a binder from a Web site, and when it arrived he was troubled that it was so difficult to fit into. After doing more research online, he found a technique that worked for him. He found the binder to be tight but not painful. He put a shirt over it, and when he looked in the mirror he was shocked at the results. His chest had a flat appearance, and he wasn't able to see any signs of breast growth.

Nathan immediately started to have more confidence. He had previously been wearing very baggy clothes to hide his body but now wore clothing that he felt more comfortable in and liked. He still had some problems, however, including when he and his friends went to the local lake. Although his close friends were aware of his gender identity, there would also be strangers present and they would question him about why he wore a shirt when swimming. Some of the other boys at school teased him about using a stall in the restroom to change for gym class. Occasionally, his binder could be seen through his T-shirts, and acquaintances would ask him why he was wearing two layers of clothing. Nathan also noticed that during the summer months the binder was very hot and made him sweat a lot. Although it provided relief from some dysphoric symptoms, it had its drawbacks, too.

NO SURGERY

Not everyone wants top surgery. There are some trans men and gender-nonconforming people who don't care about having a flat chest. There are some who do want a flat chest, even those who bind, who would rather not have a surgical procedure. As you will learn in the following section, although top surgery is generally safe and is performed often, it is not without scarring. Top surgery for men of trans experience is an optional service just like all the other gender-affirming procedures and treatments discussed in this book. There are no rule books about which surgeries make someone more masculine that gender diverse patients need to follow. The preference of having top surgery is an individual and personal decision. In addition, clinicians should be aware of their own feelings about their patients and these procedures.

TOP SURGERY

Top surgery for a man of trans experience is the removal of breast tissue to provide a flat and traditionally masculine chest. The first known top surgery on a trans man occurred around 1940 when Dr. Michael Dillon, a physician, was able to talk a plastic surgeon into providing him with the procedure (FTM Phalloplasty 2016). Dr. Dillon had been taking testosterone and living for some time as a man, and he wanted to proceed with surgical intervention.

Since that time, top surgery has become more available. A mastectomy is the general clinical name for the removal of breast tissue; top surgery is different from a mastectomy in that top surgery leaves some breast tissue behind. With a mastectomy, most or all of the breast tissue is removed. Most surgeons know how to perform a mastectomy, but many aren't trans competent and won't do top surgery on a trans man. There are plastic surgery techniques used to shape a chest in the appearance of a cis male's chest. As you will see, these techniques change depending on the amount of breast tissue involved. In the recent past, even when trans men were able to convince a surgeon to perform the operation, they had to endure insults from and being misgendered by hospital staff, and they were treated without dignity or respect. There have been trans-affirming surgeons, but they remain few and far between.

Types of Top Surgery

When sculpting a chest to look more typically male than female, the surgeon visualizes the angle or shape of the pectoral muscle. The axilla, more commonly known as the armpit, forms an angle that places the cis male nipple in a particular location (Figure 16–3). The location and size of the nipple and size of muscle present give further cues and send automatic messages that make a chest look more traditionally male (Figure 16–4).

There are multiple types of top surgery, and they go by a handful of different names depending on the surgeon and the surgeon's particular technique. The variations of surgery can typically be summed up by what type of scarring it leaves and how much or little the areola, or pigmented tissue around the nipple, is adjusted. Which surgery is recommended is highly dependent on the amount of breast tissue present and the size of the areola. The elasticity of the skin is also taken into account and may dictate which type of surgery is recommended.

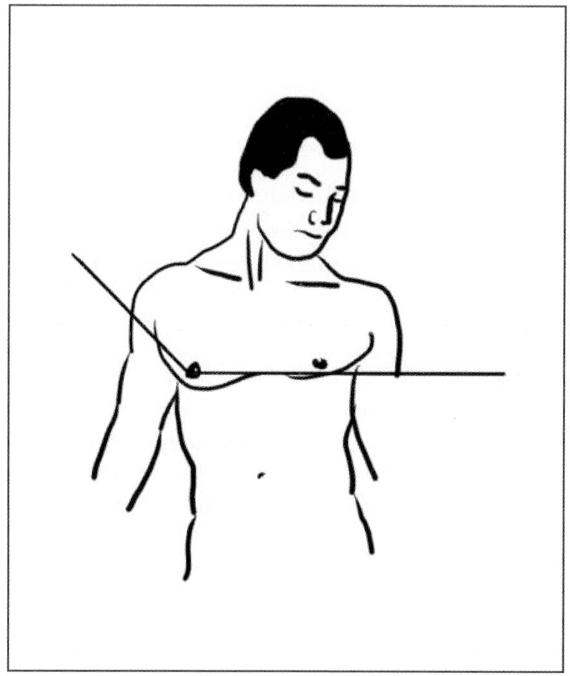

FIGURE 16–3. Cis male nipples are generally more lateral on the angle of the pectoral fold.

If there is a small amount of breast tissue and the areola is smaller than average, the surgeon my attempt what is called a semicircular technique (FTM Surgery Network 2017). This involves creating a small semicircular incision around the base of the areola (Figure 16–5). Breast tissue is removed through this small opening, and the only scar that is left is camouflaged so that any scar tissue follows the natural pattern of the areola. This technique is frequently used with cis males who have gynecomastia.

If there is a small amount of breast tissue but a larger areola, a concentric circle technique will reduce the size of the areola and confine the scarring to the area around the newly formed areola. This surgery can also be referred to as a periareolar technique.

Larger amounts of breast tissue will require a more extensive procedure in which more tissue is removed, needing larger incisions. Larger incisions lead to more scarring. These surgeries are generally divided on the basis of how the nipple is positioned. Some surgeries keep the nipple attached to its blood supply and nervous tissue (Figure 16–6). This maintains sensation. The T-anchor and buttonhole techniques both accomplish this (FTM Surgery

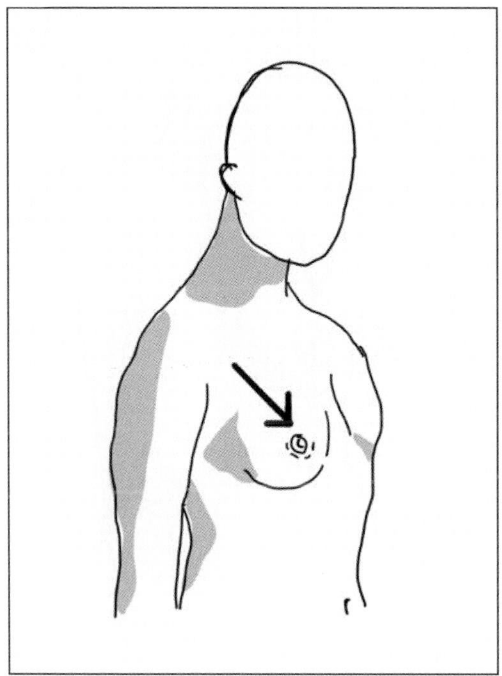

FIGURE 16–4. The areola of a cis man is generally smaller than that of a cis woman (as indicated by the dashed line).

Network 2017). In the T-anchor technique, the surgeon uses a T-shaped incision to cut around and lift the nipple into position. In the buttonhole technique, the surgeon cuts a hole in the newly sculpted chest where the nipple should be and brings the attached nipple up to this hole from underneath, just like a button on a shirt.

The free nipple graft technique can also be used if there is a large amount of breast tissue. In this technique, the surgeon first removes the nipple from its nervous tissue and blood supply. The nipple and areola are resized and grafted into location (Figure 16–7). Because the nerve supply is cut, there is no sensation. The remaining scar can be quite noticeable, especially in the year following surgery. Because of the size of the incision, the amount of time spent in the operating room can be reduced.

Case Example (*Continued*)

When Nathan turned 18 years old, he decided to have top surgery. He had been taking testosterone for several years and was ready to stop binding. Luckily, he had moved to a larger city for college and found a local surgeon

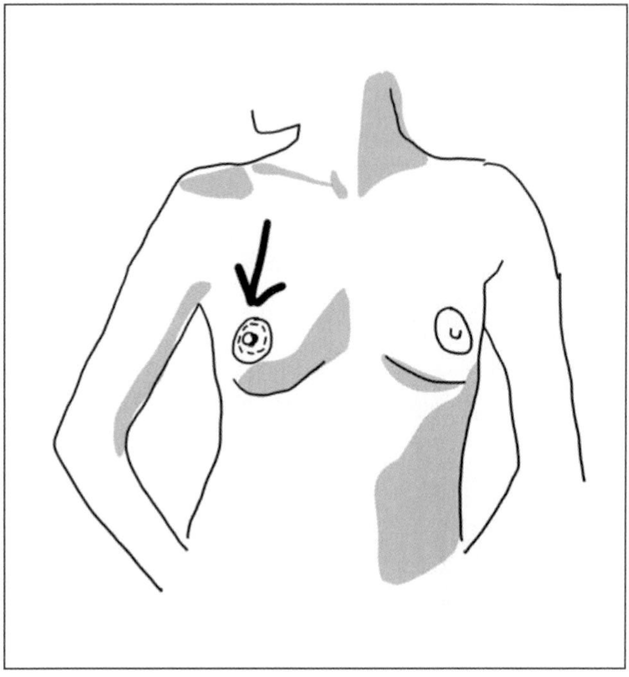

FIGURE 16–5. The incision location when removing a smaller amount of breast tissue.

who was known to provide top surgeries to trans men. After consultation, the surgeon recommended the T-anchor technique because of the amount of breast tissue present. The surgeon also said he would resize the areola.

Nathan's mother traveled to meet him the day of the surgery in order to take him back home for rest and recovery. While Nathan was being admitted to the hospital the morning of surgery, the intake staff kept referring to him as Natalie because that was the name on his insurance card. Despite repeated correction, the staff continued to call him Natalie and addressed him by the pronoun she. Nathan was already anxious about the operation, and now he was hurt that the staff wouldn't use his correct name. Even though a surgeon agrees to a procedure, the trans-sensitivity of staff cannot be guaranteed.

After the operation, Nathan awoke in recovery to a nurse still calling him Natalie. He was sedated and had tubes coming out of the bandages wrapped around his chest. He had expected this, but with the combination of the nurse calling him by the wrong name, the bandages, and the tubes, he felt more isolated. Once he was alert and there was no major bleeding, Nathan was allowed to leave with his mother. On the long car ride home, neither of them talked about the experience at the hospital. Nathan was glad that the day was over.

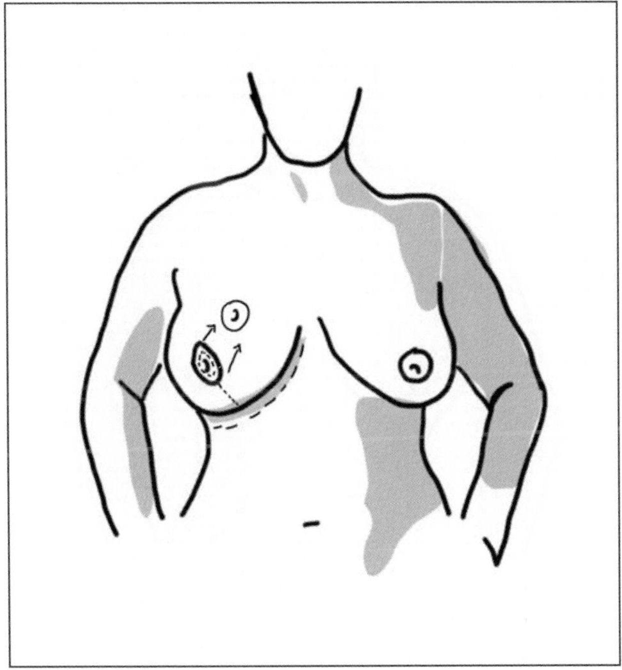

FIGURE 16–6. **With the T-anchor and buttonhole techniques, the nipple remains attached to its blood supply and is moved up into a new position through the surgical opening.**

Surgical Follow-Up

After top surgery, the recovery time can last from around 2 weeks to a month. It is usually recommended that patients take at least 2 weeks off work. Many people report that they have a significant decrease in the range of motion in their arms following surgery, and it is difficult for them to take care of activities of daily living, such as bathing or going to the bathroom. Help from someone they trust is generally needed. Pain can be an issue, but it highly depends on the person. Tubing is often placed at a small hole at the end of each incision to remove excess fluid (Figure 16–8). These drains are necessary but can be a challenge during recovery. In some rare cases, a hematoma or collection of blood can form under the incisions, and urgent medical care to drain the site may be needed.

At the follow-up visit with the surgeon, the drains are removed and the dressing is taken off. This is also an anxiety-producing visit, but one mixed with excitement at seeing the results of the surgery. There are some stitches in place that need to be removed before taking the drains out, and both re-

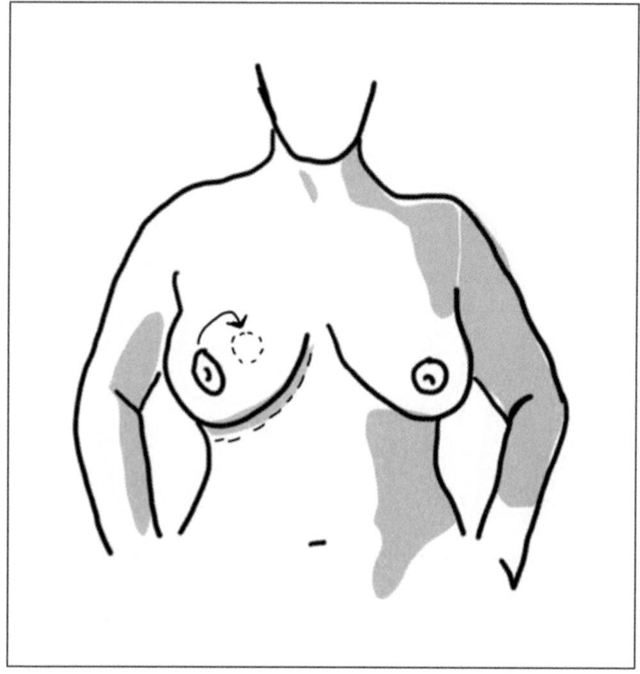

FIGURE 16–7. With the free nipple graft technique, the nipple is removed from its blood supply and grafted back onto a new location.

moving the stitches and taking out the drains are generally painless. Some patients report that removal of the bandages actually is more painful because they can stick to hair on the chest or under the arms.

Scarring will be more visible and will look red and inflamed in the beginning. It can take months to years for the scarring to fade. The amount of scarring and how visible it is will again depend on the person, their skin type, and what type of surgery was performed. In general, people are very happy with the results, and top surgery for trans men tends to be one of the more successful procedures that helps with gender dysphoric symptoms.

Case Example (*Continued*)

Nathan was able to find a surgeon near his parents' house to remove the drains and bandages. Although it was somewhat painful to have the wrapping taken off, any discomfort was overshadowed by the happiness he experienced when he saw the results of his surgery. In the following weeks, Nathan noticed that his scars started to heal. He wasn't wearing a binder anymore and was comfortable in his clothing. His friends noticed his increased confidence. The scars took some time to start to fade. It was about a year be-

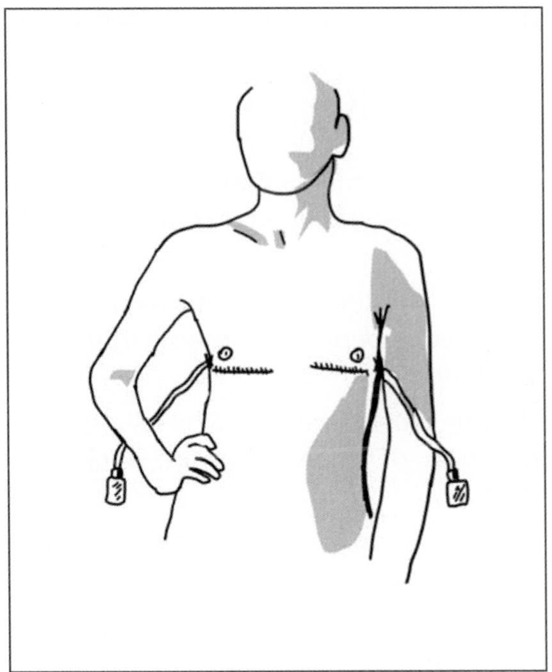

FIGURE 16–8. Drainage tubes are left in for at least a week after top surgery.

fore Nathan felt comfortable going without a shirt in front of strangers. When people asked him about his scars, he had trouble coming up with a reason as to why they were there. Overall, he was very satisfied with the results and began volunteering with the local LGBTQ center to help educate staff at medical facilities about pronouns and basic trans competency.

SUMMARY

Top surgery for trans men is a very common procedure. Prior to having surgery, many trans men decide to use binders as a way to flatten their chest. Although binding is mostly safe, you may need to review basic practices with your patients. Should a patient elect to have top surgery, the technique used will depend on the amount of breast tissue present. It is also important to find a trans-competent surgeon who has knowledgeable staff. Follow-up to top surgery can be painful for some patients. Scarring can be extensive depending on the procedure used, but it generally fades over time. Patients need to be prepared for these situations, and discussions should take place around the scarring and how the patient will explain it to strangers if they ask. Patients also may choose not to explain the scarring, but they should have a way to remove themselves from situations that may feel unsafe.

Key Points

- Top surgery for men of trans experience is the removal of breast tissue and reshaping of the chest region.
- Binding, in which tight garments made of spandex or other synthetic fibers are worn to flatten the chest, is a common practice in trans men.
- Binding can provide beneficial results if worn safely, but the length of time binders are worn daily should be limited.
- Top surgery is an optional procedure and not a requirement for anyone getting gender-affirming care.
- There are several techniques for top surgery, depending on the amount of breast tissue present and the size of the areola.
- After top surgery, patients will need help during the recovery process because mobility of their arms can be limited.
- Scarring can be mild to extensive depending on the surgery.

QUESTIONS

1. Jacob is a 15-year-old teenage boy of trans experience. He has been having symptoms of gender dysphoria for several years but has had to keep his gender identity hidden from his parents and most of his friends at school. He lives in an area where multiple trans-identified people have been assaulted, and his parents would likely disown him if he outed himself to them. You've been seeing him for therapy, which his parents understand to be focused around depression. Jacob does have symptoms of depression, but he has also been confiding in you his gender identity. He said he read online about binders and had a spandex one delivered to a

friend's house. He was excited about wearing it and the relief it brings him and would like to keep it on all the time. What would you advise?

A. Jacob probably shouldn't be wearing a binder without discussing it with his parents first. Explain to him that he should not be wearing it.
B. You tell him you support his decisions around his gender identity but want to make sure he is safe. Explain to him that binders should be worn only for limited periods and should never be slept in.
C. Binders can cause severe physical problems and should never be worn.
D. If Jacob is wanting to wear a binder, he should probably come out as trans and let all his friends, teachers, and family know about his identity.

2. Seth is a 19-year-old man of trans experience who comes to see you in an outpatient clinic after being referred for a top surgery consultation. When you ask him about the procedure, he understands the risks and benefits and can't wait to stop binding. He has been using duct tape for periods of time because he had access to some from his father's garage. What concerns do you have about his binding?

A. Tape is a realistic replacement for spandex or fiber binders when they are unavailable.
B. Seth shouldn't be using tape to bind. It can cause rashes on his skin, although there are no other major concerns.
C. Binding shouldn't be done before surgery. In addition, it is meant more for younger people of trans experience.
D. Using a material like duct tape to bind can be very dangerous. It can cause fluid collection and even broken ribs in some cases because it doesn't move with the body.

3. Gregory is a 21-year-old man of trans experience. He has been seeing you in therapy for more than a year and is planning to have top surgery in the coming months. He has been reading online about the different procedures. He says that he has a large amount of breast tissue and will probably need to have his areola resized. Given this information, which surgical technique do you think his surgeon will opt for?

A. Semicircular technique.
B. Periareolar technique.
C. Buttonhole technique.
D. Radical mastectomy.

4. Sean is a 28-year-old trans man who found it hard to understand his gender identity and sexual orientation. Because he was raised and went to school with no identified out TGNC people, he wasn't sure how to explain his feelings that he was born a boy. Over time and with therapy, he was able to identify his feelings and slowly came out as a trans man. Over the course of 2 years, he started testosterone and wanted to have top surgery. The surgeon used a T-anchor technique, and after surgery, Sean is distressed about the scarring the surgery produced. The scars are red and inflamed, and Sean wonders how people wouldn't know what surgery he has undergone just by seeing the incisions. How should you counsel Sean?

   A. Help Sean process his ideas about the surgery and scarring. Tell him the scars will likely fade, but time will tell.
   B. Remind Sean that the scars were a consequence of the operation and he was informed of them being a certainty.
   C. Brush off the scars as nothing important and emphasize that he should focus on the progress he has made.
   D. Tell him the surgeon probably botched the surgery and he should seek legal counsel.

5. Why is tubing generally left in both sides after top surgery?

   A. It prevents the skin from puckering.
   B. It allows the scars to heal better.
   C. It drains excess fluid buildup from the surgery.
   D. Drainage is collected and tested for infections.

ANSWERS

1. The correct response is option B.

Jacob has made it clear he doesn't want to inform his parents about the binder. Asking him to out himself before he is ready, to his family, friends, or teachers, would not be helpful and could be potentially dangerous. Binders are safe when used correctly and can provide a great deal of relief of gender dysphoria. Support Jacob's choice and discuss the safe use of a binder.

2. **The correct response is option D.**

    Binders are safe when made of the right material. They need to fit snugly but move with the body. Using tape can constrict the body and even lead to severe complications such as broken ribs. If a patient informs you they have been using tape, explain to them the possible risks.

3. **The correct response is option C.**

    The buttonhole technique is a good choice for patients with a larger amount of breast tissue and a need to resize the areola. The semicircular and periareolar techniques are for patients with less breast tissue. Radical mastectomy wasn't covered in this chapter but is used more for treatment of breast cancer.

4. **The correct response is option A.**

    Sean is in distress over the scarring from the surgery. He needs time to process his feelings and get supportive interventions. Those interventions can involve you explaining what you know about the healing process and that scars can fade over time. It's important to remain empathic and knowledgeable. Scarring is a well-known result of the procedure. Referring Sean to legal counsel would only complicate the issue.

5. **The correct response is option C.**

    Tubing is generally left in place following top surgery in order to drain excess fluid from the surgery sites. These drains are typically taken out after 2 weeks in a surgical follow-up visit.

REFERENCES

Asexual Visibility and Education Network: All about binders. The Asexual Visibility and Education Network. Available at: www.asexuality.org/en/topic/47170-all-about-binders/. Accessed May 16, 2017.

FTM Phalloplasty: The first transsexual phalloplasty, 2016. Available at: http://ftmphalloplasty.tumblr.com/post/132288782293/first-transsexual-phalloplasty. Accessed May 16, 2017.

FTM Surgery Network: FTM top surgery guide, 2017. Available at: www.topsurgery.net. Accessed May 16, 2017.

TransGuys.com: Chest binding 101—updated for 2017. Updated July 7, 2017. Available at: http://transguys.com/features/chest-binding. Accessed December 1, 2017.

17

TRANSFEMININE TOP SURGERY

People always ask me if they're mine. Yes, they are...all bought and paid for.

Dolly Parton

TOP SURGERY for a woman of trans experience is usually defined as breast augmentation or breast implants. Just like top surgery for trans men, top surgery for trans women is a commonly elected procedure that leads to positive results in most cases. Many trans women are happy with the surgery, and the benefits of the procedure generally far outweigh the risks.

In thinking about the general shape of binary men and women, the presence of breasts, especially in a person who is thinner, sends an automatic unconscious signal of female. For women of trans experience, having breasts is a daily reminder of their femininity. Many trans women report that although they appear to be female in the way they dress, wear their hair and makeup, and interact with people, it's still very painful at the end of the day to look into a mirror with no clothing on and see a flat chest. The lack of breast tissue is dysphoric in many trans women, and many who don't have access to breast augmentation will pad a bra with socks or other materials to give the appearance of breasts. Cis women have also been stuffing and padding their bras surely as long as bras have existed.

Why do cis women have breasts? The presence of breasts is a sign not only of a woman's femininity but also her fertility. Ancient statues, like the Venus of Willendorf from the Paleolithic period, indicate that certain cultures place value on large breasts as a sign of fertility (Figure 17–1). Depending on the era and culture, larger breasts mean a woman is more womanly. Today, the size, shape, and amount of cleavage a woman has are under scrutiny, with unrealistic images of perfectly shaped large breasts saturating advertisements, movies, and pornography.

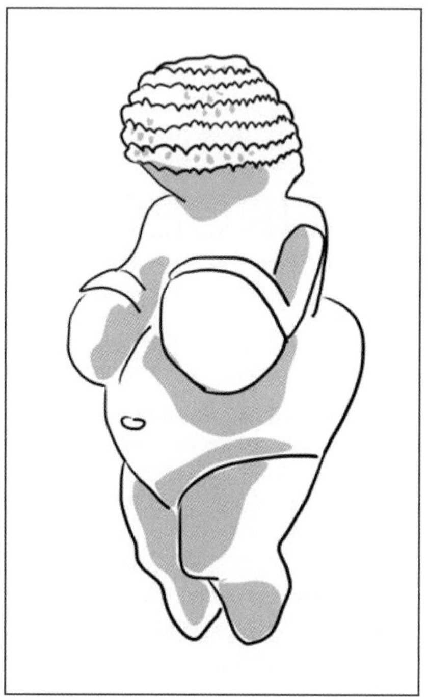

FIGURE 17–1. Ancient image of the female body.

It is thought that breasts developed to larger sizes after people started to walk upright. The formation of the breasts served several purposes. First, they are a place to store fat. Women of child-bearing age need extra calories in order to breastfeed their young. Breasts also provide a place to store milk and can change in size after childbirth to accommodate breastfeeding. Last, from a sexual arousal standpoint, it is hypothesized that breasts mimic the buttocks. When prehumans walked on all fours, sexual arousal, as in much of the animal kingdom, would occur from approaching someone from behind. Over time, as humans started to walk on two legs, that changed, and face-to-face attraction and arousal started to take precedence. Since attraction needed to happen from the front, larger breasts would mimic the buttocks as seen from the back, thus attracting mates (Shlain 2014).

Given this brief survey of evolutionary breast development, it is easy to understand why women of trans experience can have dysphoric symptoms around having a flat chest. They sometimes describe themselves as feeling less womanly or even as an imposter for using padding. Whatever the particular reason, many trans women opt for top surgery, and the results usually leave them very satisfied (Weigert et al. 2013).

NO SURGERY

Just because parts of society link the importance of breast size to femininity, that does not mean all transgender and gender-nonconforming (TGNC) people feel the need or want to have top surgery. Gender continues to be present on a spectrum and is not a binary, so a person may identify as female and choose not to have any surgical procedures, including breast augmentation. In addition, estrogen used for medicinal treatment and hormone therapy will create a small amount of breast tissue, and this may be perfectly adequate for some people. Remember that breast augmentation is an option available for TGNC people but is not a requirement.

PUMPING PARTIES

Top surgery for women of trans experience can be expensive. Only recently have insurance and managed care companies started paying for the procedure. For many trans women, having breast augmentation is not possible. This might be due to lack of insurance coverage or lack of access to care. Those who greatly desire to have breasts and do not have access to a surgeon might turn to a more dangerous means to reach their goals.

Pumping parties is a colloquial term referring to events in which people obtain commercially available products and inject them into their bodies in order to achieve a desired physical shape. Silicone is found in certain products that are easily purchased and then injected into the face, breasts, buttocks, or other places depending on personal preference. Cis women have also been known to do this, and some cis men inject silicone in order to increase penis girth. Other oily substances such as olive oil have been used as well.

Although some people might tell you that the injection of silicone has helped them reach their desired body goals, the process is very dangerous and can be deadly (Murariu et al. 2015). Breasts that have been "pumped" with silicone can eventually become hard and appear to have nodules. Some even get to the point that the skin stretches and has what is known as a peau d'orange (skin of an orange) appearance. It can also give the skin a rough leathery appearance. The silicone may travel to different parts of the body such as the heart and lungs and do irreparable harm.

Mental health professionals should readily talk to their patients, particularly women of trans experience, about pumping parties. Patients should be warned of the risks and long-term complications. The risks far outweigh the benefits, and it is a practice that should be discouraged. The presence of pumping parties only further illustrates the need for increased insurance coverage of gender-affirming procedures. There are multiple reasons why trans women would want to have breast tissue, the most common being dysphoric symptoms around their body. TGNC people should be given safe options for treatment so that they don't need to resort to injecting silicone to reach their desired state.

Case Example

Amy is a 42-year-old woman of trans experience. She previously served in the military and lived most of her life with a secret that she knew from an early age: she was a woman and always had been. She went into the military as reaction to her true feelings and thought that maybe a very "manly" job would help her overcome her feelings of being female.

Around the age of 37, Amy started to slowly come out as transgender and started to dress in female clothing and grow her hair out. She had moved from a job in the military to a job in construction and was still having a difficult time processing her gender identity. When she was asked in detail about it, the core of her ambivalence was around her parents not being accepting. She had attempted to have the conversation at one point, but her parents made it very clear that they disapproved of her gender identity and that if she wanted to remain part of the family, she should drop the discussion.

Amy grew out her hair but kept it up in a hat when she visited her parents. She did the same with clothing, wearing typical male attire when she was around her parents. When with her support network, however, she let her hair down, put on makeup, and wore dresses. She had a group of TGNC-identified friends who provided her with emotional support and became her family of choice.

Amy had symptoms of major depression secondary to years of a repressed gender identity. These symptoms included insomnia, depressed mood, lack of energy, hopelessness, and occasional thoughts of death with no plan or intent to hurt herself. She was attending sessions at a local LGBTQ clinic and found the people there to be affirming and helpful. Her therapist had discussed surgical options with her, and Amy was particularly interested in top surgery. She reported that seeing herself in the mirror every morning and evening was somewhat traumatizing because it was a reminder of her past, her family's disapproval, and her continued feelings of not feeling feminine enough.

BREAST AUGMENTATION

Breast augmentation is a surgical procedure that has been around since the late nineteenth century. For a long time, cis women have had either body fat or implants to repair their breasts for medical reasons such as cancer treatment or for purely aesthetic choices. The first implants were used in the 1960s and are typically made of either silicone or saline. Silicone implants are generally preferred because of a more natural feel, although saline is thought to be safer in the rare event of an implant rupture. Implants can be spherical in shape or elongated and tapered to produce a more natural shape.

Implants range in size from around 200 cc to 400 cc or more. One study found that between 1976 and 1996, the average size of breast implants doubled (Weigert et al. 2013). The size of the implants will come up in sessions, and trans women may want to opt for a larger breast size in order to feel more feminine. This is not always the safest option, however, and the size of a person's implants will depend on overall body type; body mass index; skin elasticity; and, for trans women, the amount of breast tissue that developed during hormone treatment. Larger breasts may lead to stretching and even back pain from carrying the extra weight. When discussing breast size with women of trans experience, it is important to have them visualize not what the perfect woman would like on the basis of cultural and media standards but how they would appear if breasts had developed on their body during puberty. As a mental health professional, you should try to have your patients think about the outcomes from all angles. Whatever decision the patient and surgeon agree on, it needs to be well informed.

The actual operation is most commonly an outpatient procedure with a quick recovery time. The placement of the incision is in such a place that it falls under the inframammary fold and is concealed in the end result. A skilled surgeon will place particular emphasis on aligning the size of the breasts as well as where the nipples fall. Patients are raised to a sitting position midoperation to give the surgeon an idea of how the breasts will appear when the patient is standing up. Slight differences in the symmetry of the breasts or the nipple placement can be very noticeable. Because of this, the implant might be placed either under the glands of the breast or even under the pectoral muscles to hold it in place (Figure 17–2) (Maycock and Kennedy 2014). Placement of the implants will depend on the surgeon's preference as well as the person's body type.

Recovery after the operation can be just a few weeks, but there are some potential complications. Ruptures are rare, and if they occur, they will be different depending on whether the implant is saline or silicone. Saline deflates and is reabsorbed into the body. A silicone implant can rupture or leak and spread to surrounding tissue, most commonly the axilla. The leaked silicone may lead to granulomas, or collections of inflammation tissue, or it could spread to other parts of the body as described in the previous section, "Pumping Parties." Another somewhat rare complication occurs when the implants cause physical stimulation of the intercostal nerves, leading to galactorrhea, or breast milk production. Your patients may be more likely to discuss complications they are experiencing in a therapy session with you rather than in a hurried surgical follow-up. Don't hesitate to ask them questions about their experience and reconnect them to medical or surgical treatment if necessary.

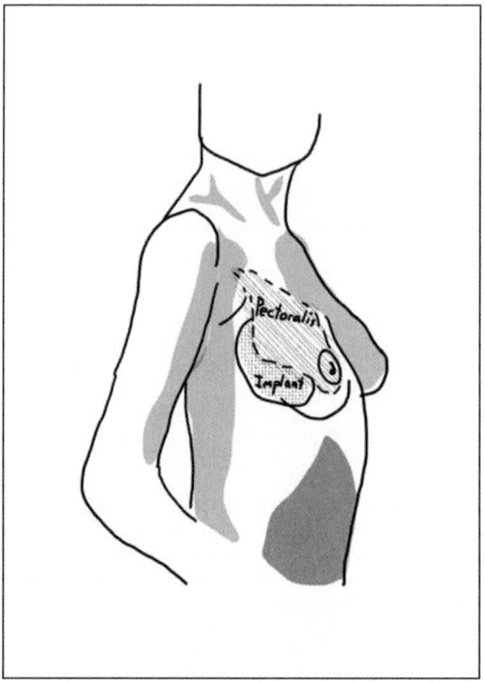

FIGURE 17–2. Implants are frequently placed under the pectoral muscle.

Case Example (*Continued*)

Amy asked her therapist to write a letter advocating for her to get top surgery. She had been taking estrogen for more than 3 years at the time she requested the procedure and had minimal breast tissue growth. Her insurance company initially rejected the request, saying that breast augmentation isn't a necessary treatment for trans women and that hormone treatment is enough. Amy's therapist, psychiatrist, and primary care physician provided support letters to say that minimal tissue growth had occurred with hormone treatment and that breast augmentation was necessary to help with symptoms of gender dysphoria. The insurance company rejected the claim again, saying that the patient's gender marker was female on the insurance card and breast augmentation was a purely cosmetic procedure. Amy was frustrated with the entire process and become more despondent and depressed because her cis female friend had had a mastectomy after a diagnosis of breast cancer and was able to get augmentation without her primary care doctor's approval or letters from mental health professionals. Amy was experiencing discrimination within the health care system, and her suicidal thoughts increased with the idea that her body would never be in line with who she has felt to be for so long.

With the help of case management and further support letters from her treatment team, Amy was finally approved for top surgery. She discussed with her surgeon the right type of implant and size and found her recovery to be only somewhat painful. She was very happy with the results and found it easier to look in the mirror every day. The presence of breasts gave her confidence and helped her to feel more feminine. Amy continued to have other stressors, however, because her parents continued to refuse to refer to her as female, use appropriate pronouns, or call her their daughter despite the fact that Amy now showed up in female attire with her hair down. The rest of the world saw Amy as female, but her parents continued to insist on calling her Alex, their son.

SUMMARY

Breast augmentation is a common procedure that has been around for more than a century. It is readily available to cis women without any mental health evaluation requirements. Trans women are required to go through multiple steps to get top surgery, and insurance companies will frequently deny approval of the procedure for multiple reasons. Some women of trans experience may choose not to have top surgery, but for those who do it is important to discuss with them the size and type of implants, making sure they understand potential risks and benefits.

Key Points

- Top surgery for women of trans experience is breast augmentation.
- Top surgery is not for everyone and isn't a requirement in the treatment of women of trans experience.
- Pumping parties are when people without access to care obtain silicone from commercially available products and inject it into their body to change their shape. It is dangerous and can lead to death.
- The size and type of implant should be discussed with patients who are seeking top surgery.
- Potential complications include rupture of the implant or galactorrhea from intercostal nerve stimulation.
- Patients may need advocacy on the part of their mental health professional in order to get their insurance company to approve top surgery.

QUESTIONS

1. Rhonda is a 22-year-old woman of trans experience. She has been coming to therapy for the past 6 months for help with symptoms of post-traumatic stress disorder following an assault 3 years ago. She has been receiving hormone treatment for 2 years and has had some breast development, but she still has dysphoric feelings about her chest and lack of more breast tissue. Her mental health team and primary care clinician advocated for her insurance company to pay for top surgery, but they denied it as an unnecessary procedure. Rhonda tells you that she is feeling desperate and that her friends told her she could have silicone injected another way. She was connected with a person who can provide the silicone injections at an affordable price. What should you say to Rhonda?

   A. Since insurance isn't paying for breast augmentation, silicone injections might be the only way for her to achieve the body she pictures herself in.
   B. Explain to her that silicone injections might be dangerous, but she will have to accept the fact that her insurance won't pay for her top surgery. Provide supportive interventions.
   C. Explain to her that silicone injections are dangerous and could lead to serious complications, including death. Reassure her that you will continue to advocate for her to get top surgery.
   D. Tell her that since you aren't a surgeon you can't comment on silicone injections. She will need to seek out information elsewhere to see if it is safe or not.

2. Tanya is a 45-year-old woman of trans experience. She has been identifying as female for many years and has been taking estrogen for at least 5 years. She is very excited about finally having access to top surgery through her managed care provider. After initial consultation with her surgeon, she was somewhat upset because of the size of the implants the surgeon recommended. She was hoping to get the largest size possible, but the surgeon explained to her that given her smaller body frame he didn't recommend it. How would you approach this matter with Tanya?

   A. Discuss with Tanya what the top surgery means to her. Explore what it means for her to be female and how breast size factors into her concept of femininity.

B. Encourage Tanya to listen to the surgeon's recommendation. Have her consider any long-term implications of breast implants that might be too large.
C. Reflect back to Tanya that you hear her disappointment and want to help her.
D. All of the above.

3. Rebecca is a 30-year-old woman of trans experience you've been seeing for therapy for several years. She has agoraphobia secondary to multiple traumatic assaults due to her TGNC identity and living in an unsafe neighborhood. Since having top surgery, her anxiety has improved somewhat as well as her confidence level. During her most recent session she tells you that she had noticed some milk leakage from her breasts and was wondering if that was a common part of breast augmentation. What should you say?

   A. It's a common side effect and there is nothing to worry about.
   B. Evaluate her for psychosis because people born male can't produce breast milk.
   C. Advise her to revisit with her surgeon. She seems to be having a rare complication of breast augmentation and needs further evaluation.
   D. Tell her that medications can cause galactorrhea and she should speak with her prescriber.

4. Jacey is a 20-year-old gender-nonconforming person who was assigned male at birth. They use the pronouns they and she. Jacey has been seeing you for medication management for the treatment of social phobia. They understand that more gender-affirming surgeries are being paid for by insurance companies and wanted to explore options with you that might be available to them. A few of her friends have had top surgery, and she is feeling pressure to have it as well. When she thinks about her body, she thinks top surgery might not be right for her. Jacey is also feeling pressure because the state she lives in requires a "complete transition" before she can have her gender markers changed on government-issued identifications. How should you proceed?

   A. Top surgery is not a requirement for anyone, but it is an option available to TGNC people. Refer Jacey to legal services and tell her you will advocate for her in any way you can.
   B. They will need to have top surgery if they want to have their state identification changed.

C. Top surgery probably isn't right for Jacey. They should also reconsider their gender identity because of this.
D. Top surgery is required only if the person plans to have bottom surgery too. Prepare Jacey for these requirements and explore with them their fear of surgery.

ANSWERS

1. **The correct response is option C.**

It's important for patients to know that pumping parties can be dangerous and can lead to death. Rhonda wants top surgery, and it seems she will go through whatever means are necessary. On the basis of her presentation, she needs top surgery. Advise her that you will continue to advocate for her and that you would like her to achieve her body goals through safe means. Legal representation may even be necessary to further appeal the decision of the insurance company.

2. **The correct response is option D.**

The size of breast implants that Tanya gets is a very personal decision. That being said, it is also necessary for her to understand the long-term implications of having breast implants that might be too large. In the end, she might still insist on the large size because it fits her concept of who she is as a woman. Your job as a mental health professional is to help her understand the different implications of her decision.

3. **The correct response is option C.**

Galactorrhea is an uncommon but potential side effect of top surgery in women of trans experience. It's likely due to intercostal nerve stimulation. People born male can have milk production for a variety of reasons. This may be due to a tumor in the pituitary gland or a side effect of antipsychotic medication. Given Rebecca's recent top surgery, the galactorrhea is probably due to the surgery, and she should schedule a follow-up visit with her surgeon for consultation.

4. The correct response is option A.

Surgery is always an option for people of trans experience. Ultimately, each individual will need to decide which gender-affirming options are right for them and their body. State laws may dictate a person's identification, but these laws will need to be changed by people who understand TGNC culture.

REFERENCES

Maycock LB, Kennedy HP: Breast care in the transgender individual. J Midwifery Womens Health 59(1):74–81, 2014 24224502

Murariu D, Holland MC, Gampper TJ, Campbell CA: Illegal silicone injections create unique reconstructive challenges in transgender patients. Plast Reconstr Surg 135(5):932e–933e, 2015 25700296

Shlain L: Sex, Time, and Power. New York, Penguin, 2014

Weigert R, Frison E, Sessiecq Q, et al: Patient satisfaction with breasts and psychosocial, sexual, and physical well-being after breast augmentation in male-to-female transsexuals. Plast Reconstr Surg 132(6):1421–1429, 2013 24281571

18

TRANSMASCULINE BOTTOM SURGERY

> Where the mind cannot be made to fit the body, the body should be made to fit, approximately at any rate, to the mind.
>
> *Michael Dillon*

WHEN IT COMES TO bottom surgery, there are a variety of options available to men of trans experience. Transmasculine bottom surgery can refer to any number of interventions described in this chapter, but the main focus tends to be on the construction of a phallus. Mental health professionals don't need to be Freudian to appreciate the emphasis society has placed on this one particular body part. However, of all the gender-affirming procedures available to transgender and gender-nonconforming (TGNC) people, transmasculine bottom surgery seems to be the one that mental health professionals have the least knowledge of.

The importance one puts on a phallus varies, of course, from person to person. Men of trans experience are no different. For some trans men the presence of a phallus is of central importance to their gender dysphoria, and their distress around not having one will continue until they have a surgical intervention. Other trans men might not focus on the phallus as much. For them, the effects of testosterone are their primary goal of treatment. Other people who identify as men of trans experience may have no interest in any surgical procedures and may decline testosterone as well. Within the range of choices regarding transmasculine bottom surgery, trans men will need to weigh the pros and cons of surgical intervention.

When working with men of trans experience in exploring surgical options, it is important to remember that these are just that, options. Patients may feel the need to go through with surgery out of a pressure to conform to what society believes a male to be. When providing supportive therapy or evaluating a trans man for bottom surgery, be careful to tease apart what is ambivalence about the surgery from anxiety about the surgical procedure itself. Some patients have waited much of their lives for these procedures, and just because they get anxious in the months prior to surgery does not mean they don't want it or aren't ready for it. Bottom surgery can be highly invasive and, as you will see, is not without its drawbacks. The possibilities of complications remain high, and the visible scarring left is quite noticeable. Each person will need to make a decision about what is right for them in having their body reflect who they are.

NO BOTTOM SURGERY

Always remember that surgical interventions are an option, not a requirement. There are many reasons why men of trans experience would not want to have bottom surgery. First, it is very expensive, and only in recent years have some insurance companies started to pay for the procedure. Even when it is covered, the choice of a surgical provider can be limited to those who have little experience working with TGNC patients. Second, it is invasive. The creation of a neophallus is difficult, and postoperative body scarring can be a major deciding factor in which surgical intervention is chosen. Last, there can be difficulty with recovery, and some neophallus structures will have their own complications with strictures and necrosis. There are a group of men of trans experience who reject the notion that bottom surgery is necessary and advocate that people accept a range of trans bodies (Schilt and Windsor 2014). All of that being said, the majority of patients who choose bottom surgery are quite happy with the results, regardless of the drawbacks (Song et al. 2011).

Strap-Ons

A strap-on is a phallus-shaped device that can be strapped around the pelvis and functions like an erect penis during sexual activity. There are many varieties, including some with clitoral stimulation to provide more sexual pleasure for the person wearing the strap-on. A strap-on is not unique to trans men but is used by many people in sexual activity. For many gender diverse people, this option is perfectly acceptable for sexual activity and is preferred over surgical interventions.

Stand-to-Pees and Packers

A stand-to-pee (STP) is a phallus-shaped device that works almost like a funnel and gives a person without a penis the ability to urinate while stand-

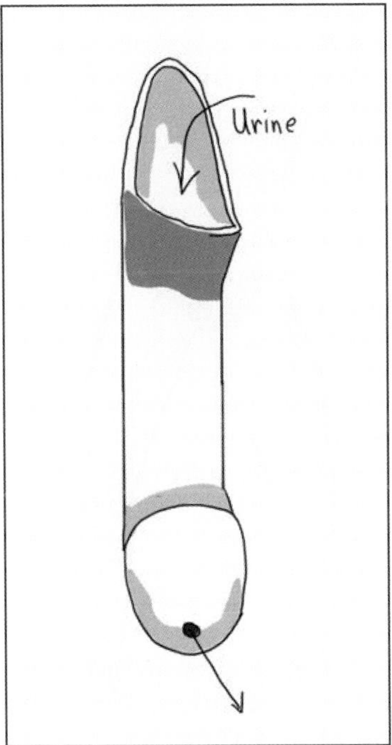

FIGURE 18–1. Typical phallic appearance of an STP device.

ing up. Given the realistic nature of some STPs, most people in a restroom will not notice if an STP is being used (Figure 18–1).

A packer is a device generally in the shape of a flaccid penis with testicles attached (Figure 18–2). It is soft and is usually worn with tight underwear to keep it in place. A lot can be said, and has been said in volumes, about the presence of the penis between a cis male's legs and how human culture has ascribed a great deal of meaning and power to it. There are studies that show that cis men, whether they are straight, gay, or somewhere in between, tend to look at and notice other men's packages (Ruel 2007). The downside to a packer is similar to issues with having a cis male penis: it can be uncomfortable at times or in an awkward position. In addition, packers cannot be worn with loose-fitting underwear.

Case Example

Rodney is a 24-year-old man of trans experience. He grew up in the Midwest and has a family who are not supportive of his sexual orientation or gender identity. Around the age of 12, Rodney was still using feminine pronouns and came out as a lesbian. He grew up isolated from the lesbian, gay, bisexual,

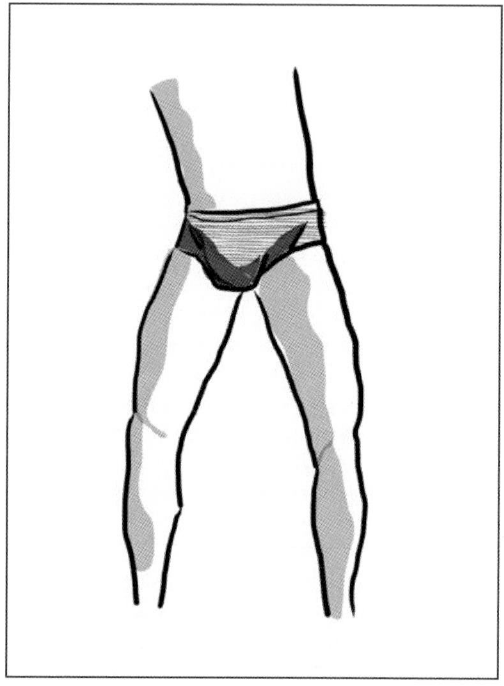

FIGURE 18–2. Packers are meant to create the illusion of cis male genitals.

transgender, and queer/questioning (LGBTQ) community and didn't have a way to describe his gender identity other than as being "butch." As Rodney approached adolescence, however, symptoms of gender dysphoria became more apparent. He started to bind and found a local LGBTQ-affirming physician who helped him start injectable testosterone. His physical appearance started to change over the course of 1–2 years. His voice became deeper, he grew a beard, and he legally changed his gender markers to male.

At this point Rodney had developed a friendship circle with people who were supportive of his gender identity. He had met other trans men and started to identify as a straight man. Around the age of 21 he had top surgery, which involved bilateral breast reduction with chest reconstruction, and he was very happy that he no longer had to bind and felt comfortable in his clothing and without a shirt. Sexually, he described himself as versatile. He enjoyed both topping (penetrating) and bottoming (being penetrated). He had no dysphoria around having a vagina and enjoyed receptive vaginal intercourse. He and his cis female partners used strap-ons and other toys to engage in penetrative sex. Rodney was clear that although he enjoyed a variety of sexual activities, he was happy with his body after top surgery and thought that phalloplasty wasn't the right option for him.

Rodney did have a desire to engage in more male-stereotypical behavior and explore his male side. One area that men of trans experience tend to focus on is the traditional male ritual of standing up to urinate. In a male restroom, the majority of the facility is typically made up of urinals. Trans men can feel pressure and a desire to want to conform. The ability to stand up to urinate can provide relief of dysphoric symptoms. Rodney's friends told him about STPs, which would allow Rodney to use the urinals unobtrusively. Rodney also found that some days he feels the desire to use a packer, which provides him with some psychological relief from his dysphoric symptoms. When Rodney wears a packer, he feels the difference and may notice other people checking it out. This can reinforce his sense of maleness and provide positive psychological benefits.

Rodney now at 24 years is in a place where he is comfortable with his body. He has thought about phalloplasty but is still happy with his body the way it is now and feels very masculine. With men of trans experience, the presence of a vagina or the absence of a penis may have little bearing on their gender identity.

METOIDIOPLASTY

Metoidioplasty is a term used for a surgical procedure for men of trans experience. The name can be translated from Latin as "formation toward male organs." It involves surgical release of clitoral tissue from the labia minora and the ligament that hold the clitoris in place. Testosterone enlarges the clitoris over time. The surgery is less expensive than phalloplasty, has fewer complications, and leaves less scarring because it is minimally invasive. Many trans men opt for this procedure because it is less invasive and provides them with a phallus from their present genitals without major surgical intervention (Perovic and Djordjevic 2003). A potential drawback is the limited size of the phallus: once the clitoral tissue is released, it can be around 1–2 inches erect (Figure 18–3). Patients can choose to have urethroplasty as well, which lengthens the urethra to the end of the neophallus, making it possible to urinate while standing. Penetrative sex is possible with metoidioplasty but is not guaranteed.

Case Example

Harry is a 35-year-old man of trans experience. He spent the majority of his life living as female and suffered for many years with gender dysphoric symptoms that were hard for him to verbalize. He developed major depression secondary to gender dysphoria and had to be treated with antidepressant medication, which helped only minimally.

Through insight-oriented psychotherapy, Harry started to discover the basis of his symptoms and came to realize he had felt male since a young age but was unable to express his gender identity. After he was able to articulate this in therapy, his depressive symptoms improved, and he and his therapist

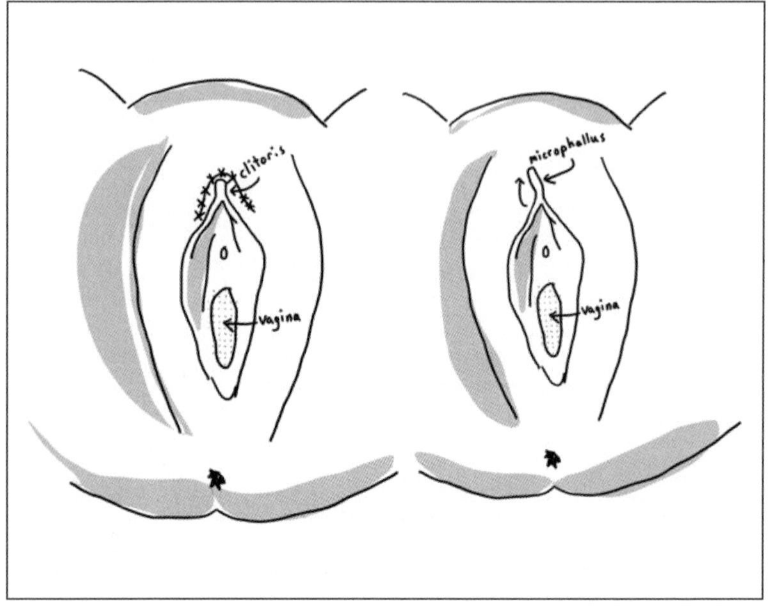

FIGURE 18–3. A metoidioplasty releases clitoral tissue, making an erection possible.

started to explore gender-affirmative options and how he could change his exterior to reflect his internal feelings.

Harry started taking testosterone with the help of his local primary care physician, changed his name and gender markers, and started to explore his masculine side. His sexual attraction has been primarily toward other men of trans experience, and he identifies as a homosexual male. After having top surgery at the age of 33, he started to explore the possibility of bottom surgery. With his particular symptoms, he wanted to have some version of a phallus to complement how he viewed himself internally, and he desired to have penetrative sex. He thought that phalloplasty would be too invasive, and he wanted to have minimal scar tissue.

Harry had a metoidioplasty in two stages. The first part was an incision of existing clitoral ligaments and the creation of a neophallus. The second stage involved urethroplasty. Harry decided he wanted to have two stages of surgery, as recommended by his surgical provider, so he could have a good chance of being able to stand up to urinate postoperatively. This was an important outcome for Harry.

After surgery, Harry had to recover over the course of 4 weeks. There was minimal scar tissue, although he was sore from the procedure. After a month or two he was able to both urinate standing up and have penetrative sexual intercourse with his partner. He was happy with the results of both the top and the bottom surgeries he had received.

PHALLOPLASTY

Phalloplasty, construction of a neophallus specifically for trans men, is probably one of the most complicated and invasive procedures a trans man can elect to undergo. Surgical techniques related to construction of a phallus have been around for almost a century (FTM Surgery Network 2017a). This area of surgical expertise came about mainly because of war veterans who sought repair after being injured in combat.

The first identified phalloplasty on a man of trans experience occurred in the early 1940s on Michael Dillon, a patient who was himself a doctor. Dr. Dillon had been living in a masculine role for several years and was able to get a colleague, Dr. Harold Gillies, to perform the procedure. It took many stages, but the outcome was successful. Dr. Dillon ultimately had to leave the country because of harassment that occurred as rumors circulated about his procedure.

There are a few versions of phalloplasty available, and which procedure is chosen depends on the specific outcomes a patient desires. The two main types of phalloplasty procedures are abdominal flap and free-flap phalloplasty. The abdominal flap technique developed by Dr. Gillies is also referred to as the Gillies technique. Both techniques have a variety of detailed options.

Abdominal Flap Phalloplasty

The procedure used by Dr. Gillies involves the incision of an abdominal flap from just above the pubic region, which is then folded and rolled over to form the neophallus. This surgery can be more or less complicated depending on whether the patient desires to involve urethroplasty. The abdominal flap phalloplasty can be done in such a way as to conceal some of the scarring and doesn't have a complicated recovery time like that required of the free-flap phalloplasty described in the following subsection. The patient will have sensation of the neophallus during sexual intercourse, but it will likely not be erotic in nature. Clitoral tissue remains, and stimulation can provide erotic sensation (FTM Surgery Network 2017b).

The flap used to create the neophallus can be extended from the abdomen, thigh, or suprapubic region. Which technique is used is a matter of aesthetics and body type. Although this is no longer the most popular form of phalloplasty because of the aesthetic surgical outcomes of the phallus, the lack of sensation, and lack of a urethroplasty, the surgery was a staple of treatment for several decades after its development.

Free-Flap Phalloplasty

A free-flap phalloplasty is, by far, the most common form of phalloplasty now performed because this procedure provides the most physical sensa-

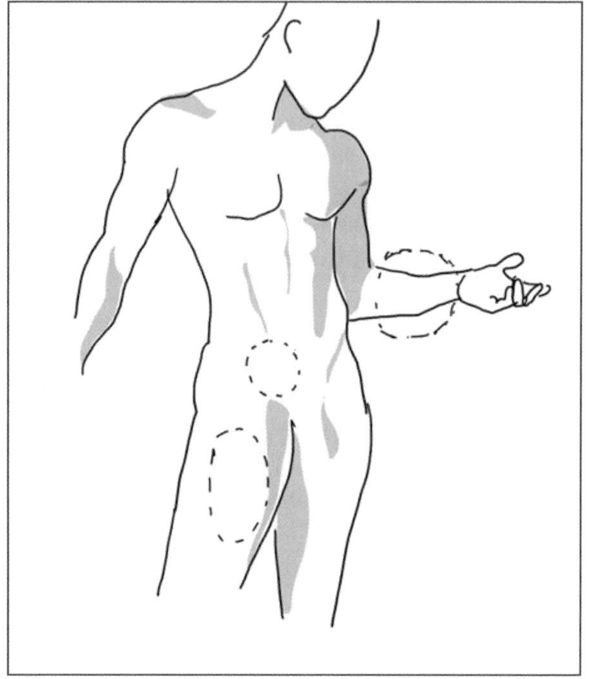

FIGURE 18–4. Skin for the neophallus can be taken from the arm, stomach, thigh, or back.

tion, the ability to urinate while standing, and a neophallus that most closely resembles a cis male penis (Morrison et al. 2015). The surgery, however, can have complications and drawbacks. The procedure may require several operations, and the person's ability to stand while urinating afterward is not certain (Van Caenegem et al. 2015).

The free flap comes from a donor site on the body, most commonly the radial forearm of the nondominant hand (Figure 18–4). The main reason for this particular site is because of both the physical sensation and the blood flow it provides (Song et al. 2011). The underside of the arm is very sensitive, and the creation of a neophallus from this region can provide adequate sensation during sexual intercourse. The flap taken from the forearm is extensive and leaves the patient with a very noticeable scar (Figure 18–5). So much tissue is removed that an additional donor skin graft is taken from the upper thigh and transplanted on the arm to help it recover.

If not taken from the forearm, the free flap can also come from the upper back, but this is frequently not an option or is not ideal for most patients because subcutaneous fat can make the donor flap too thick, and the result

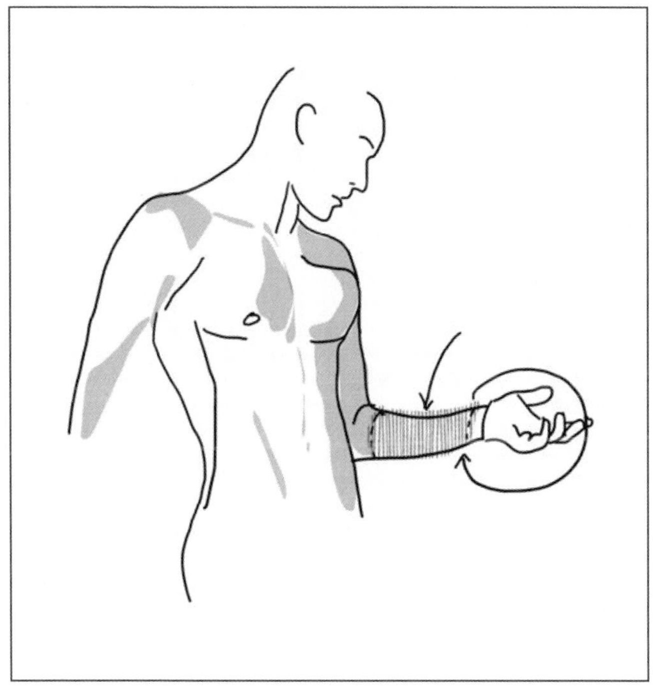

FIGURE 18–5. With free-flap phalloplasty, a sizable amount of tissue is typically removed from the circumference of the nondominant forearm.

might not resemble a typical cis male penis. Although the scarring on the upper back is easier to conceal, most trans men still elect to go with the radial arm flap because of the physical sensation this donor site provides. The majority of patients who elect to have the radial forearm flap are generally neutral about or satisfied with the appearance of the scar (Van Caenegem et al. 2015).

The free-flap phalloplasty technique is also sometimes referred to as a *tube-within-a-tube* technique (Figure 18–6). This means that a smaller tube of skin is made that will eventually become the neourethra inside the neophallus (Selvaggi and Bellringer 2011). The arteries, veins, and nerves taken from the forearm flap are connected to the iliac and groin regions. Some of the nervous tissue is connected to the same nerves that supply the clitoris, which is generally left intact under the neophallus (Figure 18–7) (FTM Surgery Network 2017b). This helps to provide erotic sensation during sexual intercourse. A urinary catheter is left inside the new urethra for a least a few weeks postoperatively to keep it patent and prevent it from closing. Creation

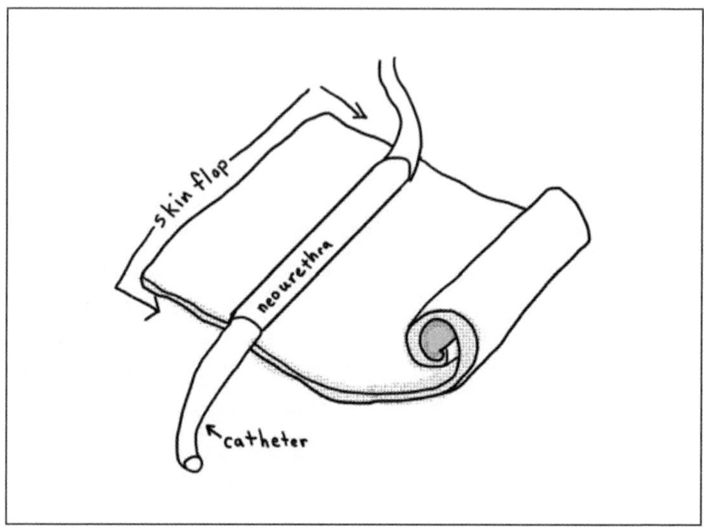

FIGURE 18–6. A catheter helps form the neourethra: the skin is rolled over and onto itself to create the neophallus shaft.

of a urethra is still considered one of the more complication-prone aspects of phalloplasty (Zhang et al. 2010).

Sculpting, or *glansplasty,* of the neophallus is typically done in the first stage of phalloplasty to create a head or glans. It is mainly for aesthetic reasons, to make the neophallus resemble a cis male penis. A second stage can be done a year later to implant prosthetics that can become erect for sexual intercourse (Morrison et al. 2015).

Case Example

Juan is a 28-year-old man of trans experience. He started his transition at an early age, and his parents supported his transition even from childhood. As a child, Juan engaged in typical "boyish" behavior and wanted only boys as friends. His parents supported his decision to wear typical boy clothing to school and asked his teachers to refer to him by male pronouns. All of his teachers and classmates referred to Juan as male.

When Juan turned 11 he started to go through puberty, and his symptoms of gender dysphoria became more apparent. He began to develop breast tissue, and his body wasn't developing like other boys around his age. Despite the support Juan received from his family and friends, his body wasn't changing to match who he felt he was supposed to be. He started wearing a binder for his chest and used packers to feel more like the other boys in his class.

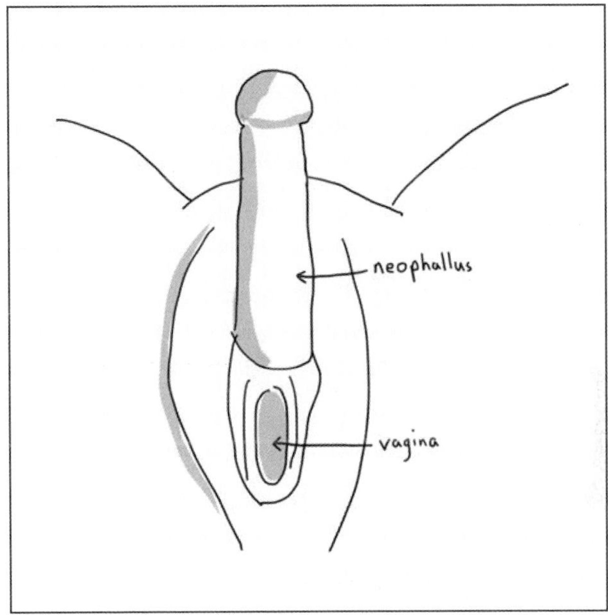

FIGURE 18–7. The clitoral nerve endings can lend to sexual stimulation in the neophallus, and the vagina is typically left in place under the neophallus.

During Juan's late teenage years, his parents consented for him to get top surgery. Juan was very happy with the results and was glad he didn't need to wear a binder anymore. He was taking testosterone, and his body was starting to transform the way he had wanted it to earlier during puberty. He began doing research on phalloplasty surgeries and decided that the radial arm flap was the best choice for him. Although he was concerned about scarring, the neophallus he envisioned could be obtained only through this procedure. He wanted erotic sexual activity and the ability to urinate while standing. Furthermore, Juan wanted to have a vaginectomy to remove his vagina and a scrotoplasty to create a neoscrotum from labia tissue. Implants would be used to create testicles. Juan was of legal age, and his parents also supported these procedures. After meeting with his surgeon, however, he decided not to have the vaginectomy because of potential complications. Given that vaginal tissue is lined with glands and secretes fluid, a vaginectomy must remove all vaginal tissue because of the potential for cysts to form should any tissue be left. A skilled surgeon is necessary for the complete removal of vaginal tissue. Juan was already concerned about the risks of phalloplasty and didn't want to worry about further complications.

The phalloplasty that Juan elected to have did include an oophorectomy and salpingectomy to remove his ovaries and fallopian tubes, respectively. Because this procedure would result in loss of fertility, Juan needed to see a psychotherapist for a period of time in order to get the surgical procedure covered by his insurance provider. Juan used the therapy sessions mostly to talk about his relationships and problems with school, although he did speak about his ambivalence about surgery and his understanding of the risks and benefits of the procedure. He had identified as male from an early age and was well aware of the potential complications from surgery.

After the first stage of his phalloplasty, Juan took some time to recover. He had to spend a few days in the hospital so his surgeon could make sure he was healing appropriately and monitor blood flow with an ultrasound. Blood flow is of the upmost importance because the neophallus tissue can start to die if the blood supply is cut off. Juan's arm was very sore and bandaged in a temporary cast to protect it for healing. The leg that provided the donor tissue for his arm was healing, but there was a noticeable scar. After a few weeks of rest, Juan was able to urinate, and the blood supply to the neophallus was sufficient. Six weeks after surgery, he felt mostly "back to normal" and was very happy with his phalloplasty results. He started to explore his sexuality more and was looking forward to the second stage of the operation, which would include erectile implants and would take place 1 year later.

The scar on Juan's arm did cause him some distress because he was unable to hide it without wearing long sleeves. Many people who saw it asked him why he had the scarring, and telling them a truthful answer would mean outing himself as a trans man. He and his therapist came up with a story that would divert people's curiosity without the need to out himself to strangers. His family and friends were aware, however, and continued to support him throughout the different stages of his transition.

SUMMARY

Transmasculine bottom surgery consists of multiple surgical procedures to help a trans man's body reflect who he sees himself to be. Many trans men may elect not to pursue bottom surgery for a variety of reasons. Some of these reasons include potential complications of procedures, cost, or simply that they don't feel they need a surgical procedure to complement their already masculine view of themselves. If a man of trans experience decides to have bottom surgery, he can elect to have metoidioplasty, phalloplasty, scrotoplasty, vaginectomy, oophorectomy, and/or saplingectomy.

Bottom surgery has many pros and cons. The psychological presence of a phallus can provide a great deal of symptom relief to a trans man who has gender dysphoria, and this can be obtained through different options. Which procedure is chosen will depend on such factors as aesthetics, the desire for erotic sensation, the need to stand to urinate, the amount of scarring, and financial limitations.

Key Points

- Bottom surgery is an elective procedure and is not a requirement for men of trans experience.
- Trans men may use devices called STPs or packers to help with dysphoric symptoms.
- The presence of a phallus is not equivalent to masculinity or maleness.
- Metoidioplasty is a surgical option with minimal scarring that works with clitoral tissue already present and enlarged from testosterone use.
- Phalloplasty has evolved over time, and various techniques are available.
- Recovery from phalloplasty can be extensive, with some significant scarring from donor sites such as the forearm.

QUESTIONS

1. David is a 25-year-old man of trans experience who comes to see you for psychotherapy and evaluation for phalloplasty. He has been taking testosterone for more than 1 year and understands many of the risks and benefits of the operation. His surgeon has recommended radial free-flap phalloplasty and has explained to him about the extensive scarring he will have on his nondominant hand. David is somewhat concerned about the loss of erotic stimulation and clitoral tissue postoperatively. How should you advise David?

   A. Clitoral tissue and erotic sensation are typically lost with phalloplasty. It's one of the drawbacks to the procedure.
   B. You don't really know anything about phalloplasty, and any questions David has should be directed back to his surgeon.
   C. From your knowledge, clitoral tissue is typically preserved in phalloplasty, and nerve endings are even connected into the neophallus. David may not need to have cause for concern, but you can consult with his surgeon to make sure.
   D. Clitoral tissue will absolutely be preserved, and he has nothing to worry about. There will be no change in erotic sensation.

2. Lewis is an 18-year-old man of trans experience who comes to see you to talk about bottom surgery. He is very ambivalent about surgery and makes several statements to you while in session, saying that he doesn't understand why people can't accept him the way that he is. How should you respond?

   A. Phalloplasty is a necessary requirement for men of trans experience to complete transition. Explore his anxiety about the surgery.
   B. Explore his ambivalence. Discuss with Lewis what he thinks it means to be masculine and to be male. Help him understand that surgery is one of many options available to him, but ultimately, he gets to decide what changes, if any, to make to his body.
   C. He probably doesn't want bottom surgery. You should tell him he doesn't need it and it will likely not lead to good results given the potential for complications.
   D. Go over the options of bottom surgery with him. Make sure he understands what phalloplasty and metoidioplasty are.

3. What is an STP, and what is it used for?

   A. STP is a form of special dressing used in the healing process after a phalloplasty.
   B. STP, also known as a standard packer, is a penis-like device that trans men wear to create a psychological phallus.
   C. STP, or standard protocol, refers to basic steps a patient should take after bottom surgery to remain healthy.
   D. STP, or stand-to-pee, is a device trans men might use to allow them to stand up to urinate at a traditional male restroom urinal.

4. What are the advantages of using a radial forearm flap in free-flap phalloplasty?

   A. The forearm skin provides a lot of sensation as well as a blood supply that is ideal for making a neophallus.
   B. It is a good place to remove tissue and will lead to little scarring.
   C. With regard to recovery, radial forearm free-flap phalloplasty is probably the least painful of the procedures.
   D. The forearm free-flap site doesn't really have any advantages and is rarely used in phalloplasty procedures today.

5. Jun is a 32-year-old man of trans experience. He has been seeing you in psychotherapy to help with symptoms of bipolar disorder I, which runs in his family. He has been stable on medication for 3 years and is now in a place to pursue gender-affirming procedures. He has identified as male since childhood. His symptoms of bipolar disorder started around the age of 28. Today he is talking about phalloplasty and the potential for other surgical procedures. He is considering vaginectomy but has heard there can be complications. What should you tell him?

    A. A vaginectomy is a very safe procedure, and few complications have been reported.
    B. With a vaginectomy there can be some complications, such as the formation of cysts postoperatively. Advise Jun to ask his surgeon about the procedure during consultation.
    C. A vaginectomy is not an option for men of trans experience because it isn't covered by insurance plans.
    D. Discuss with Jun the possibility that his manic symptoms are causing his desire to have a vaginectomy.

ANSWERS

1. **The correct response is option C.**

    Clitoral tissue is generally left in place during a phalloplasty, and the particular surgery for which David is being evaluated is known for good erotic sensation as one of its selling points. However, guaranteeing erotic sensation is going too far, and patients should understand that although these surgeries generally have good outcomes, nothing is certain. If you are going to work with men of trans experience, you should understand the basic pros and cons of bottom surgery options. Simply deferring to the surgeon without any knowledge is not trans-competent care. If you are confused about the basics, you can consult with David's surgeon to understand the procedure so you can discuss these issues with David.

2. **The correct response is option B.**

   Lewis tells you himself that he doesn't understand why people can't accept him the way that he is. The crux of your treatment may be around how he views masculinity, maleness, and himself. Phalloplasty is definitely not a requirement for trans men and there is no such thing as a transition being "complete." Everyone has their own journey, and surgeries are options available to patients, not steps for them to take. It might be worth going over the potential bottom surgery procedures with Lewis, but his ambivalence is related to people accepting him for who he is, not the types of surgery.

3. **The correct response is option D.**

   STP ("stand-to-pee") is a common device used to allow people to stand for urination. Men of trans experience will know what STPs are, and you should, too.

4. **The correct response is option A.**

   The main advantages of a radial forearm free-flap phalloplasty is that it provides good sensation and a strong blood supply to the neophallus. It causes extensive scarring on the forearm and can be one of the more difficult procedures to recover from. However, given the advantages, it is still one of the most commonly used techniques for phalloplasty.

5. **The correct response is option B.**

   A vaginectomy is one option of many available to men of trans experience for bottom surgery. It does have potential complications, just as with any procedure. One complication involves the formation of cysts should any vaginal tissue be left after the operation. These types of risks and benefits can be discussed with the surgeon, but as Jun's therapist, you can offer to help him clarify any concerns he might have.

REFERENCES

FTM Surgery Network: FTM phalloplasty surgery procedures, 2017a. Available at: www.phallo.net/procedures/. Accessed June 6, 2017.

FTM Surgery Network: FTM top surgery guide, 2017b. Available at: www.topsurgery.net. Accessed May 16, 2017.

Morrison SD, Perez MG, Carter CK, Crane CN: Pre- and post-operative care with associated intra-operative techniques for phalloplasty in female-to-male patients. Urol Nurs 35(3):134–138, 2015 26298948

Perovic SV, Djordjevic ML: Metoidioplasty: a variant of phalloplasty in female transsexuals. BJU Int 92(9):981–985, 2003 14632860

Ruel L: Eyetracking points the way to effective news article design. Online Journal Review, March 12, 2007. Available at: www.ojr.org/070312ruel. Accessed 1 December 2017.

Schilt K, Windsor E: The sexual habitus of transgender men: negotiating sexuality through gender. J Homosex 61(5):732–748, 2014 24392744

Selvaggi G, Bellringer J: Gender reassignment surgery: an overview. Nat Rev Urol 8(5):274–282, 2011 21487386

Song C, Wong M, Wong CH, Ong YS: Modifications of the radial forearm flap phalloplasty for female-to-male gender reassignment. J Reconstr Microsurg 27(2):115–120, 2011 21049401

Van Caenegem E, Wierckx K, Taes Y, et al: Body composition, bone turnover, and bone mass in trans men during testosterone treatment: 1-year follow-up data from a prospective case-controlled study (ENIGI). Eur J Endocrinol 172(2):163–171, 2015 25550352

Zhang Y, Lu L, Zhang W, et al: A simple and effective method for phalloplasty in female-to-male transsexuals. Plast Reconstr Surg 126(5):264e–265e, 2010 21042084

19

TRANSFEMININE BOTTOM SURGERY

When you become the image of your own imagination,
it's the most powerful thing you can ever do.

RuPaul

TRANSFEMININE BOTTOM SURGERY is essentially the creation of a neovagina with a surgical procedure called a vaginoplasty. When considering cis female anatomy, sculpting an external feminine appearance out of cis male anatomy is as artistic as it is surgical. To create a neovagina, a vaginal canal needs to be made, as well as a clitoris, labia majora, and labia minora. Several techniques have been developed to accomplish this, but the penile inversion technique appears to be the most popular and has been for many years.

Vaginoplasty is an expensive and invasive procedure. For many women of trans experience, especially those without access to health care, the time and money required make having a vaginoplasty impossible. Recently, insurance companies have started to pay for the procedure, giving surgical access to thousands of women of trans experience. This access gave rise to a new problem: lack of providers. Although many surgeons are trained in doing breast reduction or breast augmentation, few know the subtle art of vaginoplasty. The need for the surgery outweighs the number of providers, and many women of trans experience continue to have no access to vaginoplasty for this reason in particular.

Even if a woman of trans experience does get access to both coverage and a surgeon for the procedure, the actual operation and recovery can be difficult. There are electrolysis requirements leading up to surgery, the surgery is performed in a number of stages, and there are manual or device-related dilation needs following the procedure. Regardless of the cost, time commitment, and complications, many women of trans experience are still very satisfied with the results.

SEXUALIZATION OF TRANS WOMEN

Western culture has historically sexualized women of trans experience. They are seen as living in between the worlds of masculine and feminine. Despite society's historical and continued homophobia and transphobia, there is a sexuality space that has been created for trans women who appear very feminine on the surface but have had no gender-affirming procedures. There are many cis men and some cis women who are attracted to trans women who have not had a vaginoplasty. It's important not to use the term "pre-op" because that implies that all women of trans experience without a vaginoplasty are pre-operation and will have an operation eventually. Remember that all of these gender-affirming procedures are optional, and individuals decide which surgeries, if any, are best for them and their bodies.

There may be a number of reasons that certain cis men are attracted to women of trans experience who still have their penis. Some would say it's another form of sexual orientation. Just as some people are attracted solely to men or women, some people might also be attracted to those who live as both or neither male or female on the basis of their physical anatomy. There is also a group of cis men who have struggled with their sexuality and are unable to accept their homosexual feelings. A woman of trans experience may provide them with enough femininity so as not to disturb their ideas about their perceived sexuality and enough masculinity to meet their sexual urges.

NO SURGERY

All people have a feminine side, however hidden it might be. What makes someone female? Is it enough to have long hair and a feminine face, dress in feminine clothing, have breasts, and carry oneself in a feminine way? For many women of trans experience, the ability to have breast augmentation and facial feminization is enough to help with symptoms of gender dysphoria. Not all trans women feel dysphoric about their penis. Some embrace gender nonconformity and their body as is. Others want to keep their penis for sex and sexuality reasons. That being said, many trans women feel very dysphoric about their penis and very much desire a vaginoplasty.

TUCKING

Tucking refers to the act of tucking a person's penis and testicles so they are not visible through the clothing. It is a practice done by both women of trans experience and some gender-nonconforming people, but it has been made known in popular culture by drag queens. Tucking can be somewhat painful

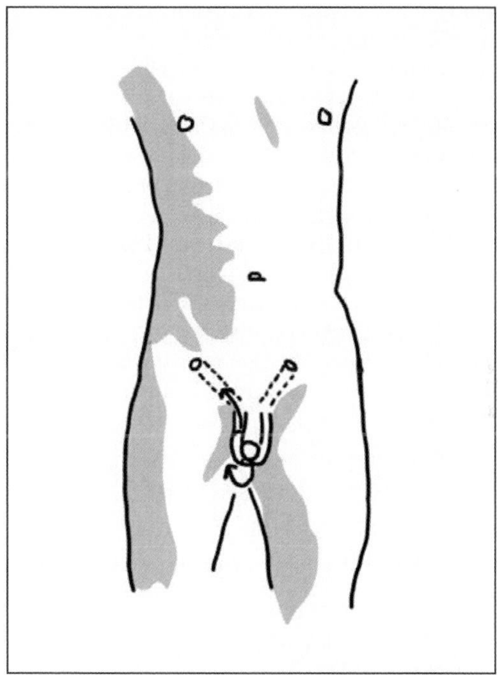

FIGURE 19–1. Tucking involves moving the testicles into the inguinal canals and tucking the penile shaft between the legs.

for some, but it accomplishes the goal of creating a flat front and giving the appearance of a cis female body form. The penis is typically pulled under the perineum and held in place with tape or tight underwear. The testicles are sometimes pushed into the inguinal canals to further create a flat contour (Figure 19–1). Just as with binding, tucking should be done only for a limited time. Constriction of tissue for too long can cause fluid buildup and potential tissue damage. There are some who believe it to cause sterility as well. These potential risks should be discussed with patients. Although most of the people who engage in tucking are well aware of the potential risks and benefits, it is important for a trans-competent provider to understand this practice.

Case Example

Leslie is a 37-year-old woman of trans experience. She has what many mental health practitioners would describe as a "textbook case" of gender dysphoria. At the early age of 3, Leslie, then called Lester, played with dolls, wanted to wear dresses, and spent most of her time with cis females. Her parents were open to letting her explore and be herself and thought that her feminine inclinations would pass over time. They did not. She asked to be called Leslie around the age of 8. During puberty, she started to develop more masculine characteristics, including a deepening voice and changes to her face and body. She was upset by these changes and wanted to have more feminine features to match who she felt she was inside. Regarding her genitals, Leslie didn't have any dysphoric feelings. It was her outward appearance, particularly around her face, that brought about dysphoric symptoms. She wanted to have puberty suppression treatment, but no experienced providers practiced in the state where she lived. In her early 20s, she obtained access to health care that would provide gender-affirming procedures. For Leslie, facial feminization and breast augmentation were the most important procedures. After these procedures, she was satisfied with the alignment of her body and mind and never thought vaginoplasty to be necessary. She enjoyed sexual activities with cis men, cis women, and other women of trans experience.

BRIEF HISTORY OF TRANSFEMININE BOTTOM SURGERY

Bottom surgery for trans women has existed in some form since the early twentieth century. The first documented person to receive a vaginoplasty was Dora Richter in 1922 (Goddard et al. 2007). This was made possible with the support of Magnus Hirschfeld, a pioneer in the understanding and support of diverse human sexuality and gender identity. Lili Elvenes (also known as Lili Elbe), whose story was fictionalized and made famous by the book and movie *The Danish Girl*, had her procedure shortly after.

It was Georges Burou, a gynecologist, who developed the now popular penile inversion technique in the 1950s. He ran a clinic called Clinique du Parc out of Casablanca and reported that had performed some form of the procedure on no fewer than 3,000 people (Burou 1973). The techniques that Dr. Burou developed have become what is referred to as the gold standard in vaginoplasty today (Ettner et al. 2016).

PENILE INVERSION TECHNIQUE

Surgical Steps

The penile inversion procedure goes by several names, but essentially, it creates a neovagina from the external tissue of the penis. Although the procedure may appear complicated at first, the stages can be broken down into steps, and understanding these steps will help with an understanding of how the neovagina functions after completion and recovery (MTF Surgery 2017).

Before having surgery, many patients will need electrolysis. Because the tissue will be inverted and folded over in some places, the presence of hair follicles can lead to complications. Some patients may require several weeks of electrolysis treatment prior to surgery. Others will have the electrolysis completed during the operation and need few, if any, previous treatments. Different surgeons have their own opinions about electrolysis, and requirements may vary depending on who performs the procedure.

Some vaginoplasty procedures are done all in one operation. Others require a multistep process. This is also at the preference of the surgeon. Regardless of how many steps are needed, the first surgical procedure is usually an *orchiectomy*, or removal of the testicles. The testicles are removed via an incision down the midline of the scrotum, and the scrotal tissue is left in place for use as part of the neovagina and potentially the labia majora in later steps. Because orchiectomy is a sterilizing procedure, a clear discussion about the patient's desire for children is needed prior to the surgery. Many women of trans experience have low to no sperm secondary to previously taking estrogen and the testosterone blocker spironolactone. An orchiectomy, however, is permanent, and some patients may elect to have their sperm frozen and stored prior to the procedure.

Once the testicles are removed, resection of the penis occurs. It's important to understand the anatomy of the penis at this step. The majority of the shaft of the penis is made up of a spongy material that can fill with blood to create an erection. This spongy material is removed during a vaginoplasty. An incision is made at the base of the glans, or head, of the penis, and the skin around the shaft is pushed down, almost like pushing up the sleeve of a long-sleeved shirt. All the nervous innervation is on the dorsal, or top side, of the penis and remains untouched so that it can eventually be used to form the neoclitoris. The two elongated spongy sections on each side of the penis are removed, leaving the nerve pedicle attached to the glans (Figure 19–2).

Two openings are created just above the top of the penis shaft base. The upper opening will become the neoclitoris by means of a clitoroplasty, and the lower opening will be the new urethral meatus, or opening. The glans is still attached to its nervous supply and is sculpted to fit into the upper opening. This means that what was once the head of the penis is converted into the neoclitoris. This makes it possible for women of trans experience to continue to experience erotic stimulation during sexual activity postsurgery.

The urethra is then brought up and through the second opening. There will be extra urethral tissue because of the length of the penis. The urethra is cut along its length up to the new urethral meatus. The extra tissue will be added to the wall of the neovagina. At this point, the neovagina is made up of tissue from the external shaft of the penis and the extra tissue from the

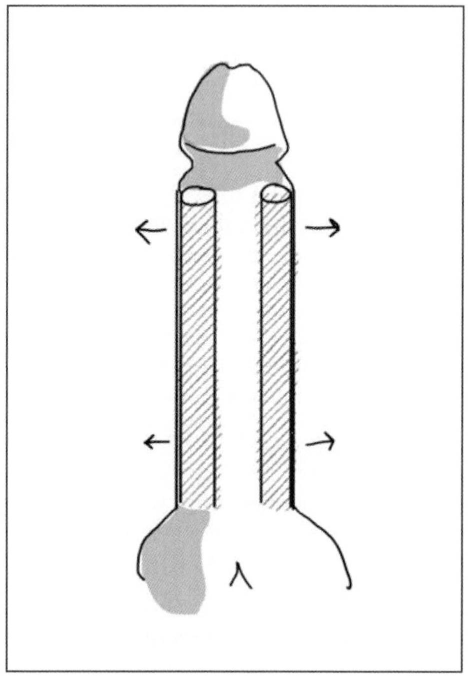

FIGURE 19–2. The spongy tissue is removed, leaving the nerves and arterial supply intact.

urethra. The urethral tissue is generally folded over and closes the end of what will be the inside of the neovagina.

Next, the perineum, or skin between what was the scrotum and the anus, is incised, and the surgeon manually locates the sacrospinous ligament deep within the pelvis. This structure will serve as the anchor for the neovagina to hold it in place and prevent it from prolapsing, or extruding outside the body (Figure 19–3). The tissue that was once the penile shaft and the extra urethral tissue are then inverted and anchored to the sacrospinous ligament. The tightening of the tissue as it is anchored brings the opening of the neovagina down, creating the external appearance of cis female genitalia. After the neovagina is anchored, there will be extra skin present externally. This skin will be sculpted along with remaining scrotal tissue to make the labia majora and minora, a process also known as a vulvoplasty. Sculpting of the external neovagina may also need to be done in later stages, and further tissue might be needed to achieve optimal aesthetic results. Because the neovagina is made from the still innervated shaft of the penis, sexual stimulation should be possible from inside the neovagina.

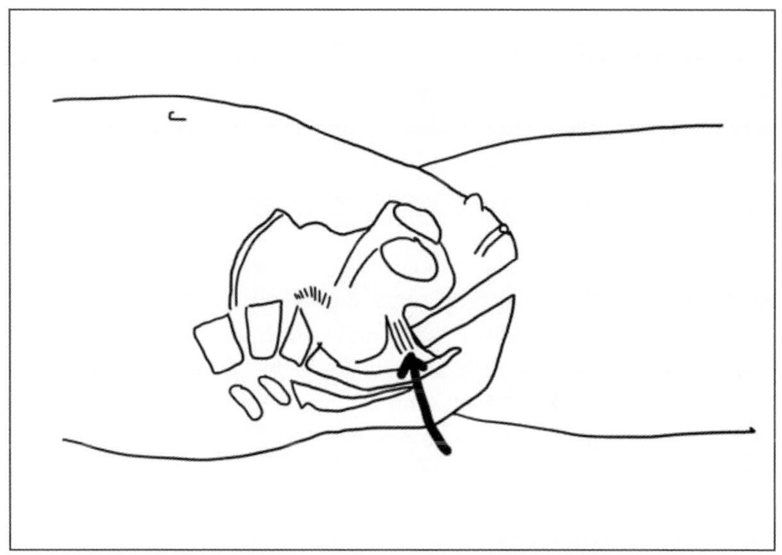

FIGURE 19–3. **The sacrospinous ligament serves to anchor the neovagina.**

Surgical Follow-Up

After the surgery, patients are expected to stay in the hospital for about 3 days. The most common complication of vaginoplasty is stricture, or closing, of the neovagina. Because of this, frequent and daily dilation is required with devices known as dilators. Some surgeons recommend at least 20 minutes of dilation up to three or four times per day. Dilation of some sort should continue daily for several months. Weekly dilation either with a dilator or through sexual intercourse is recommended permanently.

Pain can be an issue, but many trans women report that the recovery is tolerable. Sitting or walking can be uncomfortable, and loose-fitting clothing is needed to allow for blood flow and the healing process to take place. The tilt of the urethral opening is critical because the stream of urine that comes out needs to point down. If patients report that the stream of urine points outward instead of downward, they should consult with their surgeon.

Pain may also be expected with vaginal dilation. The multiple daily dilations are necessary to prevent the neovagina from closing. If patients are unable to complete the daily dilation requirements, they must consult with their surgeon quickly to prevent further complications. Patients should understand that dilation will be uncomfortable in the beginning, but most people report an improvement and ease with dilation over time.

COLON GRAFT

The colon graft procedure can go by several names, such as rectosigmoid vaginoplasty or sigmoid colon vaginoplasty. It is an alternative method for vaginoplasty that essentially creates a neovagina from part of the sigmoid colon. It involves an abdominal incision that is made to remove about 20 cm, or close to 8 inches, of colon. This section of colon is internally moved to the new perineal opening.

Like any other surgery, the colon graft procedure has pros and cons. One potential reason for choosing this procedure is lack of sufficient penile shaft skin. Individuals with a shorter penis might not have enough skin to create a neovagina of sufficient length, around 3–6 inches. The colon segment can create a neovagina that is 8 inches on average. The mucosa or lining of the colon can also create its own secretions, providing lubrication during sexual intercourse.

There are also a few drawbacks to this procedure. The first is lack of sensation. Much of the penis is removed, although the glans can still be used to create the neoclitoris. The inside of the neovagina, however, will not have the same sexual stimulation as with the penile inversion technique. Aesthetically, people report that they do not like the external look of the neovagina after a colon graft. The inside of the colon is red mucosa, which is visible from the neovagina meatus, or external opening. There are also reports of a malodorous smell that can continue for months after the procedure (Schechter 2016).

NONGENITAL SKIN GRAFTS

One other technique that is rare but could potentially be used more often in the future involves taking a skin graft from another part of the body, sometimes the buttocks, and molding it into a neovagina. A foam mold is sculpted in the form of a vagina and wrapped with a condom. The new skin graft is wrapped around the foam mold and sutured into a cylinder (Wheeless and Roenneburg 2017). The neovagina is put in place much like the colon graft technique described above, and the foam mold and condom are removed once the neovagina is secure. This procedure has many of the same drawbacks as the colon graft, with lack of sensation being one of the biggest.

Case Example

Maria is a 39-year-old woman of trans experience. She grew up in a rural area and spent 10 years in prison. At the age of 25, she was assaulted by a man who was attempting to rape her while she was walking home. She struck him over the head with a rock in self-defense. She hit him in such a way that the man died of his injuries. Once the police discovered that Maria was born male, she was prosecuted and sent to prison even though she had acted in self-defense.

While in prison, Maria was placed with other men and referred to by her birth name, Mario. She was denied access to hormones and spironolactone, which made her symptoms of gender dysphoria worse. She was assaulted both sexually and physically several times in prison. The other prisoners took her to be a gay man, and the guards had no interest in protecting her given their views on transgender and gender-nonconforming (TGNC) people. She knew the only way to get out of prison was to keep quiet and not complain. She suffered in this environment for many years.

After 10 years, Maria was released early for good behavior and left the rural town she grew up in to seek TGNC-affirming care in a major urban area. Although she would have rather lived in the town where she was raised, her friends and family didn't want to speak with her, and other locals had threatened her while she was walking around town.

Once in the city, Maria had a hard time finding work. She could make some money as a dog walker, but most places wouldn't employ her with her criminal record and because her gender identity did not match her identification and legal documents. Having no major source of income, Maria was homeless and was forced into a men's shelter, where she was harassed by the men there.

Maria got connected to a local lesbian, gay, bisexual, transgender, and queer/questioning (LGBTQ) clinic and was given a primary care doctor who started her on hormones and spironolactone. With medicinal treatment in place, she started to feel better emotionally and went to therapy weekly with a gender-affirming therapist to help with symptoms of posttraumatic stress disorder. Maria also got connected with a case manager who helped her change her legal name and gender marker on her identification. After this, it was easier for her to get work because she was able to better conceal her trans identity from employers.

About a year into treatment, Maria got breast augmentation with the help of her primary care doctor and therapist. Her symptoms of gender dysphoria were greatly improving because her body was starting to align more with who she had always felt to be. Some months after breast augmentation, Maria was ready for vaginoplasty. The only problem was that there were no surgeons in her city to perform the procedure because none of them had been trained. Maria began to feel frustrated and hopeless, thinking she would have to live for the rest of her life in a body she was not comfortable with.

Fortunately, Maria didn't have to wait too long because a local hospital hired a trained surgeon who could perform the penile inversion procedure. Maria started electrolysis and asked to have an orchiectomy done as the first stage of the procedure. She was happy that she could stop spironolactone after the orchiectomy. During the second stage of the procedure, Maria underwent a penile inversion vaginoplasty, clitoroplasty, and vulvoplasty. Maria found the recovery pain tolerable and was able to follow the dilation recommendations given by her surgeon.

Now Maria is working and has her own apartment. She is much happier with her physical appearance and is working with her therapist and primary care doctor to explore facial feminization as another step in her treatment. She spends her time advocating with her local LGBTQ center for education of clinicians so that more providers can provide gender-affirming care.

SUMMARY

Transfeminine bottom surgery is a combination of several procedures but largely is the creation of a neovagina during vaginoplasty. Some women of trans experience may choose not to have a vaginoplasty for a variety of reasons. If they do, the current gold standard vaginoplasty is a penile inversion technique that uses the external skin of the penis shaft to line the inner part of the neovagina. Depending on the surgeon and the amount of tissue available, another common procedure is a colon graft, which uses a section of the sigmoid colon to create a neovagina. Some frequent drawbacks to a colon graft are aesthetics and a malodorous smell. Other types of skin grafts are less popular but have been used.

Key Points

- Transfeminine bottom surgery is the process of making a neovagina through vaginoplasty.
- Trans women have historically been fetishized by some cis men.
- Some trans women may not desire vaginoplasty for various reasons.
- The penile inversion technique is the gold standard vaginoplasty procedure.
- Patients may need to have multiple rounds of electrolysis before having vaginoplasty.
- Vaginoplasty can be a multistep procedure but typically is done in one surgery.
- Daily dilation of the neovagina, multiple times a day, is essential to prevent stricture.
- Women of trans experience continue to have a lack of access to gender-affirming surgeons who can perform vaginoplasty.

QUESTIONS

1. Amber is a 27-year-old woman of trans experience who was disowned by her family at an early age. She was homeless for many years but started to make money by doing sex work. As she entered treatment, she started hormones and had top surgery, and now she is ready for vaginoplasty. When she told some of her clients that she was going to have the procedure, several of them threatened to stop using her services because they are attracted to her only while she still has a penis. She asks you for advice on what to do.

    A. Amber should consider her source of income and probably put off the vaginoplasty procedure.
    B. Amber's ambivalence about vaginoplasty means she doesn't really want it.
    C. Explore Amber's goals in treatment and focus on helping her find income that will support her gender identity.
    D. Tell Amber that you'll need to report her to the authorities if she continues sex work.

2. Why is electrolysis necessary prior to vaginoplasty?

    A. During vaginoplasty, the skin is folded in over itself, and it is essential that hair follicles do not become embedded in the neovagina or neovulva.
    B. It's more aesthetically pleasing.
    C. Removal of hair is necessary for all surgical procedures.
    D. All of the above.

3. In the penile inversion vaginoplasty technique, after the urethra is separated from the penis, what happens to the extra urethral tissue?

    A. There usually isn't any extra urethral tissue.
    B. It's cut away because it serves no purpose.
    C. It is incised and added to the wall of the neovagina.
    D. It is used to create the neovulva.

4. During a penile inversion vaginoplasty, what prevents the neovagina from prolapsing?

    A. Muscular tensions from the perineal wall hold the neovagina in place.

B. The inside is anchored to the sacrospinous ligament.
C. Erectile tissue from the former penis holds it in place.
D. It is attached to the sigmoid colon to keep it in place.

5. Which of the following is *not* true about colon graft vaginoplasty?

   A. It is an option for patients who do not have a lot of penile tissue.
   B. The neovagina from a colon graft is short, about 4 inches in length.
   C. The mucosa can provide lubrication during sexual activity.
   D. Some patients report a malodorous smell for several months after surgery.

6. Maria, the patient from a case example earlier in this chapter, is seeing you in psychotherapy weekly for gender-affirming care and for treatment of posttraumatic stress disorder symptoms. Two weeks after vaginoplasty, she comes to your office in recovery. She has been dilating three times a day as the surgeon recommended, but now she thinks she is recovered and no longer needs to dilate. What do you tell her?

   A. If she thinks the vaginoplasty is healed, she can stop dilation and follow up with her surgeon.
   B. She needs to dilate three times a day for the rest of her life after a vaginoplasty procedure.
   C. She can hold off on dilation, then follow up with her primary care doctor regarding what to do next.
   D. Dilation following vaginoplasty typically needs to occur every day and up to three times a day in the first month. Even months after the procedure, weekly dilation is usually necessary.

ANSWERS

1. The correct response is option C.

Amber has been pretty clear with her goals. She said she wanted vaginoplasty, and only after her clients threatened her did she doubt her decision. Her goals in gender-affirming treatment are to have vaginoplasty, and she needs help finding income that won't require her to live in a body she is uncomfortable with. Breaking confidentiality (e.g., by reporting someone to the police) is allowed only when a patient poses a serious risk to self or others.

2. **The correct response is option A.**

    The shaft of the penis and scrotal tissue are folded to make the neovagina and neovulva. It's important that no hair follicles are present because they can lead to infection later in recovery.

3. **The correct response is option C.**

    The extra urethral tissue is incised open and attached to the penile shaft tissue to create the neovagina.

4. **The correct response is option B.**

    The neovagina is prevented from prolapsing by anchoring it to the sacrospinous ligament located at the base of the pelvis deep within the pelvic cavity.

5. **The correct response is option B.**

    The colon graft is an option for patients without much penile tissue. The neovagina from a colon graft is long, up to 8 inches or more. One of the main pros to having a colon graft vaginoplasty is the creation of a long vaginal canal. The mucosa can provide lubrication during sex, and a foul odor has been described by some patients in the months of recovery after the surgery.

6. **The correct response is option D.**

    Daily dilation is absolutely essential to prevent stricture of the neovagina. Some surgeons recommend up to 20 minutes three times a day. If Maria is concerned with inflammation or pain, she should consult her primary care clinician or surgeon for physical examination.

REFERENCES

Burou G: Male to female transformation, in Proceedings of the Second Interdisciplinary Symposium on Gender Dysphoria Syndrome. Edited by Laub DR, Gandy P. Stanford, CA, Division of Reconstructive and Rehabilitation Surgery, Stanford University Medical Center, 1973. Available at: http://ai.eecs.umich.edu/people/conway/TS/Burou/Burou.html. Accessed June 6, 2017.

Ettner R, Monstrey S, Coleman E (eds): Principles of Transgender Medicine and Surgery, 2nd Edition. New York, Routledge, 2016

Goddard JC, Vickery RM, Terry TR: Development of feminizing genitoplasty for gender dysphoria. J Sex Med 4(4 Pt 1):981–989, 2007 17451484

MTF Surgery: MTF vaginoplasty: what patients need to know before choosing a technique. MTF Surgery, 2017. Available at: www.mtfsurgery.net/mtf-vaginoplasty.htm. Accessed December 1, 2017.

Schechter L: Gender confirmation surgery: an update for the primary care provider. Transgender Health 1(1):32–40, 2016

Wheeless CR Jr, Roenneburg ML: McIndoe vaginoplasty for neovagina, in Atlas of Pelvic Surgery, Online Edition, 2017. Available at: www.atlasofpelvicsurgery.com/2VaginalandUrethra/13McIndoeVaginoplastyforNeovagina/chap2sec13. Accessed June 6, 2017.

20

OTHER GENDER-AFFIRMING PROCEDURES

I have just as much woman in me as I have man. It's just a matter of channeling the energy into which way you use it.

Grace Jones

IN CHAPTERS 16–19, I focused on top and bottom surgery options, which are some of the most commonly requested interventions by the transgender and gender-nonconforming (TGNC) community. Although these procedures can have a big impact on a TGNC person's quality of life, self-esteem, and body image, dysphoric symptoms may manifest in relation to other parts of the body besides the genitals and the chest, and these symptoms may actually be more distressing for patients.

One thing that is different about top and bottom surgery and some of these other procedures is the fact that top and bottom surgeries affect body parts that can typically be concealed. Unless people are getting into or out of the shower or bath or unless they spend time nude at home or in open places, direct visual sight to their chest or genitals is covered. Although the presence of certain shapes may suggest the particular body parts that are under a person's clothing, it is still left largely to the imagination of the perceiver. For instance, a woman of trans experience who wants top surgery can use padding and/or bras to help communicate to others a feminine shape with the contours of her body. Although she may have intense dysphoric symptoms when she sees herself, she is somewhat able to hide these body concerns from others until she is able to have gender-affirming surgery.

There are other areas of a person's body, namely, the face and neck, that are usually visible for people to see and develop opinions about, both con-

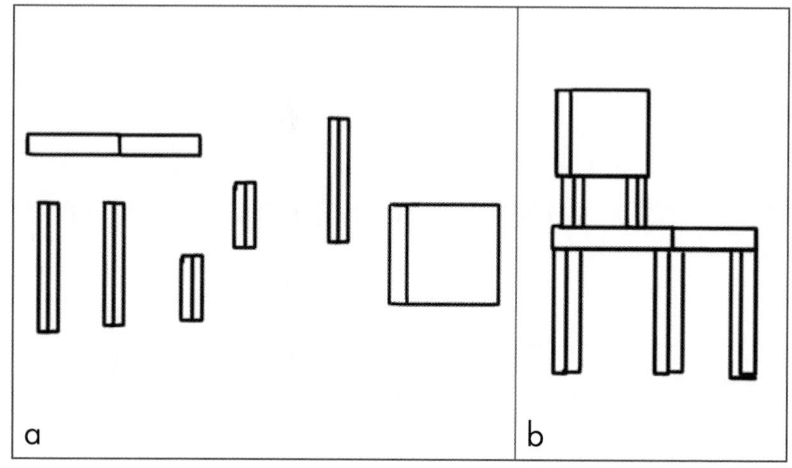

FIGURE 20–1. (a) Shapes alone communicate no particular meaning. (b) The arrangement of shapes can create meaning based on their location.

sciously and unconsciously. To see how automatic the brain is at forming an option, look at Figure 20–1a. The shapes don't really mean anything to the viewer except that they are simple geometric figures. However, if these shapes are arranged and spaced in a certain way, the individual objects start to take on meaning, and the mind identifies the conjoined objects as something new (Figure 20–1b). Now you see a chair: four legs, a seat, and a back compose a chair, and regardless of the material that it is made of, you'd still label it as a chair.

The same automatic labeling takes place with gender, particularly with aspects of the face. We look at people all day long and assign them a gender, age, race, ethnicity, and even a mood. The ways in which a face is shaped defines how masculine, feminine, or androgynous it appears (Figure 20–2). Take some time to study some of the major differences in the facial representations. Explore the hairline, the brow, the eyes, nose, cheeks, lips, jaw, and chin. Appreciate the shapes that are formed. Some of these shape stereotypes are based on biology and hormones, whereas others are more culturally assigned. The face can be one of the first places that communicates gender to other people, and some gender diverse patients may want to alter this aspect of themselves before anything else. For many TGNC people, being automatically and correctly identified as their true gender identity is one of the most transformative and validating moments they can have (Raffaini et al. 2016).

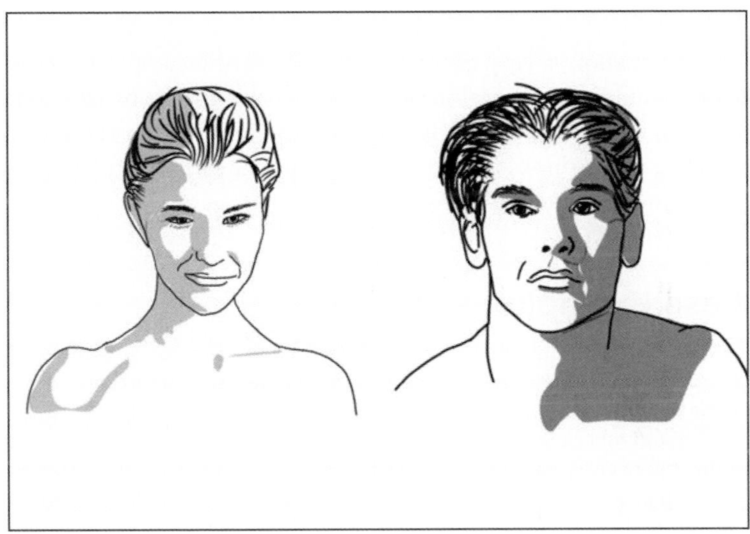

FIGURE 20–2. **General facial features of cis women and cis men.**

In this chapter, I discuss facial feminization and other surgical and nonsurgical procedures that can help TGNC people physically affirm their gender. The majority of the chapter will focus on feminizing techniques, although there is brief mention of masculinizing options. Testosterone typically changes the body in many ways that will masculinize the body. However, although estrogen feminizes the body, those assigned male at birth typically need further gender-affirming procedures to help with specific gender dysphoric symptoms. As you will see, a cis male body has more hard angles and additional tissue that cannot be changed with hormone treatment alone. Many of these procedures are currently not covered by insurance companies, but this is slowly changing with the evidence of how beneficial they can be to the mental health of the TGNC individual.

NO SURGERY

As stated in previous chapters, gender-affirming procedures are always options for TGNC people and should never be requirements. What is considered masculine or feminine largely remains tied to cultural norms, and how people identify regarding their gender does not mean that they want their body to look a certain way. The shapes of human bodies are very diverse, and whether or not a gender diverse person wants to conform to cultural norms is a personal decision.

TRANSFEMININE FACIAL FEMINIZATION

Facial feminization is very different from standard facial plastic surgery. When cis women have facial plastic surgery, their goal is usually to look younger but in the end still look like themselves. For a woman of trans experience, the goal is to look like a different person. The surgeon and the patient work together to develop a new face that resembles the patient's gender identity (Spiegel 2008).

Case Example

In Chapter 15, "Transfeminine Hormones," we met Patricia, a 36-year-old woman of trans experience who was in the process of going through hormone therapy and supportive psychotherapy. Patricia had been taking estrogen for a number of years and was happy with some of the results, but her main concern was with her face. Looking in the mirror exacerbated most of her dysphoric symptoms. She was excited to be talking about top surgery and bottom surgery, but for her, her face was the most important thing that needed to be changed.

Patricia did not have unrealistic ideas about how she wanted to look. When talking about the specific areas of her face that caused her worst dysphoric symptoms, Patricia was immediately able to point to her nose, jaw, chin, and eyes. Her nose, she reported, was too broad and had a hooked shape on the end. She would prefer a narrower and more feminine-shaped nose. Her jaw protruded in a box shape and was very square; her chin was also square and cleft. Her eyes, she reported, were spread too far apart, and she thought she had too many wrinkles forming.

All of the conditions Patricia mentioned are classic examples of locations on the face that contribute to our automatic perception of someone being masculine or feminine. With the exception of the wrinkles around Patricia's eyes, all of the relevant surgeries are directly related to gender dysphoria and should be provided if the patient desires. For some people, facial feminization can be a life-changing and life-preserving procedure that benefits their overall mental health more than medications or therapy. The wrinkles Patricia wanted changed would fall more under cosmetic surgery and are not necessarily associated with gender dysphoria. Regardless of a person's gender identity, we all age.

The easiest way to think about facial feminization is to examine the possible procedures one by one (Altman 2012). Rather than starting at the top of the head and moving down, we will view the gender facial differences from areas most frequently noticed first when meeting someone, starting with the eyes and moving on to the nose, brow, forehead, lips, cheeks, chin, jaw, and hair.

Eyes

A person's eyes can be altered in a gender-affirming way. In cis women, the eyes generally have more lashes and are more oval in shape. In cis men, they are set deeper in the face and are more rectangular (see Figure 20–2). The eyes can be feminized through orbital-reshaping surgeries, such as orbital rim contouring, which is generally done with a brow lift. The shape of the eyes can also be altered with the application of cosmetics. If cosmetics are their only option, women of trans experience may need help learning from other trans women how to apply makeup to create a more feminine look.

Nose

Patricia's nose was very upsetting to her. She said it was too wide and had a hump in the middle. These aspects are very common for a cis man's nose (Figure 20–3). To make a nose more feminine, the bridge of the nose needs to be narrowed, with an inward curvature rather than a hump. The top of the nose also tends to stick up in cis women, exposing the nostrils more.

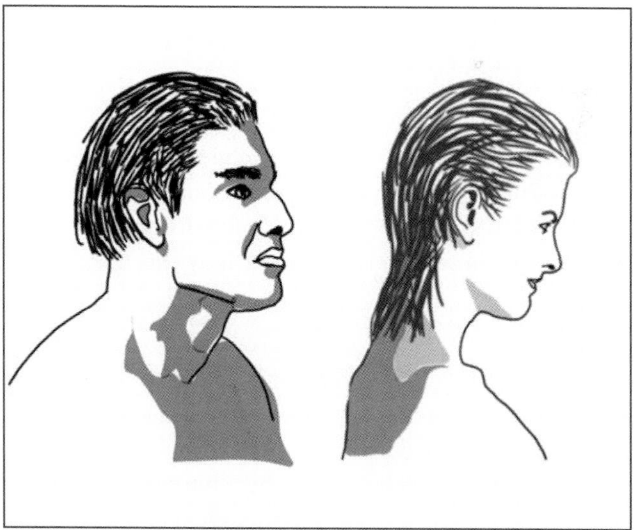

FIGURE 20–3. **General profile features of cis men and cis women.**

Brow

The eyebrows on cis women are thinner and more arched, whereas in cis men, they tend to be thicker and straight across with a square shape (see Figure 20–2). Most people can change the shape of their eyebrows on their own by tweezing or by applying cosmetics, but electrolysis may be an option for some who would like to make permanent changes. The location of the eyebrows in cis women tends to be over the orbital ridge just above the eyes, whereas with cis men, they sit right on the orbital ridge (Figure 20–2). A brow lift can elevate the eyebrows to a more feminine place and give a more open and feminine look to the eye orbits.

Forehead

The forehead in a cis male typically has significant bossing or protruding roundness to it (see Figure 20–3). With a cis female, there is typically a gentle slope down from the hairline to the top of the nose. Forehead shaving or a bone reduction can be done to give the forehead a more feminine shape. This can be done while repositioning the hairline (see subsection "Hair" below).

Lips

In cis women, the lips tend to be fuller, more curved up, and with a shortened distance between the upper lip and the base of the nose (see Figure 20–3). Surgery can specifically lift the upper lip and curl it up at the same time (Ettner et al. 2016).

Cheeks

Feminine cheeks tend to be fuller and sit higher on the face just under the eyes (see Figure 20–2). Cis men are known for having flatter cheeks. Cosmetics can be used to create the illusion of more feminine contours. If surgery is desired, cheek implants can be particularly effective.

Chin

Cis men have a chin that is more prominent, with sharper edges and a box-like appearance (see Figure 20–2). To make the chin more feminine, either it can be shaved down or pieces can be removed and the bone grafted back together. Patricia had a very large cleft in her chin that she felt contributed to an overall masculine appearance. She attempted to hide it with makeup, but cosmetics can do only so much.

Jaw

Cis men are known to have more of an angle to their jaw, which can be very prominent in some people. The angle from the ear to the chin drops down like a box. With cis women, there is a natural curve from the ear to the chin and a lack of prominence (see Figure 20–3). The excess jaw bone can be removed through surgery or shaved down. Patricia was particularly unhappy with the shape of her jaw, which was very noticeable.

Hair

Cis women have a hairline that falls farther forward on the forehead (see Figure 20–2). The space between their eyebrows and hairline is shorter, particularly on the sides. The hairline may need to be brought forward and can be done in such a way that the scar tissue is hidden by the hairline itself.

Adam's Apple

Cis men have a prominent and well-known piece of cartilage in their neck commonly known as the Adam's apple. Cis women have it too, but there isn't as much tissue, making it less noticeable. This extra tissue can be removed via a tracheal shave. The cut to get to the trachea cartilage is generally done through a natural crease in the neck, which makes it easier to hide any scar tissue. The presence of an Adam's apple has traditionally been a known cultural reference to identify people who were assigned male at birth. It is yet another example of a subtle body shape that can consciously and unconsciously communicate gender.

FEMININE BODY PROCEDURES

Abdominoplasty and Body Contouring

When estrogen has failed to significantly help with fat distribution during hormonal treatment, a persistent and larger amount of belly fat may remain, and there may be little change to the hips and buttock region. Because of this, fat may need to be moved from one area and applied to another. This is referred to as body contouring. If an extreme amount of belly fat is present, an abdominoplasty or tummy tuck may be needed. This will provide the patient with more of an hourglass figure and a traditionally feminine appearance.

Implants

When estrogen has not worked for fat redistribution and surgeries such as tummy tucks and bony contouring are not possible, implants may be used. Implants can be inserted into the cheeks, hips, or buttocks regions to help sculpt the body.

Voice Therapy

Voice therapy is not necessarily a procedure, but voice lessons can help women of trans experience learn through coaching how to feminize and raise the pitch of their voice (Gelfer and Van Dong 2013). People's quality of life can be greatly affected by how they perceive their own voice to sound. Many symptoms of gender dysphoria can focus on the sound of a person's voice and whether or not it is perceived to be at the typical gender pitch (Hancock et al. 2011). Although the perception of a person's voice as being masculine or feminine is typically in the ear of the beholder, the way TGNC people's voices sound can affect whether and how often they are misgendered over the phone and even in person.

There are surgical options that can shrink the size of a person's vocal cords, but these procedures can lead to complications (Selvaggi and Bellringer 2011). For men of trans experience, the vocal cords generally respond to testosterone therapy and lengthen over time.

TRANSMASCULINE BODY PROCEDURES

Case Example

Neil is a 28-year-old man of transgender experience who has been going to a gender-affirming clinic for the past 4 years. He has been taking testosterone and also completed top surgery and a phalloplasty procedure. He has grown some facial hair, although it didn't come in very thick. Neil has dressed in more masculine clothing for many years. Despite all this, he continues to be misgendered. He says it is mostly due to his face. Even with the facial hair, the curves in his face remain soft, and his face has more feminine features. If he had been able to start testosterone earlier, things might have turned out differently. His face might have matured just like that of a cis male for whom testosterone was present during that crucial time around puberty and adolescence when so many changes take place. People typically refer to him as male when he talks on the phone because his voice dropped to a lower pitch while he was taking testosterone. Despite this, his facial features continue to create significant distress.

Facial Masculinization

In some ways, facial masculinization can be easier than facial feminization. With facial feminization, the goal is primarily to remove bone structures, but facial masculinization is about having structures added to give more angles to the face. Implants can be used to provide a more masculine appearance to the jawline, chin, and forehead. A person's hairline, on the other hand, usually responds well to testosterone, resulting in a forehead that is larger overall with temporal hair recession.

Body Masculinization

Masculinizing the body can be done in three major ways. The first way is weightlifting. Having more defined muscles and not curvy arms and legs will give a more masculine appearance to the body. Depending on the outcome of top surgery, pectoral implants may be needed if muscle growth cannot be achieved. These implants can also create enough of a lift and curve to the pectoral region to hide scar tissue from top surgery. Last, the hips and buttock area may need body contouring to produce a flatter shape to the hip area. This would largely focus on the removal of fat from those areas.

Hair Grafting

Sometimes, facial hair won't grow from hormone treatment. If a patient is certain about wanting facial hair, hair grafting is a possibility. Grafting takes a person's own hair from areas such as the scalp, harvesting the hair follicles and transplanting these follicles to different parts of the body, such as on the face to make a beard.

SUMMARY

Reshaping the face and body are additional procedures that one can use to achieve a more gender-affirming body. Which procedures are selected and why is a personal decision on the part of the patient. Although many of these procedures are not covered by insurance, this will likely change in the future as more evidence emerges to show the benefits both to treating gender dysphoria and to general psychological wellness. Clinicians should be knowledgeable about all potential procedures because they will need to provide psychoeducation to their patients regarding their options.

Key Points

- Many body or facial procedures and treatments for gender dysphoria are not covered by insurance companies because they are deemed "not medically necessary."
- There are several locations on the face that signal a more masculine appearance or a more feminine appearance.
- Gender-signaling location points on the face include the eyes, brow, nose, cheeks, forehead, lips, hairline, jaw, and chin.

- Body and/or facial procedures should be made available to patients who get less than optimal results from hormone therapy.
- Facial feminization or masculinization is creating a new face for patients so their appearance matches their gender. It is important that there be a solid surgeon-patient bond with a shared realistic vision of what will be done.
- As technology evolves, more options will be made available to TGNC people to create an alignment of their body and their mind.

QUESTIONS

1. How is the general distance from the upper lip to the nose different for cis males and cis females?

   A. The distance in cis women is shorter.
   B. The distance in cis men is shorter.
   C. The distances are the same.
   D. The distance can vary dramatically from person to person.

2. Patricia, the 36-year-old woman of trans experience from the case example earlier in the chapter, is ready to have facial feminization. Her surgeon plans to do work on her nose, lips, jawline, hairline, and forehead. Although Patricia is very excited about the surgery, she is somewhat nervous about having a scar on her forehead. All the other procedures seem to have a place to hide the scar tissue, but she doesn't seem to understand how this can happen with her forehead being reshaped. What should you say?

   A. There will be a small scar across the forehead, but it's an unfortunate side effect of having the procedure.
   B. The surgeon will enter through the nose to get to the forehead and reshape it.
   C. An incision is usually made above the hairline. Confirm with Patricia's surgeon, but the scar will likely be hidden.
   D. Cuts are made above the orbits of the eye to get access to the forehead. This will hide the scar tissue.

3. Patricia is also worried about her Adam's apple. She says she forgot to mention it to the surgeon when they discussed her procedures because they were so focused on her face. People are going to know she was born male when they see it. She is unclear what can be done.

    A. Nothing can be done about the Adam's apple. She will have to get used to it.
    B. The surgeon can take out Patricia's Adam's apple, but he will have to remove her thyroid as well.
    C. It's still unclear what is available. Only experimental studies have been done.
    D. Tracheal shaving can help with Patricia's Adam's apple. She should talk to her surgeon during the next visit.

4. What is body contouring?

    A. Body contouring is removing hair from one site on the body and placing it on another.
    B. Body contouring is moving fat from one area to another to create a more masculine or feminine physique.
    C. Body contouring is shaping the body by using weight machines to give a masculine appearance.
    D. Body contouring is the application of pressure to certain parts of the body, such as with a girdle, in order to create a feminine shape.

5. Patricia has had facial feminization and is very happy with the results. Her surgeon told her to come back in 2 months for tracheal shaving. When the 2 months were over, her insurance company sent her a letter saying that tracheal shaving is not a medically necessary procedure. Patricia is very anxious because although many people in her small town are aware of her gender identity, strangers will see her Adam's apple and know she was assigned male at birth. What should you do?

    A. If the insurance company has rejected the claim, there is nothing Patricia can do. Conduct therapy with her to try to decrease her focus on it.
    B. Work with her to raise funds from friends and family. That's the only way the surgery will ever happen.
    C. Explain to her that the Adam's apple isn't very noticeable and the surgery probably isn't needed.
    D. Call the insurance company and advocate for Patricia, saying this is a medically necessary procedure for her mental health.

ANSWERS

1. **The correct response is option A.**

   In general, the distance from the upper lip to the base of the nose is smaller in cis women.

2. **The correct response is option C.**

   Surgeons are usually pretty good about hiding or disguising scars from plastic surgery on the face. The scar for the forehead will likely be hidden behind the hairline, but you can call the surgeon with the patient present to confirm. This will go a long way to helping decrease patients' anxiety level. They typically have enough to worry about.

3. **The correct response is option D.**

   Tracheal shaving removes extra tissue to decrease the size and appearance of what is known as the Adam's apple. As a trans-affirming mental health clinician, you should be aware of the procedures that are available to your patients.

4. **The correct response is option B.**

   Body contouring is specifically moving tissue or fat from one area of the body to another in order to create a more masculine or feminine shape. This is not yet covered by insurance but may be medically necessary if hormones have had little to no effect.

5. **The correct response is option D.**

   This is a moment where you, as the mental health professional, can truly advocate for your patient. This surgery is medically necessary. The patient is having severe dysphoric symptoms and needs further treatment. Make all possible efforts to get the surgery approved. If the insurance company continues to deny the procedure, involve legal services.

REFERENCES

Altman K: Facial feminization surgery: current state of the art. Int J Oral Maxillofac Surg 41(8):885–894, 2012 22682235

Ettner R, Monstrey S, Coleman E (eds): Principles of Transgender Medicine and Surgery, 2nd Edition. New York, Routledge, 2016

Gelfer MP, Van Dong BR: A preliminary study on the use of vocal function exercises to improve voice in male-to-female transgender clients. J Voice 27(3):321–334, 2013 23159032

Hancock AB, Krissinger J, Owen K: Voice perceptions and quality of life of transgender people. J Voice 25(5):553–558, 2011 21051199

Raffaini M, Magri AS, Agostini T: Full facial feminization surgery: patient satisfaction assessment based on 180 procedures involving 33 consecutive patients. Plast Reconstr Surg 137(2):438–448, 2016 26818277

Selvaggi G, Bellringer J: Gender reassignment surgery: an overview. Nat Rev Urol 8(5):274–282, 2011 21487386

Spiegel JH: Challenges in care of the transgender patient seeking facial feminization surgery. Facial Plast Surg Clin North Am 16(2):233–238, viii, 2008 18355710

21

CONCLUSION

By doing the work to love ourselves more, I believe we will love each other better.

Laverne Cox

NOW THAT YOU'VE reached the end of this guide, I would like to summarize some of the main points that you should take away. Although the details about hormone treatment and gender-affirming therapy may, at times, be overwhelming, the information provided in these chapters is necessary. However, knowledge alone does not make you a good mental health provider for gender diverse people. What will, in my opinion, make all practitioners good providers for transgender and gender-nonconforming (TGNC) people are an open mind, an open door, and a strong voice.

ACCEPTANCE OF PATIENTS' IDENTITIES

As stated in Chapter 1, "Introduction," the majority of the learning needed to work with gender diverse patients is accomplished by breaking down lifelong personal and cultural stereotypes about what is male and what is female. Letting go of boxes and allowing patients to be free to be who they are may seem easy, but it is probably one of the most challenging things all mental health practitioners must do. Only by doing so can you start to appreciate the true individual nature of gender. When you are able to see people in the way they wish to be seen, you will be able to function as a healer and provide care for gender diverse people in the same way you are already doing with others. Years of marginalization and stigma have made the TGNC community skeptical of mental health providers. Now is our chance to heal those wounds and approach gender variant individuals from a place of acceptance and compassion.

ACCESS TO CARE

The overarching theme through all the chapters in this book has been access to care. We cannot help gender diverse people without TGNC-competent clinicians. TGNC people continue to have limited access to trans-competent providers, and places such as inpatient psychiatric units, emergency rooms, and outpatient offices are still in many ways unsafe. Knowing the information provided in these chapters will put you in a place to start treatment with gender diverse people. It is important for you to make yourself available to TGNC people to provide access to care where it is sorely needed. Access to care includes providing gender-affirming therapy, helping TGNC people with gender marker changes, and writing letters for gender-affirming procedures. Wherever you provide mental health care, that can be a place that is safe and affirming for TGNC people.

ADVOCATING FOR CARE

TGNC people need more advocates. As someone who now has a general understanding of TGNC care, you can help advocate for your gender diverse patients. There are so many areas where voices are needed, and depending on your location, your one voice can make a world of difference for gender diverse people. Many state laws discriminate against TGNC people, and it is a mental health care provider's responsibility to advocate for TGNC people in the hopes of improving their overall mental health. We cannot expect our therapies or medications to provide any healing without first helping make the world a safer and more affirming place for TGNC people. Just as it is our duty to write evaluations, prescribe medications, fill out forms, and make phone calls, it is also our duty to do the same for our TGNC patients. Although the forms and phone calls you make will initially be of a different nature than what you are used to, you will quickly see that your voice in the matter can make a difference.

TEACHING

Last, it is our responsibility to take the information we have about TGNC people and teach it to those who do not have that knowledge. Now that you are more informed about gender diversity, you will start to notice where injustices and treatment failures take place within mental health care and the larger health care system. When you see these treatment failures taking place, it is important that you speak up and provide feedback to your colleagues. It is also equally important that you do so in a supportive way. If your colleagues feel shamed when you correct them, you will likely only alienate them and cut off the potential to foster a TGNC-competent provider. Mental health clinicians should be approached with the attitude that everyone can learn about gender diversity and apply it to their practice.

THANK YOU

Thank you for taking the time to take in this information and learn about gender diversity. My writing is just one perspective among others. Although I am not a TGNC person myself, I do consider myself part of the queer community. Having worked with gender diverse people for the past decade, I have made an attempt to put down on paper the stories I have heard and the lessons I have learned. Mental health professionals know that with each patient we meet, we learn lessons and adapt to become better therapists and providers. The more gender diverse people you meet and interact with, the more gender affirming and knowledgeable you will become. Be the healer you were trained to be by continuing your education and learning. You now have an opportunity to provide compassion, care, and understanding to a population that has been lacking in support for far too long.

Index

Page numbers printed in **boldface** type refer to tables or figures.